NLMDUP

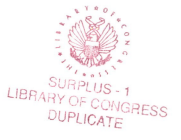

Urological Disease in the Fetus and Infant

Urological Disease in the Fetus and Infant

Diagnosis and Management

Edited by

D.F.M. Thomas MA FRCP FRCS

*Consultant Paediatric Urologist, St James's University Hospital
and the General Infirmary, Leeds;
Honorary Reader in Paediatric Surgery, University of Leeds*

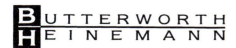

BUTTERWORTH
HEINEMANN

Butterworth-Heinemann
Linacre House, Jordan Hill, Oxford OX2 8DP
A division of Reed Educational and Professional Publishing Ltd

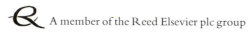 A member of the Reed Elsevier plc group

OXFORD   BOSTON   JOHANNESBURG
MELBOURNE   NEW DELHI   SINGAPORE

First published 1997

British Library Cataloguing in Publication Data
Urological disease in the fetus and infant: diagnosis and
  management
  1. Pediatric urology   2. Fetus – Diseases
  I. Thomas, D.F.M.
  618.9′2′6

ISBN 0 7506 0768 8

Library of Congress Cataloguing in Publication Data
Urological disease in the fetus and infant: diagnosis and management
  /edited by D.F.M. Thomas.
     p.   cm
  Includes bibliographical references and index.
  ISBN 0 7506 0768 8
  1 Pediatric urology.   2 Fetus – Diseases.   3 Infants (Newborn) –
  – Diseases.   I Thomas, D.F.M.
  RJ466.U76   97–26049
  618.92′6–dc21   CIP

Typeset by BC Typesetting, Bristol BS18 1NZ
Printed and bound in Great Britain by The Bath Press, Somerset

Contents

Contributors

J.D. Atwell MB ChB FRCS
Hon. Emeritus Consultant Paediatric Surgeon,
The Wessex Centre for Paediatric Surgery,
Southampton

A.P. Barker MBBS FRACS
Paediatric Surgeon and Urologist,
Princess Margaret Hospital for Children,
Perth, Western Australia

S. Bewley MA MD MRCOG
Director of Obstetrics, Guy's and
St. Thomas's Hospital, London

P.A. Borzi MB BS FRACS FRCS
Consultant Paediatric Urologist, Mater and
Royal Children's Hospitals, Brisbane,
Australia

J.T. Brocklebank MB FRCP(Ed) FRCP(Lond)
Consultant Paediatric Nephrologist, St. James's
University Hospital, Leeds; Reader in
Paediatric Nephrology, University of Leeds

P.M. Cuckow FRCS
Senior Registrar, Department of Paediatric
Urology, Hospital for Sick Children, Great
Ormond Street, London

C. Cullinane MB MAO BCh FRCPath
Consultant Pathologist, St. James's University
Hospital, Leeds

D. De Mello MD
Professor of Pathology and Paediatrics,
St. Louis University School of Medicine, USA

B.R. Elejalde MD
Clinical Professor of Obstetrics and
Gynaecology, University of Wisconsin
Medical School, Madison, USA

M.J. Ellison MRCP
Consultant Paediatrician, Singleton Hospital,
Swansea

M.M. Fitzpatrick MD MRCP
Consultant Paediatric Nephrologist, St. James's
University Hospital, Leeds

A.L. Freedman MD
Pediatric Urology Fellow, Children's Hospital
of Michigan, Detroit, USA

Y.L. Homsy MD FRCSC FAAP
Professor of Urology and Paediatrics,
University of South Florida, Tampa,
Florida, USA

H. Irving MB BS FRCR
Consultant Radiologist, St. James's University
Hospital, Leeds

F. Jewkes MRCP
Consultant Paediatric Nephrologist, Cardiff
Royal Infirmary, Cardiff

R. Lambert MD FRCPC
Clinical Associate Professor of Nuclear
Medicine, Université de Montréal, Quebec,
Canada

R.J. Lilford PhD MRCP FRCOG
Professor of Health Services Research,
West Midlands Regional Health Authority,
Birmingham

M. Maizels MD
Professor of Urology, Northwestern
University Medical School, Children's
Memorial Hospital, Chicago, USA

G.C. Mason MD MRCOG
Consultant in Feto Maternal Medicine,
General Infirmary, Leeds

P.D.E. Mouriquand MD FEBU
Consultant Paediatric Urologist, Hospital for
Sick Children, Great Ormond Street, London

L.M. Reid MD FRCP FRCPath FRACP MA
(Hon. Harv)
Wolbach Professor of Pathology, Pathologist-
in-Chief, Children's Hospital, Boston, USA

A.M.K. Rickwood MA FRCS
Consultant Paediatric Urologist, Royal
Liverpool Children's Hospital, Liverpool

C.H. Rodeck DSc FRCOG
Professor of Obstetrics and Gynaecology and
Head of Department, University College,
London

E. Shapiro MD
Professor – Director of Pediatric Urology,
New York University Medical Center,
New York, USA

R. Squire FRCS DCH
Consultant Paediatric Surgeon, St. James's
University Hospital, Leeds

D.F.M. Thomas MA FRCP FRCS
Consultant Paediatric Urologist, St. James's
University Hospital and The General
Infirmary, Leeds; Honorary Reader in
Paediatric Surgery, University of Leeds

J.G. Thornton MD MRCOG DTM&H
Reader in Obstetrics, University of Leeds

K. Verrier Jones FRCP
Laura Ashley Senior Lecturer in Paediatric
Nephrology, Cardiff Royal Infirmary, Cardiff

R.H. Whitaker MD MChir FRCS
Formerly Consultant Paediatric Urologist,
Addenbrooke's Hospital, Cambridge

D.M. Williams MB MRCP
Consultant Paediatric Oncologist,
Addenbrooke's Hospital, Cambridge

Preface

'Ultrasonic echo sounding has much to offer in the field of obstetrics, for which this technique is extremely suitable because of the very powerful echoes with which fetal parts, and in particular the fetal head, within the medium of liquor amnii, can provide.' This, the opening sentence of Professor Ian Donald's chapter devoted to obstetric ultrasound in the 1968 edition of his textbook *Practical Obstetric Problems* was my introduction to the concept of prenatal ultrasound diagnosis. At a time when technology had been devised to beam images of the Apollo missions back from the moon, it seemed incongruous that the more immediate world of the fetus had largely defied exploration. The concept of adapting sonar to explore the fluid environment of the fetus was both logical and exciting. In itself the idea was not new, but it was not until the late 1960s and early 1970s that ultrasound began to fulfil its promise as a practical diagnostic tool in clinical obstetrics. Ultrasound has been one of medicine's major success stories in the closing quarter of the 20th century. No other technological innovation has been so rapidly developed nor found such widespread application.

Inevitably, some of the benefits claimed for obstetric ultrasound have been questioned, but not even the most hardened sceptic could realistically advocate turning the clock back to the pre-ultrasound era – so firmly is ultrasound now rooted in the practice of obstetrics. The task confronting radiologists, obstetricians and paediatric clinicians has been to learn how best to utilize and apply the information derived from prenatal ultrasound for the benefit of our patients.

Urological Disease in the Fetus and Infant summarizes some of the important lessons learned from more than a decade of detecting urinary tract malformations *in utero*. The scope of the book extends to encompass the first twelve months of life – reflecting the physiological continuum from fetal to post-natal life. It is important to acknowledge the limitations of prenatal ultrasound, particularly when confined to a single fetal anomaly scan before 20 weeks of gestation. Even clinically significant urinary tract malformations such as posterior urethral valves, may not give rise to detectable dilatation at this stage in pregnancy and may thus remain unrecognized. For this reason *Urological Disease in the Fetus and Infant* addresses the diagnosis and management of clinically presenting genitourinary disorders as well as those detected prenatally.

Current understanding of the basic science underpinning the diagnosis and management of urological disorders of the fetus and infant is considered, for example, in the chapters on embryological development of the genitourinary tract, the lung–kidney axis and fetal and neonatal renal function. The principal aim of the book, however, has been to draw together the various strands of this multidisciplinary field in contributions from respected clinicians in diagnostic imaging, obstetric and perinatal medicine, neonatal and paediatric medicine and surgery.

Ideally the parents of any fetus with a pre-natally identified urological anomaly would have the benefit of ready access to authoritative counselling from experts in all the relevant disciplines in the dedicated environment of a prenatal counselling clinic. In practice, the increasing demands on busy clinicians, coupled with problems of rescheduling conflicting timetables, can make this a difficult goal to achieve. For clinicians faced with the task of counselling parents on the implications of prenatally detected urological disease, I hope that much of the information they require can now be found within the covers of *Urological Disease in the Fetus and Infant*.

Working as a paediatric urologist in Leeds has provided me with the opportunity to collaborate closely with obstetricians and radiologists with a shared interest, and in many cases nationally recognized expertise in the field of prenatal diagnosis. Several of these colleagues have contributed to this book and to them I am particularly grateful. I would also wish to acknowledge the radiologists, obstetricians and paediatricians in district hospitals throughout the Yorkshire Region who have contributed directly and indirectly to prospective and follow-up studies undertaken by myself and colleagues in Leeds. Finally, and most importantly, I am indebted to Mrs Judith Ball for her invaluable contribution to *Urological Disease in the Fetus and Infant*, from its inception through to the preparation of the final manuscript.

1

Epidemiology and genetics of genitourinary malformations

J.D. Atwell

Introduction

In the future when gene mapping is current practice the fate of every individual, excluding accidents, will be predictable. At the present time we are only partially along that road and much remains unknown, particularly concerning the aetiology of congenital defects within the genitourinary system. In some conditions such as polycystic kidneys the method of inheritance is understood, in others, the coexistence of certain anomalies and features has allowed the identification of syndrome complexes, some of which have a known genetic basis, whereas in others the causation is unknown.

Factors such as maternal age, birth order, season of birth, intrauterine infections, vitamin deficiencies, and drugs may have an effect upon the developing fetus. In the urinary tract genetic factors and obstruction within the urinary tract are probably the two most important factors and may even be interrelated. For example, renal dysplasia is associated with obstruction in double ureters with an ectopic ureterocele and multicystic renal dysplasia is associated with an atretic pelviureteric junction. Intermittent obstruction such as severe fetal vesicoureteric reflux is associated with dysplasia. However, many examples exist of the genetic cause of dysplasia: it therefore seems that the aetiology of a condition may be multifactorial, with genetic and other factors affecting the intrauterine environment. In congenital genitourinary tract anomalies genetic factors probably play a more important role than environmental factors. Only time and the accumulation of further data and research will provide the answers which we seek.

The following conditions will be discussed.

Renal disease:
   Renal agenesis
   Dysplasia: hypoplasia
   Horseshoe kidney: ectopia
   Polycystic disease.
Pelvicalyceal collecting system anomalies:
   Duplex pelvicalyceal system
   Vesicoureteric reflux
   Paraureteric diverticulum
   Megaureters
   Pelviureteric junctional hydronephrosis
   Ectopic ureteroceles.
Outflow tract anomalies:
   Bladder exstrophy: epispadias
   Posterior urethral valves
   Hypospadias.
Chromosomal disorders.
Syndrome complexes.
Neoplastic disease.

Renal disease

Renal agenesis

Renal agenesis may be unilateral or bilateral, in the latter it is incompatible with life, the newborn dying from pulmonary hypoplasia or renal failure. Although bilateral and unilateral renal agenesis will be discussed separately, there are examples of both types occurring in the same family [1].

Bilateral renal agenesis

The incidence is 1 in 3–4000 births [2,3]. The clinical features are characterized by Potter's syndrome of a flattened face with epicanthic folds, low-set ears, spade-like hands and talipes [4]. The talipes and pulmonary hypoplasia are related to the oligohydramnios. Cytogenetic studies have been normal [5].

Although the method of inheritance is unknown, genetic factors play a role. Studies in twins have shown that bilateral renal agenesis may be either concordant or discordant and in two other sets of monozygous twins the renal agenesis was bilateral in one and unilateral in the other [6]. Familial occurrence has often been reported [7]. In a series of 199 patients seven had siblings similarly affected [8]. As bilateral renal agenesis is incompatible with life, it is not a clinical problem for the practising paediatric urologist despite the progress in renal transplantation.

Unilateral renal agenesis

Essentially there are two types of unilateral renal agenesis, first those associated with a ureteric bud and, second, those where the ureter is absent and there is asymmetry of the trigone of the bladder.

Unilateral renal agenesis is commoner than bilateral renal agenesis, with an incidence of 3 per 1000 after ultrasonography of 682 adults [9]. The incidence from autopsy studies is reported as 1 in 551 [10].

There is a high incidence of renal and other anomalies of the urogenital tract affecting the solitary kidney [11,12]. The anomalies found in the contralateral solitary kidney include renal dysplasia, renal ectopia, vesicoureteric reflux, pelviureteric junctional hydronephrosis, ipsilateral anomalies of the mullerian system and cysts of the seminal vesicle [13]. Unilateral renal agenesis is often seen in patients with high anorectal agenesis and oesophageal atresia and tracheo-oesophageal fistula: in both of these anomalies the vertebral column may be abnormal, suggesting that the 'insult' occurred

early in intrauterine life at between 29 and 32 days of gestation. This observation is supported by the spectrum of caudal regression [14] and confirmed by the production of renal agenesis by irradiating the caudal somites in the experimental animal [15].

Other intrauterine environmental factors such as congenital rubella [16] and thalidomide [17] have been associated with unilateral renal agenesis. The role of ureteric obstruction is relevant, especially in patients with an ipsilateral ureteric remnant in whom renal dysplasia may occur. The possible reabsorption of such a hypoplastic dysplastic remnant may occur if there is obstruction on that side. In the experimental situation obstruction to the mesonephric ducts leads to renal agenesis [18]. However, genetic factors do play a major aetiological role in renal agenesis whether unilateral or bilateral [1,19]. Familial examples have been described in brothers [20], in sisters [21] and in monozygous twins [22]. One of the earliest reports [23] described a boy and his uncle both with renal agenesis. There is insufficient evidence to determine the method of inheritance, but it is probably dominant as it has been described in three generations of one family [24].

Chromosomal anomalies and syndrome complexes have all been associated with renal agenesis (Table 1.1), but again there appears to be no definite pattern. There is also a higher incidence of other renal anomalies such as horseshoe kidney, duplex pelvicalyceal collecting system, pelviureteric junctional hydronephrosis and vesicoureteric reflux, in other members of the families (Figure 1.1a).

Table 1.1 Genetic disorders and syndrome complexes associated with renal agenesis

Turner's syndrome
Trisomy 13 syndrome
Trisomy 18 syndrome
18g Syndrome
Rubinstein–Taybi syndrome
Marfan's syndrome
Aniridia, and psychomotor retardation syndrome
Extrahepatic biliary atresia syndrome
Klippel–Feil deformity
VATER association

Familial Interrelationship of Congenital Renal Anomalies

(a)

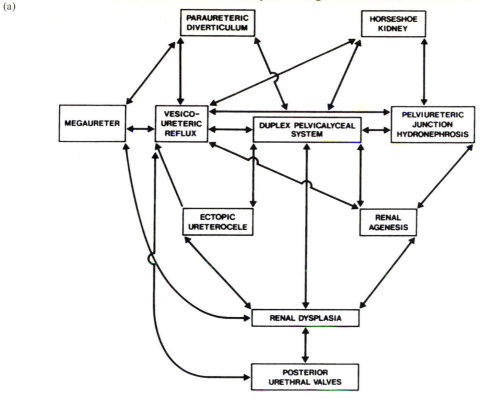

Duplex Pelvicalyceal System: Vesico-ureteric Reflux, Para-ureteric Diverticulum
Familial Interrelationahip

(b)

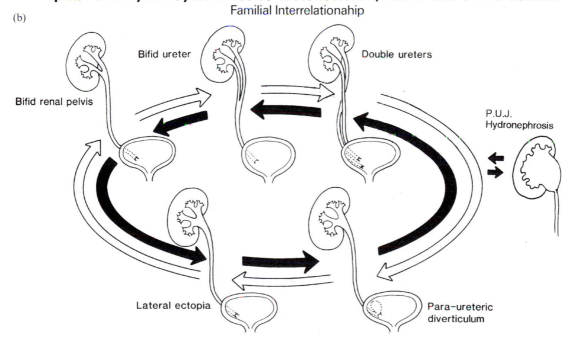

Figure 1.1 (a), (b) Interrelationship between different congenital urinary tract anomalies.

Renal dysplasia: hypoplasia

Renal dysplasia is classified into three main groups [25]. In group I there is obstruction of a ureter so the whole kidney is affected. In group II the dysplasia is segmental, e.g. with double ureters and an ectopic ureterocele the upper pole is affected, and in group III with obstruction to the outflow tract, such as posterior urethral valves or the prune belly syndrome which may result in bilateral dysplasia or hypoplasia. It can be seen from this classification that obstruction within the urinary tract during intrauterine life is of aetiological significance.

Genetic factors may also be important, as segmental dysplasia is associated with double ureters and double ureters are probably inherited as an autosomal dominant gene of variable penetrance [26,27]. The other factor which is important is the timing of the obstruction during intrauterine life, e.g. if early in gestation renal dysplasia may be the result whereas a later onset of obstruction may result in hydronephrosis. This is supported by the finding of contralateral problems in 20 patients with a multicystic kidney in whom the opposite kidney was hydronephrotic in 11 and hypoplastic in five [28]. This clinical observation has been supported by experimental work in the pregnant ewe. Early obstruction to the ureter in the fetal sheep resulted in multicystic renal dysplasia whereas later obstruction was associated with hydronephrosis [29]. The use of maternal and infant ultrasonography has led to a better understanding of the natural history of renal dysplasia before and after delivery of the infant.

There is an association with renal dysplasia and nephroblastoma [30] and pelviureteric junctional hydronephrosis, both of which have a familial tendency or chromosomal anomaly as part of the interrelationship. This, together with the common association of double ureters with segmental dysplasia, supports the view that genetic factors as well as obstruction are important in the aetiology of renal dysplasia.

Familial examples of renal dysplasia in siblings have been reported [31–33]. There has only been one review of a family survey, using ultrasound for the investigation of first-degree relatives [34], which found two affected siblings in 1 in 21 families investigated.

Table 1.2 Genetic disorders and syndrome complexes associated with renal dysplasia and hypoplasia

Trisomy 18
Cerebro-hepato-renal syndrome (Zellweger's)
Meckel's syndrome
Laurence–Moon–Biedl syndrome
Exomphalos-macroglossia-gigantism syndrome
Polydactyly with neonatal chondrodystrophy
Renal dysplasia and asplenia

The association of multiple congenital defects such as oesophageal and rectal atresia with renal dysplasia is well known and suggests local environmental effects as a causative factor. Other anomalies found in association with renal dysplasia and hypoplasia are listed in Table 1.2.

Horseshoe kidney: renal ectopia

The incidence of horseshoe kidneys varies between 1 in 400 to 1 in 1000 [35,36]. There is a preponderance of males and in approximately 20% there are other congenital genito-urinary tract anomalies (16/96) and other system anomalies were often found (51 in 32 patients from a series of 96) [37].

Horseshoe kidneys associated with chromosomal anomalies (Turner's syndrome) and other syndrome complexes (Table 1.3) (Figure 1.2), and in association with double ureters, vesicoureteric reflux, posterior urethral valves and pelviureteric junction (PUJ) hydronephrosis, have been seen by the author.

Monozygotic twins, one with a horseshoe kidney and one with crossed renal ectopia, has

Table 1.3 Genetic disorders and syndrome complexes associated with horseshoe kidney and renal ectopia

Turner's syndrome
Trisomy 13 syndrome
Trisomy 18 syndrome
18g Syndrome
Trisomy 9p syndrome
Meckel's syndrome
Facio-cardio-renal syndrome
Oro-cranio-digital syndrome
13 Ring syndrome
Exomphalos-macroglossal gigantism syndrome
Marfan's syndrome
Klippel–Feil deformity
Vater association

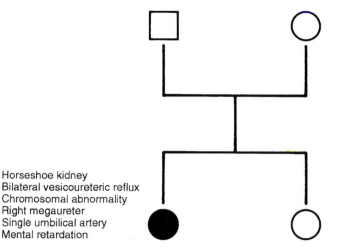

Horseshoe kidney
Bilateral vesicoureteric reflux
Chromosomal abnormality
Right megaureter
Single umbilical artery
Mental retardation

Figure 1.2 Family history of a patient with a horseshoe kidney and multiple anomalies.

been reported [38]. I have treated monozygotic concordant twins with horseshoe kidneys whose parents had normal renal outlines on pyelography. The interrelationship between renal anomalies is well recorded in a family in whom the mother had right double ureters, the daughter left renal agenesis and her son a horseshoe kidney [39]. In another family reported [40], three siblings had a horseshoe kidney.

In patients with vertebral anomalies the incidence of horseshoe kidney is increased, suggesting an early 'insult' to the fetus at the time of segmentation of the embryo.

In a personal series of 96 patients with spina bifida, there were the following associated renal anomalies: horseshoe kidney (three); crossed renal ectopia (two); renal agenesis (three); ectopia (three); duplex pelvicalyceal collecting system (three); renal hypoplasia/dysplasia (one). Thus a similar pattern is appearing with genetic and local environmental factors being important in aetiology, but there is no established pattern of an interrelationship between such genitourinary tract anomalies (Table 1.3).

Polycystic kidneys (Table 1.4)

Two types of polycystic disease occur, first, infantile polycystic disease (Potter type I) and, secondly, adult polycystic disease (Potter type III).

Table 1.4 Genetic disorders and syndrome complexes associated with cystic kidneys

Intestinal polyposis (Peutz–Jegers syndrome)
Turner's syndrome
Trisomy 21 syndrome
Trisomy 13 syndrome
Trisomy 18 syndrome
Klinefelter's syndrome (XXY)
Cerebro-hepato-renal (Zellweger's) syndrome
Meckel's syndrome
Laurence–Moon–Biedl syndrome
Tuberous sclerosis
Ehlers–Danlos syndrome
Exomphalos-macroglossia-gigantism syndrome
Oro-facio-digital syndrome
Polydactyly with neonatal chondrodystrophy
Marfan's syndrome
Apert's syndrome
Extrahepatic biliary atresia
Goldenhar's syndrome
Renal dysplasia and asplenia

Infantile polycystic disease (Potter Type I)

This form of polycystic disease is inherited as an autosomal recessive gene. On clinicopathological findings, it has been subdivided into four groups, perinatal, neonatal, infantile and juvenile [41]. Fortunately, the incidence is low (0.16 per 1000 live births). In severe cases the oligohydramnios is associated with pulmonary hypoplasia and early death. In the majority of patients death occurs from progressive renal failure within the first year of life. Associated genitourinary tract anomalies include a duplex pelvicalyceal collecting system, horseshoe kidney, posterior urethral valves and hypospadias. The kidneys are uniformly enlarged and there may be hypertension and hepatomegaly.

Adult polycystic disease (Potter Type III)

This form of polycystic disease is inherited as an autosomal dominant gene with high penetrance. The patient is often symptom free until the third to fifth decade, but then presents with pain in the loin, haematuria, palpable kidneys and hypertension. In one of my patients with bilateral VUR and paraureteric diverticula, the father had polycystic kidneys (Figure 1.3). Often the diagnosis is made as an incidental finding at a post-mortem examination. Cystic disease of the liver, spleen, lungs, ovaries and uterus have been reported in association with adult polycystic disease. A chromosomal anomaly is described with an α-globulin locus on the short arm of chromosome 16.

On rare occasions the adult form is seen in infancy: in one such case the renal enlargement was gross, producing respiratory difficulties, but renal function was normal. The patient grew around his enlarged kidneys and eventually the diagnosis of tuberous sclerosis was confirmed.

The pathogenesis of renal cysts is difficult to determine except by microdissection techniques. There may be dilatation through Bowman's capsule or the convoluted tubules (mesonephric origin). The cysts found in cystic dysplasia are associated with ureteric obstruction (group I), segmental (group II) or with outflow tract obstruction (group III). In these latter groups the timing of the obstruction during intrauterine life is critical, with dysplasia or hydronephrosis being the sequelae.

Pelvicalyceal collecting system anomalies

Duplex pelvicalyceal collecting system
(Table 1.5) (Figure 1.1b)

In the general population up to 5% may have one of the variants of a duplex pelvicalyceal collecting system. The commonest variant is a bifid renal pelvis (4.3%) and either bifid or double ureters (0.7%) [27]. Many of these patients remain symptom free throughout life but others are associated with urinary infection (vesicoureteric reflux), incontinence (ectopic ureter), obstruction (ectopic ureterocele) and loss of functioning renal tissue (dysplasia/hypoplasia).

In 1956 a mother and two daughters with either bifid or double ureters was reported [42] and the recommendation was made that 'once a duplication of the upper urinary tract is discovered in a patient all members of the family warrant intravenous pyelography'.

In order to determine the method of inheritance of a duplex collecting system, two groups have carried out intravenous pyelography in first degree relatives of index patients with either bifid or double ureters [26,27]. In the first series, 123 intravenous pyelograms (IVPs) were carried out in the first degree relatives of 39 index patients (M 9 : F 30) and in 8 of 52 parents and 7 out of 67 siblings and 1 of 4 grandparents duplications were found. In the second survey, 30 index patients were investigated and 21 relatives had a bifid system of whom 11 had either double or bifid ureters. As there was an equal frequency of a duplex system in parents and siblings, it would support the concept that the method of inheritance is autosomal dominant, probably with variable penetrance.

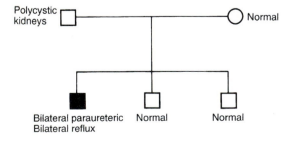

Figure 1.3 Index patient with bilateral VUR and paraureteric diverticula whose father had the adult form of polycystic kidneys.

Table 1.5 Genetic disorders and syndrome complexes associated with a duplex pelvicalyceal collecting system

Turner's syndrome
Trisomy 13 syndrome
Trisomy 18 syndrome
Rubinstein–Taybi syndrome
Exomphalos-macroglossia-gigantism syndrome
Marfan's syndrome
Spina bifida
Hypertelorism with oesophageal abnormality and
  hypospadias

In the second series an additional observation was the finding of three families with vesicoureteric reflux unassociated with either a bifid or double collecting system (Figure 1.4). A further observation is that in many patients with vesicoureteric reflux the radiologist does not report the minor degrees of a duplex system such as a bifid renal pelvis. In the older textbooks [43] there is the statement that the incidence of urinary infection in patients with a duplex system is increased 20-fold. Another significant observation is that in patients with a unilateral bifid renal pelvis, with bifid or double ureters associated, there is vesicoureteric reflux in 25% [44], which suggests that the position of the ureteric orifice may be relevant in the aetiology of vesicoureteric reflux and that this may be determined by genetic factors [45,46].

Vesicoureteric reflux (Table 1.6) (Figure 1.1b)

Familial vesicoureteric reflux (VUR) was first described in 1964 [47]. In this family a mother

Table 1.6 Genetic disorders and syndrome complexes associated with vesicoureteric reflux

Laurence–Moon–Biedl syndrome
Silver–Russell syndrome
Hypertelorism with oesophageal abnormality and
   hypospadias
Perthes disease
Preauricular sinuses

and three daughters had VUR and the maternal grandmother at 41 years of age had chronic pyelonephritis (reflux nephropathy) and a history of urinary tract infections in childhood. This author made other observations, first, all the members of the family suffered with severe constipation and, secondly, what happens to these female children in any future pregnancy with dilatation of the upper urinary tracts.

Since 1964 there have been numerous reports of familial VUR [44–46,48–54]. In two of these reports the relationship between VUR and a duplex pelvicalyceal collecting system is

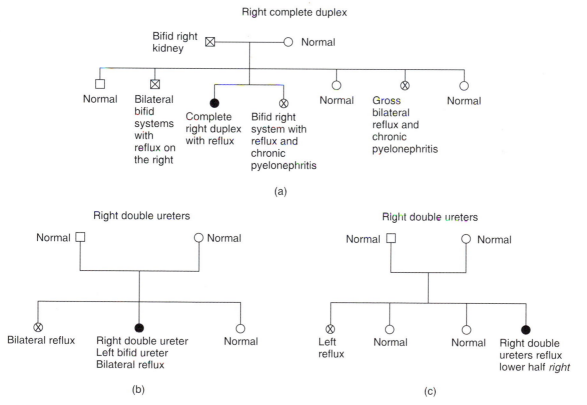

(a)

(b)

(c)

Figure 1.4 The family histories of three families with familial duplex pelvicalyceal collecting systems and VUR unassociated with a duplex system.

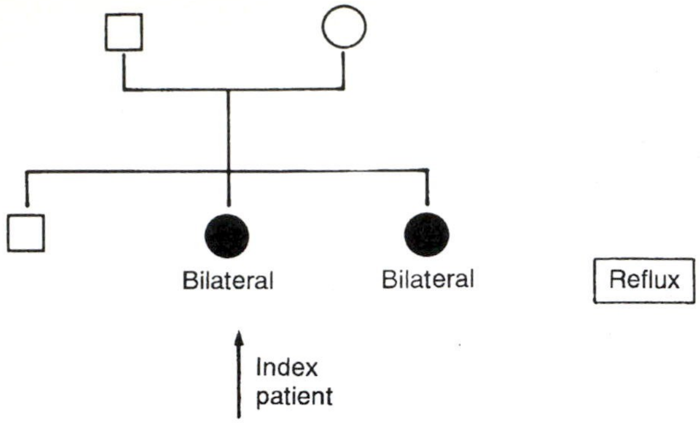

Bilateral   Bilateral   Reflux

Index
patient

Figure 1.5 A family history showing an example of familial reflux.

recorded. In the first report [49], three of eight families with VUR had an associated duplex system. In the second [44], a review of 32 index patients with VUR, in seven families there was familial VUR (Figure 1.5) and in a further six families a duplex pelvicalyceal collecting system was found in first degree relatives (Figure 1.6). These findings support the hypothesis that there is a direct relationship between VUR and a duplex collecting system and that it may be inherited as an autosomal dominant gene which in some patients may be of low penetrance.

If this hypothesis is accepted the interrelationship between a duplex collecting system and lateral ectopia of the ureteric orifice causing VUR is relevant. There is no doubt that the length of the intramural ureter is important in preventing VUR [55]. In a duplex system with double ureters, the lower pole ureter passes more directly through the wall of the bladder and the resultant shorter course predisposes to VUR and there is either renal dysplasia or, if infection occurs, reflux nephro-

pathy. Reflux to the contralateral non-duplex kidney in unilateral cases is found in 25% [44] with a symmetrical trigone. In patients with asymmetry of the trigone the VUR was unilateral, whether a bifid system was present or absent. This suggests that lateral ectopia of the ureteric orifice is the common factor in such patients.

The results of two family surveys [27,44] support the inheritance of a duplex system and primary VUR is by autosomal genes of variable penetrance and that lateral ectopia of the ureteric orifice should be considered as part of the syndrome of duplicity (Figure 1.7).

Other authors [46] suggest that the length of the intramural ureter is determined by multiple genes with a cumulative effect, and that this polygenic method of inheritance would explain the transmission within families, sexual and racial differences, and the unilateral and bilateral occurrence of VUR.

Attempts have been made to identify a marker which would highlight the genetic susceptibility to VUR. The relationship between

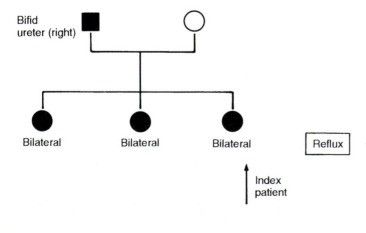

Bifid
ureter (right)

Bilateral   Bilateral   Bilateral   Reflux

Index
patient

Figure 1.6 A family history showing an example of familial reflux and its association with a duplex pelvicalyceal collecting system.

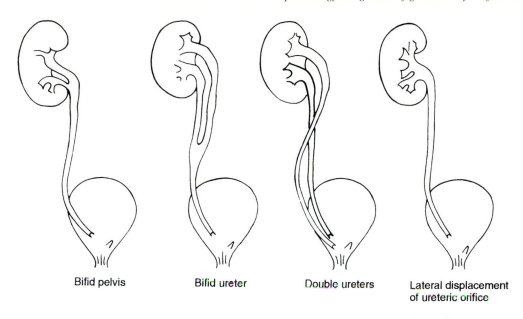

Bifid pelvis   Bifid ureter   Double ureters   Lateral displacement
                                                                     of ureteric orifice

Figure 1.7 Lateral ectopia with VUR could be considered as part of the syndrome of a duplex pelvicalyceal collecting system.

hair and eye colour and primary VUR has been investigated [56,57] and no correlation was found, with the exception of red hair in 900 children with VUR.

Antigenic specificities have also been investigated [58,59]. The HLA antigen specificities in patients with reflux nephropathy were studied in 44 patients and compared with 526 controls. In female patients with reflux nephropathy HLA B_{12} and in male patients with reflux nephropathy HLA B_8 in combination with HLA A_9 were increased. In both sexes, HLA BW_{15} was increased.

Paraureteric diverticulum (Figure 1.1b)

It is possible that the paraureteric diverticulum (PUD) represents an aborted ureteric bud [60]. In two surveys of patients with a duplex collecting system [27] and VUR [44], there was a relative of an index patient with PUD. This observation led to an investigation of the families of 22 index patients with PUD [60,61]. In three index patients the PUD was associated with either a bifid or double ureter, which is a 20-fold increase over the expected incidence. Three mothers had bifid ureters and one sister a bifid renal pelvis. One mother had bilateral reflux nephropathy, two siblings had VUR and one brother a PUD.

This high incidence of duplications of the collecting system in index patients and first-degree relatives suggests a direct relationship between the two conditions which may have a genetic basis. The increase was 20-fold for index patients and 10-fold for first-degree relatives. The formation of a PUD remains obscure, but a blind-ending ureteric bud could become everted by the normal intravesical pressure to form a diverticulum. There was also an increased incidence of VUR, suggesting that VUR, PUD and duplication of the pelvicalyceal collecting system form a syndrome complex with similar methods of inheritance (Figure 1.8).

Megaureters

Identical twin sisters have been reported, one of whom had gross bilateral VUR and the other had left VUR [62]. In another girl with gross bilateral VUR her non-identical twin sister was normal. At that time it was suggested that the dilatation of the ureters was primary and genetic in origin rather than secondary to the VUR.

This last feature causes problems in clinical practice, as in patients with fetal VUR [63,64] the dilatation of the ureters is often severe and could support a primary cause. However with

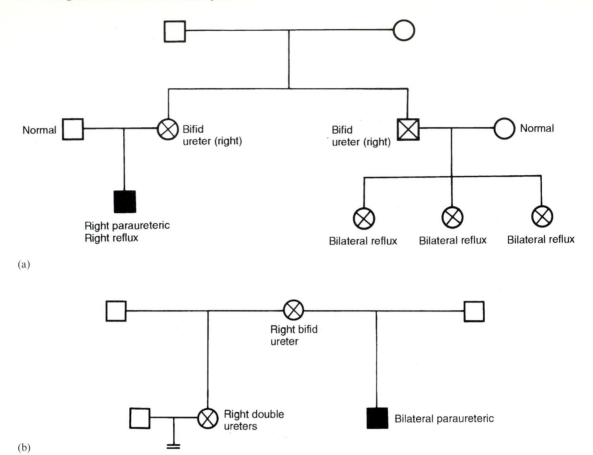

(a)

(b)

Figure 1.8 (a) Familial bilateral VUR whose father had a bifid right ureter. His sister also had a right bifid ureter and her son had a right paraureteric diverticulum associated with right VUR. (b) A mother with a right bifid ureter had a daughter by her first marriage with right double ureters and a son by her second marriage with bilateral paraureteric diverticula.

severe fetal VUR and a developing ureter, the effect is still open to conjecture. Similarly, three index patients with a PUD had megaureters [61] and it is debatable whether these are primary or secondary.

There are isolated reports of megaureters in first-degree relatives [65], but there has been no prospective survey of first-degree relatives of index patients with megaureters. In our survey megaureters were found in association with a PUD(3) [61] (Figure 1.9), and in a series with pelviureteric junctional (PUJ) hydronephrosis one father and one sibling were found with bilateral dilatation of the ureters. In another

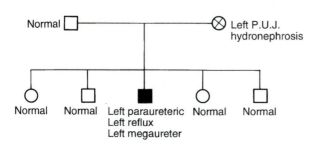

Figure 1.9 Family history with an index patient with a paraureteric diverticulum, left VUR and a left megaureter primary or secondary. Note that the mother of this child had a left PUJ hydronephrosis.

family previously presented, the VUR in one sibling was so severe that it could be classified as a megaureter [27].

Pelviureteric junctional hydronephrosis
(Table 1.7) (Figure 1.1a)

The familial nature of pelviureteric junctional (PUJ) hydronephrosis was first reported in 1948 [66]. Since then there have been six similar reports [67–72].

Table 1.7 Genetic disorders and syndrome complexes associated with dilated ureters and PUJ hydronephrosis

Turner's syndrome
Trisomy 21 syndrome
Trisomy 13 syndrome
Trisomy 18 syndrome
XXY Klinefelter's syndrome
Meckel's syndrome
Laurence–Moon–Biedl syndrome
Rubinstein–Taybi syndrome
Marfan's syndrome
Congenital generalized lipodystrophy
Extrahepatic biliary atresia syndrome

In a family survey to determine the incidence of urological conditions in a series of 19 index patients with PUJ hydronephrosis (Figure 1.10), there was a marked difference of the incidence in families with one parent affected (two of six siblings) and those with neither parent affected (3 of 33 siblings) [73]. In a review of the earlier papers on familial PUJ hydronephrosis, the authors suggested an autosomal dominant gene of variable penetrance [72], which is supported by the results of a prospective survey [73].

In that survey three fathers and one mother had PUJ hydronephrosis. Other findings included one mother with a bifid ureter and three of her six children had bifid ureters, infundibular stenosis (two), renal calculi (two), bilateral dilatation of the ureters (two) and reflux nephropathy (one).

A clinical association of PUJ hydronephrosis and VUR has not often been reported, but is said to range between 10 and 20% [74,75]. In such patients the obstruction demonstrated on intravenous pyelography and DTPA renography must be differentiated from reflux-induced hydronephrosis. The coexistence of VUR with PUJ hydronephrosis could be explained by a coexisting anomaly of a common ureteric bud, as there is a known association between a duplex pelvicalyceal collecting system, VUR, PUD and, indirectly, PUJ hydronephrosis.

Ectopic ureteroceles

Ectopic ureteroceles are associated with double ureters and renal dysplasia, both of which are known to have a genetic basis. It therefore becomes difficult to evaluate the genetic basis of the condition, although the renal dysplasia is almost certainly secondary to obstruction from the ureterocele.

Ureteroceles have been reported in identical twins [76], i.e. they were concordant. However, I have seen discordant identical twins with a left double ureter and an associated ectopic ureterocele (Figure 1.11(a)) and double ureters occurring in a grandmother and a granddaughter, the former with VUR and the latter with an ectopic ureterocele (Figure 1.11(b)). There has been one review of 26 index patients with ectopic ureteroceles, and contralateral duplicity of the calyceal collecting system was seen in 12 of the index patients. There were 12 other known relatives out of 114 who had other known urological anomalies, including a duplex system which is a 5–10-fold increase over the expected incidence.

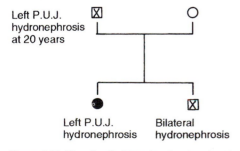

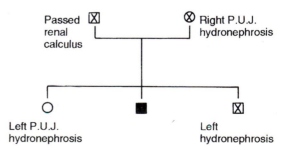

Figure 1.10 Two family histories showing familial PUJ hydronephrosis.

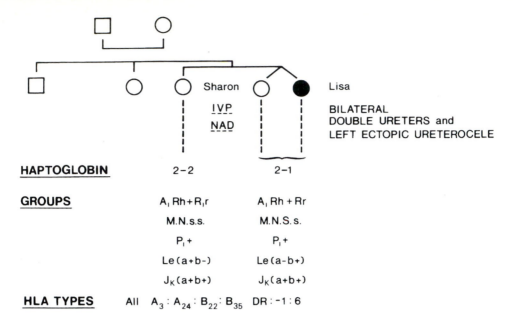

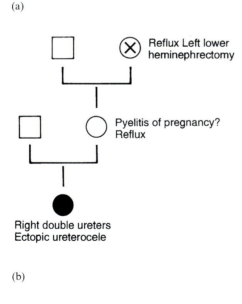

Figure 1.11 (a) Discordant identical twin girls (part of triplets), one of whom had a left double ureter with an ectopic ureter with an ectopic ureterocele. (b) Double ureters with reflux in a grandmother and with an ectopic ureterocele in her granddaughter. The mother of the granddaughter suffered with pyelitis of pregnancy but was not fully investigated.

Outflow tract anomalies

Posterior urethral valves

In the author's clinical practice, posterior urethral valves in siblings have not been encountered. Renal dysplasia in association with severe VUR is found quite commonly in patients with posterior urethral valves and it may either be related to an anomalous origin of the ureteric bud or to some, at present, unknown genetic factor.

Renal dysplasia may be genetically determined or related to obstruction during early intrauterine life [77]. In one study of renal dysplasia with ultrasonography, a family was found with two brothers with posterior urethral valves and renal dysplasia [34].

Bladder exstrophy and epispadias

Bladder exstrophy is commoner in males with an overall incidence of 3.3 per 100 000 births, whilst the incidence of epispadias is 2.4 per 100 000 births [78]. Female epispadias is rare, with a M : F ratio of 4 : 1.

The aetiology of bladder exstrophy and epispadias is unknown, but a group of infants born to women treated with progestins in early pregnancy had bladder exstrophy/epispadias anomalies [79]. The risk of recurrence of bladder exstrophy and epispadias in the same family was thought to be low, and as many patients were infertile the risk to subsequent generations was low, but in a series of 66 exstrophy patients with 215 offspring three had exstrophy. This risk of 1 in 70 is far greater than the expected incidence in the general population [80]. Exstrophy in both of monozygotic twins was found in 5 of 17 sets of twins [80].

Hypospadias

There was an increase in the incidence of hypospadias in 1969, rising to a peak in 1970–71, and then it plateaued [81,82]. The former authors found a mean incidence of 1.76 per 1000 live births and suggested that there may be an environmental cause for the observed increase, such as the use of the contraceptive pill or the use of progestagens for recurrent abortion. Other authors [83] have shown that there is an increased risk of developing hypospadias in infants born as a result of assisted reproduction technology (ART) and reported two infants with hypospadias out of 53 male infants conceived following ART. One of the infants with a penoscrotal hypospadias was one of a set of dizygote twins and the other twin had a glandular hypospadias. In another study [84] to determine whether hypospadias is associated with the maternal use of oral contraceptives, no demonstrable association was found in a series of 725 infants in Spain and 631 infants in Sweden.

There is no doubt that genetic factors play an important part in the causation of hypospadias [85]. In one large-scale family survey from Denmark, 10% of brothers of index patients were also affected, which is some 30 times the expected incidence in the population. Fathers have often been similarly affected

(Figure 1.12). The suggested method of inheritance is polygenic. In a series of 80 patients [86], five were due to progestin and five had anomalies of the sex chromosomes which included XX/XY mosaicism (three) and 10 XO/XY mosaicism (two).

The androgen receptor gene has been studied in two unrelated families. Two brothers presented with severe penoscrotal hypospadias, bilateral undescended testes and micropenis in one of the families, and in the other family two brothers had perineal hypospadias without any other associated defects. In both families androgen synthesis was normal. Androgen binding assays from the four patients with hypospadias demonstrated abnormal androgen binding affinity. Gene mutations were identified and a single base androgen gene mutation was found in both families [87].

Other congenital anomalies found in association with hypospadias include inguinal herniae and undescended testes. The association of undescended testes with a hypospadias is an indication for chromosomal investigations. Other anomalies associated with hypospadias are often within the genitourinary system and there is evidence that the more severe the anomalies the higher the incidence of other associated defects [88]. In a series of 272 patients with hypospadias (45% had penoscrotal hypospadias), 139 anomalies were found in 108 patients and included undescended testes (36), utriculus masculinus (32), prepenile scrotum (21), hypoplasia of the testis (18), PUJ hydronephrosis (six), rotation of the penis (five), vesicoureteric reflux (four) and miscellaneous anomalies (nine). This association of defects may also have a genetic origin as seen in the family history of one of my patients with a duplex system, PUJ hydronephrosis and hypospadias occurring in siblings (Figure 1.13).

Chromosomal anomalies

Chromosomal anomalies have been subdivided into three groups in this chapter, the commoner anomalies such as Turner's syndrome and trisomy 21 (group I), rare anomalies such as the 13g syndrome (group II) and a final group of very rare defects (group III) (Table 1.8).

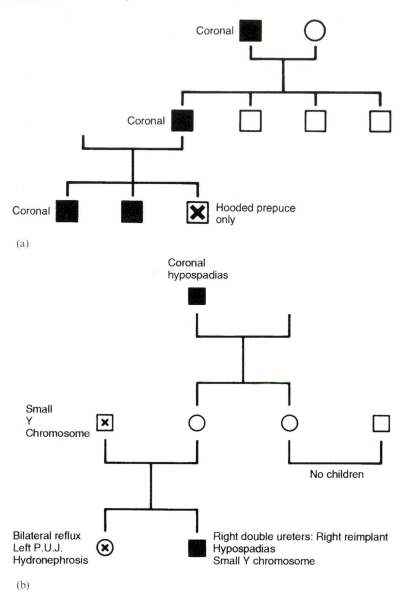

Figure 1.12 (a) Family history of coronal hypospadias through three generations. (b) Family history of hypospadias in a grandfather and his grandson. Note the chromosomal anomaly and VUR and PUJ hydronephrosis in the sister of the grandson.

Group I

Turner's syndrome

This syndrome is characterized by short stature, ovarian dysgenesis and webbing of the neck, and occurs in 1 in 5000 liveborn infants. Other signs include cubitus valgus, a broad chest with widely spaced nipples and hypoplastic nails. Cardiovascular anomalies such as coarctation of the aorta occur in up to 40% of the patients.

Renal anomalies

A variety of renal anomalies occurs in about 66% of patients and includes horseshoe kidney, cystic, duplex and ectopic kidneys, PUj hydronephrosis and renal agenesis.

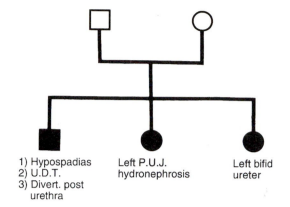

1) Hypospadias
2) U.D.T.
3) Divert. post urethra

Left P.U.J. hydronephrosis

Left bifid ureter

Figure 1.13 Family history showing a patient with hypospadias with his two sisters having a PUJ hydronephrosis and a bifid ureter.

Genetics

The chromosomes (45 XO) are said to be attributable to cytogenetic errors, such as non-disjunction or chromosomal loss during gametogenesis.

Trisomy 21 (Down's syndrome)

Patients with Down's syndrome have a variable degree of mental retardation, hypotonia, narrow and upward slope of the palpebral

Table 1.8 Chromosomal anomalies associated with renal anomalies

Group I
Turner's syndrome (45 XO)
Down's syndrome (trisomy 21)
Trisomy 13 syndrome
Trisomy 18 syndrome

Group II (see Table 1.9)
13g Syndrome
18g Syndrome
Triploidy syndrome
Cat eye syndrome
Long arm 21 deletion syndrome

Group III (see Table 1.10)
4p Syndrome
5p Syndrome
Trisomy 8
Partial trisomy 10g syndrome
Trisomy 9p syndrome 9p monosomy
Trisomy 9p mosaic
XXXXY Syndrome
XXXXX Pentax syndrome
XXY Klinefelter's syndrome

fissures, epicanthic folds, flat nasal bridge and a flattened occiput and simian creases. Prominence of the tongue, a high-arched palate, low-set ears and broad short hands are other characteristics. The IQ is usually 25–50 but can be as high as 80. The incidence is 1 in 600 live births, but increases to 1 in 50 with a maternal age over 45 years. Congenital heart disease is common and occurs in up to 40% and includes septal defects, patent ductus arteriosus and pulmonary stenosis. Duodenal atresia, obstruction and malrotation is a common associated gastrointestinal anomaly.

Renal anomalies

These are unusual in Down's syndrome, but PUJ hydronephrosis and cystic changes may be found.

Genetics

The fundamental anomaly is an extra chromosome 21 due to non-dysjunction of the chromosome during meiosis and a major predisposing cause is increasing maternal age. Some 3% of the patients have translocation inherited from the parents, therefore chromosomal analysis of the parents is necessary. Antenatal diagnosis is now an essential part of management, especially in the pregnant mother over 35 years of age when the incidence increases to 1 in 800 live births.

Trisomy 13

The syndrome is characterized by multiple congenital anomalies which include mental retardation, CNS defects such as microcephaly, cleft lip and palate, low-set ears, simian creases, polydactyly and undescended testes. In 80% of patients there are cardiovascular anomalies such as septal defects, patent ductus arteriosus and dextrocardia. The incidence is 1 in 14 500 live births. The prognosis is poor and the majority of infants die in the first year of life.

Renal anomalies

Polycystic kidneys, duplex pelvicalyceal collecting system, unilateral renal agenesis, horseshoe kidney and PUJ hydronephrosis have been reported in this syndrome.

Genetics

There are 47 chromosomes with an extra chromosome 13. This is due to non-dysjunction during meiosis.

Trisomy 18 (Edward's syndrome)

This syndrome is common in females, with an incidence of 1 in 4500 live births. The commonest associated problems are polyhydramnios, single umbilical artery, mental retardation, hypertonicity, low-set ears and micrognathia; undescended testes and inguinal and umbilical herniae are also found, as well as congenital heart defects such as a ventricular septal defect and patent ductus arteriosus. External genital anomalies include hypospadias, hypoplasia of the labia majora, prominence of the clitoris and bifid uterus. The mortality is high and only 10% survive longer than their first birthday.

Renal anomalies

These include horseshoe kidney, renal agenesis, renal dysplasia, duplex pelvicalyceal collecting system, ectopia, solitary cysts, PUJ hydronephrosis and polycystic kidneys.

Genetics

There is trisomy of all or part of chromosome 18, probably due to non-dysjunction in meiosis.

Group II (Table 1.9)

This group comprises rare syndromes with genitourinary anomalies.

Group III (Table 1.10)

This group comprises very rare syndromes with renal anomalies.

Syndrome complexes

The following syndrome complexes will be described and briefly discussed:

Rubinstein–Taybi
Apert's
Klinefelter's
Silver–Russell
Peutz–Jeger

Klippel–Trenaunay–Weber
Linear sebaceous naevus
Ehler–Danlos
Beckwith–Wiedemann
Tuberous sclerosis
Renal dysplasia and asplenia
Meckel's
Laurence–Moon–Biedl
Extrahepatic biliary atresia
Klippel–Feil
Cerebrohepatorenal (Zellweger's)
Marfan's
Vater association.

Rubinstein–Taybi syndrome

The clinical features include mental subnormality, microcephaly, downward slanting palpebral fissure and broad thumbs and first toes. The incidence is sporadic.

The renal anomalies associated with this syndrome include a duplex pelvicalyceal collecting system and renal agenesis.

Apert's syndrome

The clinical features include syndactyly, acrocephaly, craniosynostosis, facial asymmetry, flat midface, proptosis and sometimes a cleft palate. The condition is inherited as an autosomal dominant, although a fresh mutation is the commonest presentation.

The renal anomalies found include polycystic kidneys and hydronephrosis.

Klinefelter's syndrome (XXY)

The clinical features include tall stature, undescended testes and delayed fusion of epiphyses. The extra X chromosome is due to non-dysjunction from failure in meiosis of the X chromosome.

The renal anomalies found include renal cysts and hydronephrosis.

Silver–Russell syndrome

The clinical features include short stature, skeletal asymmetry, late closure of anterior fontanelle, a triangular face, down-turning

Table 1.9 Group II: rare syndromes with genitourinary anomalies

Syndrome name	Genetics	General	G.U. anomalies
13g Syndrome	Ring 13 chromosome	Mental retardation Absent thumbs Anorectal agenesis	Hypoplastic kidneys Hydronephrosis Hypospadias Undescended testes
18g Syndrome	Deletion of a $\frac{1}{4}$ or $\frac{1}{2}$ of the length of the long arm or chromosome 18 or ring 18 chromosome	Mental retardation Deafness Midfacial hypoplasia Hypertelorism Narrow palate Low-set ears Optic atrophy	Hypospadias Hypoplastic labia minora and clitoris Undescended testes Horseshoe kidney Unilateral renal agenesis Hydronephrosis
Triploidy syndrome	Full set of extra chromosomes Fertilization of an ovum by two spermatozoa	Usually stillborn or early abortion	Polycystic kidney Cystic dysplasia Hydronephrosis
Cat eye syndrome	Extra acrocentric chromosome	Coloboma of iris Anorectal agenesis Microophthalmia Congenital heart disease Biliary atresia Dislocated hips Cleft palate Mental retardation	Renal ectopia Hydronephrosis Cystic dysplasia Renal hypoplasia
Long arm 21 deletion syndrome	Deletion of the long arm of chromosome 21	Mental retardation Prominent nasal bridge Micrognathia Pyloric stenosis Thrombocytopenia	Hypospadias Undescended testes Hemivertebrae Syndactyly Renal agenesis

Table 1.10 Group III: very rare syndromes with renal anomalies

Chromosomal anomaly	Renal anomaly
4p Syndrome	Renal agenesis Renal hypoplasia Vesicoureteric reflux Hydronephrosis
5p Syndrome	Renal agenesis Horseshoe kidney Duplex collecting system
Trisomy 8	Hydronephrosis Vesicoureteric reflux Bifid renal pelvis
Partial trisomy 10g syndrome	Renal hypoplasia
Trisomy 9g syndrome	Horseshoe kidney Hydronephrosis
Trisomy 9p syndrome 9p Monosomy	Hydronephrosis Duplex collecting system
Trisomy 9p mosaic	Renal cysts
XXXXY Syndrome	Hydronephrosis
XXXXX Syndrome	Renal hypoplasia Renal dysplasia
XXY Klinefelter's syndrome	Renal cysts Hydronephrosis

angle of the mouth, syndactyly, cryptorchidism, hypospadias and a small penis. The method of inheritance is by a dominant single gene.

The renal problems encountered included PUJ hydronephrosis and VUR.

Peutz–Jegers syndrome

The clinical features include gastrointestinal polyposis and mucocutaneous melanotic pigmentation. The lesions are hamartomas and the inheritance is by an autosomal dominant gene.

The renal anomalies found include polycystic kidneys and ureteral polyposis. Malignant transformation of the polyp may occur.

Klippel–Trenaunay–Webber syndrome

The clinical feature is haemangiomas of the kidney.

Linear sebaceous naevus syndrome

The clinical features include midfacial naevus, convulsions and mental retardation, and colobomas.

The renal anomalies include nodular nephroblastomatosis.

Ehler–Danlos syndrome

The clinical features include hyperelasticity of the skin and blood vessels and hypermotility of the joints. Thus congenital dislocation of the hips, epicanthic folds and congenital heart disease are associated with this condition. Ten different types have been described [89] and the condition is probably autosomal dominant, although some types are inherited as an autosomal recessive condition.

The renal anomalies found in association include PUJ hydronephrosis, hypoplastic renal artery, polycystic disease and medullary sponge kidney.

Exomphalos: macroglossia; gigantism (Beckwith–Wiedemann syndrome)

The clinical features include macroglossia, omphthalocele, and an ear anomaly with a bilateral focal indented areas on the posterior rim of the helix. Islet cell hyperplasia is associated with hypoglycaemia. The condition is inherited as an autosomal dominant condition.

The renal anomalies found include nephroblastoma, renal medullary dysplasia, hydroureters, renal ectopia and cysts and possibly hypospadias.

Tuberous sclerosis

This condition was first described by Von Recklinghausen in 1862. The clinical features include mental retardation, epilepsy and adenoma sebaceum which appears between 2 and 5 years of age. Shagreen patches become apparent. Intracranial calcification occurs. The expected incidence is 1 in 20 000 to 1 in 300 000 live births. It is inherited as an autosomal dominant condition.

The renal anomalies found include renal angiomyolipomas and cystic disease, which resemble adult polycystic disease which occasionally presents in the neonatal period.

Renal dysplasia and asplenia

This is a condition characterized by dysplasia of the kidney, liver, pancreas and absence of the spleen. The associated anomalies include renal cystic disease and cardiac anomalies. The method of inheritance is unknown.

Meckel's syndrome

This condition was described by Meckel in 1822. The clinical features include occipital encephalocele, microcephaly, cleft lip and palate, abnormal facies, and polydactyly. Oligohydramnios occurs with Potter facies, pulmonary hypoplasia and club feet. It is inherited as an autosomal dominant.

The renal anomalies include polycystic kidneys, renal dysplasia and multicystic kidneys.

Laurence–Moon–Biedl syndrome

This condition was first described in 1866 and the clinical features include retinitis pigmentosa, mental retardation, obesity, short stature, hypogonadism and polydactyly. It is inherited as an autosomal recessive condition.

The renal anomalies are found in 70–90% of patients and include polyuria, impaired renal concentration and renal failure. The pathophysiology of the condition is not understood. Anorectal agenesis may also be found.

Extrahepatic biliary atresia syndrome

This syndrome was first described in 1964 [90], with five families with two or more siblings with extrahepatic biliary atresia, cardiac and renal malformations.

Klippel–Feil syndrome

This syndrome was first described in 1912. The clinical features include a short neck, low hairline and an abnormal radiograph of the cervical spine. Facial asymmetry, torticollis and Sprengel's deformity may be associated findings. The possible method of inheritance is autosomal dominant.

The renal abnormalities found include renal agenesis and renal ectopia.

Cerebrohepatorenal syndrome (Zellweger's syndrome)

The clinical features are gross hypotonia, dysmorphic facial appearance, high forehead and a dolicocephalic skull, narrow palatal arch, hepatomegaly and ocular changes. The cause is unknown but may be metabolic and related to disturbances of pipecolic acid metabolism and intrahepatic cholestasis.

The renal anomalies found include renal cortical cysts. The patients usually die between 6 months and 3 years of age.

Marfan's syndrome

The clinical features include spider hands and feet, a dolicocephalic skull, postural kyphosis, excessive mobility of joints, high arched palate and a funnel or pigeon chest. The ocular defects include squint, nystagmus, myopia, coloboma, cataracts and subluxation of the lens. Cardiovascular defects include atrial septal defects, coarctation of the aorta and a patent ductus arteriosus. Inheritance is by an autosomal dominant gene.

Genitourinary tract-associated anomalies include undescended testes, polycystic kidneys, renal ectopia and a duplex pelvicalyceal collecting system.

Vater association

It is well known that any serious congenital malformation is often associated with other congenital anomalies; for example, there is an association of rectal atresia with oesophageal atresia and duodenal atresia with Down's syndrome. Some of these anomalies have conveniently been grouped together to form the Vater association. The defects include vertebral, anorectal, tracheo-oesophageal and renal congenital anomalies [91–93]. This interrelationship is seen in Figure 1.14.

Neoplastic disease

Many factors are concerned with the aetiology of malignant disease. However, when a tumour develops in an infant or child, genetic factors are probably playing a greater role than environmental factors. In adults developing malig-

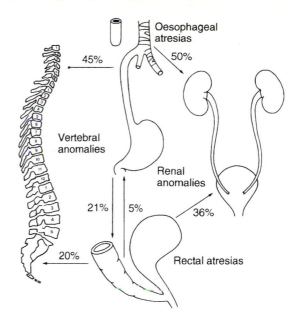

Figure 1.14 Association of oesophageal atresia and rectal atresia with vertebral and renal anomalies (VATER association).

nant disease over 50 years of age, the converse is true.

Nephroblastoma

This tumour of childhood is the second commonest tumour in this age range, with an incidence of 1 in 10 000 live births [94]. In up to 4% of patients the tumour may be bilateral. Associations with the Wiedmann–Beckwith syndrome, hemihypertrophy, horseshoe kidney and a duplex pelvicalyceal collecting system have been reported. There is also a higher incidence of hypospadias and undescended testes [95].

The triad of aniridia, genitourinary tract anomalies and nephroblastoma has been shown to be due to a chromosomal anomaly, with deletion of part of the short arm of chromosome 11 and always included band 11p 13 [96–98]. The deletion 11p 13 is not seen in either normal or tumour tissue from sporadically occurring patients with a nephroblastoma.

The majority of nephroblastomas arise sporadically. Nephroblastomas in a pair of twin boys has been reported [99]. Other familial examples include eight reports of nephroblastoma in concordant monozygotic twins and in a monozygotic twin discordant for nephroblastoma. in that family another sibling developed a nephroblastoma [100].

Nephroblastoma occurring in successive generations of a family has been reported [101]. A father and two of his three daughters developed nephroblastomas [102].

In a review of 58 familial cases [103] it was found that the tumours developed at an earlier stage and the incidence of bilateral disease was increased from the expected 4% to 21%. The probable mechanism of inheritance is by mutation of a gene which with survival of an affected individual would show dominance.

Nephroblastomatosis

Beneath the capsule of the kidney of an infant under 4 months of age there may be small microscopic nodules of primitive metanephric tissue. At times this may be diffuse and at other times it is nodular. The majority of these lesions regress as the infant gets older. These lesions may be a precursor of a nephroblastoma and evidence of their presence is found in up to 50% of nephroblastomas and in almost all patients with a bilateral nephroblastoma [104].

Acknowledgements

I thank the Department of Teaching Media and Medical Illustration of the University of Southampton for Figures 1.1–1.14.

References

1. Kohn G, Borns PF. The association of bilateral and unilateral renal aplasia in the same family. *J Pediatr* 1973; **83**: 95–97.
2. Potter EL. Bilateral renal agenesis. *J Pediatr* 1946; **29**: 68–76.
3. Leck I, Record RG, McKeown T, et al. The incidence of malformations in Birmingham, England 1950–1959. *Teratology* 1968; **1**: 263–280.
4. Potter EL. Facial characteristics of infants with bilateral renal agenesis. *Am J Obstet Gynaecol* 1946; **51**: 885–888.
5. Passarge E, Sutherland JB. Potters syndrome: chromosome analysis of 3 cases with Potters syndrome or related syndromes. *Am J Dis Child* 1965; **109**: 80–83.
6. Crawford M d'A. Renal agenesis and hypoplasia. In: *The Genetics of Renal Tract Disorders*. Oxford Medical Publications, 1988; chap 10.1.1, table 10.1, p 529.
7. Whitehouse W, Mountrose U. Renal agenesis in non-twin siblings. *Am J Obstet Gynecol* 1973; **116**: 880–882.
8. Carter CO, Pescia G. A family study of renal agenesis. *J Med Genet* 1979; **16**: 176–188.
9. Roodhooft AM, Birnholz JC, Holmes LB. Familial nature of congenital absence and severe dysgenesis of both kidneys. *New Engl J Med* 1984; **310**: 1341–1345.
10. Barakat AJ, Drougas JG. Occurrence of congenital abnormalities of kidney and urinary tract in 13 775 autopsies. *Urology* 1991; **38**: 347–350.
11. Dees JE. Prognosis of the solitary kidney. *J Urol* 1960; **83**: 550–552.
12. Holmes LB. Unilateral renal agenesis: common, serious, hereditary. *Paediatr Res* 1972; **6**: 419.
13. Lynch MJ, Flannigan GM. Seminal vesicle cyst, renal agenesis and epididymitis in a 50 year old patient. *Br J Urol* 1992; **69**: 98.
14. Duhamel B. From the mermaid to anal imperforation: the syndrome of caudal regression. *Arch Dis Child* 1961; **36**: 152–155.
15. Wolff E. *La science des monstres*. Paris: Gallimand, 1948.
16. Menser M, Robertson SEJ, Dorman DC. Renal lesions in congenital rubella. *Pediatrics* 1967; **40**: 901–904.
17. Warkany J. *Congenital Malformation, Notes and Comments*. Chicago: Year Book Medical Publishers, 1971; p 92.
18. Boyden EA. Experimental obstruction of the mesonephric ducts. *Proc Soc Exp Biol Med* 1927; **24**: 572–576.
19. Fitch N. Heterogeneity of bilateral renal agenesis. *Can med Assoc J* 1977; **116**: 381–382.
20. Gorvoy J D, Smulewicz J, Rothfield SH. Unilateral renal agenesis in two siblings: case report. *Pediatrics* 1962; **29**: 270–273.
21. Ten Berge BS, Wildervanek LS. Familiare congenitale afwijkingen van het uropoietischen genitale systeem. *Ned Tidischr V Geneeskd* 1951; **95**: 2389.
22. Waardenburgh PJ. Einseitige aplaisie der neiren und ihrer abfuhrwege bei beiden eineiigen zwillingspaarlingen. *Acta Genet med Gemellol (Roma)* 1952; **1**: 317–320.
23. Bound JP. Two cases of congenital absence of one kidney in the same family. *Br Med J* 1943; **2**: 747.
24. Schimke RN, King CR. Hereditary urogenital aplasia. *Clin Genet* 1980; **18**: 417–420.
25. Risdon RA. Renal dysplasia. *J Clin Pathol* 1971; **24**: 57–71.

26. Whitaker J, Danks DM. A study of the inheritance of duplication of the kidneys and ureters. *J Urol* 1966; **95**: 176–178.

27. Atwell JD, Cook PL, Howell CJ et al. Familial incidence of bifid and double ureters. *Arch Dis Child* 1974; **49**: 390–393.

28. Pathak IG, Williams DI. Multicystic kidney and cystic dysplastic kidneys. *Br J Urol* 1984; **36**: 318–331.

29. Beck AD. The effect of intrauterine obstruction upon the development of the foetal kidney. *J Urol* 1971; **105**: 784–789.

30. Hartman GE, Smolik LM, Schochat SJ. The dilemma of the multicystic dysplastic kidney. *Am J Dis Child* 1986; **140**: 925–928.

31. Cain DR, Griggs D, Lackey DA et al. Familial renal agenesis and total dysplasia. *Am J Dis Child* 1974; **128**: 377–380.

32. Pescia GK, Evans KA, Carter CO. The risk of recurrence of renal agenesis. In: *Vth International Congress Human Genetics (Ab)*. Excerpta Medica, 1976; p 94.

33. Williams DI, Risdon RA. Hypoplastic, dysplastic and cystic kidneys. In: Williams DI, Johnston JH (eds) *Paediatric Urology*, 2nd edn. London: Butterworths, 1982; chap 14, pp 137–150.

34. Al Saadi AA, Yoshimoto M, Bree R et al. A family study of renal dysplasia. *Am J Med Genet* 1984; **19**: 669–677.

35. Walters W, Priestley JB. Horseshoe kidney – a review of 68 surgical cases. *J Urol* 1932; **28**: 271–277.

36. Glenn JF. Analysis of fifty-one patients with horseshoe kidney. *New Engl J Med* 1959; **261**: 684–687.

37. Boatman DL, Kolln CP, Flocks RH. Congenital anomalies associated with horseshoe kidney. *J Urol* 1972; **107**: 205–207.

38. Bridge RAC. Horseshoe kidneys in identical twins. *Br J Urol* 1960; **32**: 32–33.

39. Perlman M, Williams J, Ornoy A. Familial ureteric bud anomalies. *J Med Genet* 1976; **13**: 161–163.

40. David RS. Horseshoe kidney: a report of one family. *Br Med J* 1974; **4**: 571–572.

41. Blyth H, Ockenden BG. Polycystic disease of the kidneys and liver presenting in childhood. *J Med Genet* 1971; **8**: 257–284.

42. Girsh LS, Karpinski FIE. Urinary tract malformations, their familial occurrence with special reference to double ureter, double pelvis and double kidney. *New Engl J Med* 1956; **254**: 854–855.

43. Campbell MF, Harrison JH. *Urology*, vol 2, 3rd edn. Philadelphia: Saunders, 1970; pp 1488, 1800.

44. Atwell JD, Cook PL, Strong L et al. The interrelationship between vesicoureteric reflux, trigonal abnormalities and a bifid pelvicalyceal collecting system: a family survey. *Br J Urol* 1977; **49**: 97–107.

45. Burger RH, Smith C. Hereditary and familial vesicoureteral reflux. *J Urol* 1971; **106**: 845–851.

46. Burger RH. A theory on the transmission of congenital vesico-ureteral reflux. *J Urol* 1972; **108**: 249–254.

47. Tobenkin MI. Hereditary vesico-ureteral reflux. *South Med J* 1964; **57**: 139–147.

48. Mulcahy JJ, Kelalis PP, Stickler GB, Burke EC. Familial vesico-ureteral reflux. *J Urol* 1970; **104**: 762–764.

49. Amar AD. Familial vesico-ureteral reflux. *J Urol* 1972; **108**: 969–971.

50. Mebust WK, Foret JD. Vesicoureteral reflux in identical twins. *J Urol* 1972; **108**, 635–636.

51. Bredin HC, Winchester P, McGovern JH et al. Family study of vesicoureteral reflux. *J Urol* 1975; **113**: 623–625.

52. Middleton GW, Howards SS, Gillenwater JY. Sex linked familial reflux. *J Urol* 1975; **114**: 36–39.

53. de Vargas A, Evans K, Ransley P et al. A family study of vesico-ureteric reflux. *J Med Genet* 1978; **15**: 85–96.

54. Jerkins GR, Noe HN. Familial vesicoureteral reflux: a prospective study. *J Urol* 1982; **128**: 774–778.

55. Cass AS, Ireland GW. Significance of ureteral submucosal length, orifice configuration and position in vesicoureteral reflux. *J Urol* 1972; **107**: 963–965.

56. Manley CB. Reflux in blonde haired girls. *Soc Paediatr Urol Newslett* 14 October, 1981.

57. Urrutia EJ, Lebowitz RL. Relationship between hair/eye colour and primary vesicoureteral reflux in children. *Urol Radiol* 1985; **7**: 23–24.

58. Senger DPS, Rishid A, Wolfish NM. Histocompatibility antigens and urinary tract abnormalities. *Br Med J* 1978; **1**: 1146.

59. Torres VE, Moore SB, Kurtz SB, Offord KP, Kelalis PP. In search of a marker for genetic susceptibility to reflux nephropathy. *Clin Nephrol* 1980; **14**: 217–222.

60. Atwell JD, Allen NH. The interrelationship between paraureteric diverticula, vesicoureteric reflux and duplication of the pelvicalyceal collecting system: a family study. *Br J Urol* 1980; **52**: 269–273.

61. Allen NH, Atwell JD. The paraureteric diverticulum in childhood. *Br J Urol* 1980; **52**: 264–268.

62. Stephens FD, Joske RA, Simmons RT. Megaureter with vesico-ureteric reflux in twins. *Aust N Z J Surg* 1955; **24**: 192–194.

63. Scott JES, Renwick M. Antenatal diagnosis of congenital abnormalities in the urinary tract. *Br J Urol* 1988; **62**: 295–300.

64. Najmaldin A, Burge DM, Atwell JD. Fetal vesicoureteric reflux. *Br J Urol* 1990; **65**: 403–406.

65. Mackay H. Congenital bilateral megaloureters with hydronephrosis. A remarkable family history. *Proc R Soc Med* 1945; **38**: 567–568.

66. Aaron G, Robbins MA. Hydronephrosis due to aberrant vessels: remarkable familial incidence with report of cases. *J Urol* 1948; **60**: 702–705.

67. Cannon JF. Hereditary unilateral hydronephrosis. *Ann Int Med* 1954; **41**: 1954–1060.

68. Raffle RB. Familial hydronephrosis. *Br Med J* 1955; **1**: 580–582.

69. Jewell JH, Buchert WI. Unilateral hereditary hydronephrosis: a report of four cases in 3 conservative generations. *J Urol* 1962; **88**: 129–136.

70. Martin DC, Goodwin WE. Hereditary and familial aspects of some common urological problems. *Urol Dig* 1968; **7**: 11–17.

71. Simpson JL, German J. Familial urinary tract anomalies. *JAMA* 1970; **212**: 2264–2265.

72. Gross FR, Kaveggia L, Opitz JM. Familial hydronephrosis. *Z Kinderheil* 1973; **114**: 313–321.

73. Atwell JD. Familial pelviureteric junction hydronephrosis and its association with a duplex pelvicalyceal system and vesicoureteric reflux. *Br J Urol* 1985; **57**: 365–369.

74. Lebowitz RL, Blickman JG. The coexistence of ureteropelvic junction obstruction and reflux. *AJR* 1983; **140**: 231–238.

75. Maizels M, Smith CK, Firlit CF. The management of children with vesico-ureteral reflux and ureteropelvic junction obstruction. *J Urol* 1984; **131**: 722–727.

76. Riba LB. Ureterocele: with case reports of bilateral ureteroceles in identical twins. *Br J Urol* 1936; **8**: 119–131.

77. Beck AD. The effect of intrauterine obstruction upon the development of the fetal kidney. *J Urol* 1971; **105**: 784–789.

78. International Clearinghouse for Birth Defects Monitoring Systems. Epidemiology of bladder exstrophy and epispadias. *Teratology* 1987; **36**: 221–227.

79. Blickstein I, Katz Z. Possible relationship of bladder exstrophy and epispadias with progestins taken in early pregnancy. *Br J Urol* 1991; **68**: 105–106.

80. Shapiro E, Lepor H, Jeffs RD. The inheritance of the exstrophy–epispadias complex. *J Urol* 1984; **132**: 308–310.

81. Kallen N, Winberg J, Castilla E et al. An epidemiological study of hypospadias in Sweden. *Acta Paediatr Scand Suppl* 1982; **293**: 1–2.

82. Simpkin JM, Owens JR, Harris F. Incidence of hypospadias. *Lancet* 1985; **ii**: 384.

83. MacNab AJ, Zouves C. Hypospadias after assisted reproduction incorporating in vitro fertilization and gamete intrafallopian transfer. *Fertil Steril* 1991; **56**: 918–922.

84. Kallen B, Mastroiacovo P, Lancaster PAL et al. Oral contraceptives in the etiology of hypospadias. *Contraception* 1991; **44**: 173–182.

85. Editorial. Genetics of hypospadias. *Br Med J* 1972; **4**: 189–190.

86. Aarskog D. Clinical and cytogenetic studies in hypospadias. *Acta Paediatr Scand Suppl* 1970; **203**: 1–62.

87. Batch JA, Williams DM, Evans BAJ et al. Androgen receptor gene mutation – possible etiology for severe hypospadias? In: *Abstract ESPU Meeting, Cambridge*, 1993.

88. Shima H, Ikoma F, Terakawa T et al. Developmental anomalies associated with hypospadias. *J Urol* 1979; **122**: 619–621.

89. Pinnel SR, Murad S. In: Stanbury JB, Wyngaarden JB, Frederickson DS, Goldstein JL and Brown MS (eds) *Metabolic Basis of Inherited Disease*, 5th edn. New York: McGraw-Hill, 1983; p 1425.

90. Kraus AN. Familial extrahepatic biliary atresia. *J Paediatr* 1964; **65**: 933–937.

91. Quan L, Smith DW. The Vater Association, vertebral defects, anal atresia, T E fistula with oesophageal atresia, radial and renal dysplasia. *J Pediatr* 1973; **87**: 104–107.

92. Bond-Taylor W, Starer F, Atwell JD. Vertebral anomalies associated with esophageal atresia and tracheo-esophageal fistula with reference to the initial operative mortality. *J Pediatr Surg* 1973; **8**: 9–13.

93. Atwell JD, Beard RC. Congenital anomalies of the upper urinary tract associated with esophageal atresia and tracheo-esophageal fistula. *J Pediatr Surg* 1974; **9**: 825–831.

94. Cochran W, Froggat P. Bilateral nephroblastoma in two sisters. *J Urol* 1967; **97**: 216–220.

95. Miller RW, Fraumeni JF, Manning MD. Association of Wilm's tumour with aniridia, hemihypertrophy and other congenital malformations. *New Engl J Med* 1964; **270**: 922–927.

96. Francke U, Riccardi VM, Hittner HM et al. Interstitial del (11p) as a cause of the aniridia–Wilms tumour association: band localisation and a heritable basis. *Am J Hum Genet* 1978; **30**: 81A.

97. Franke U, Holmes LB, Atkins L et al. Aniridia–Wilms tumour association: evidence for specific deletion of 11p 13. *Cytogenet Cell Genet* 1979; **24**: 185–192.

98. Riccardi VM, Sujansky E, Smith AC et al. Chromosomal imbalance in the aniridia–Wilms tumour association: 11p interstitial deletion. *Pediatrics* 1978; **61**: 604–610.

99. Draper GJ, Heaf MM, Kinnear-Wilson LM. Occurrence of childhood cancers among sibs and estimation of familial risks. *J Med Genet* 1977; **14**: 81–90.

100. Juberg RC, St Martin EC, Hundley JR. Familial occurrence of Wilms tumour: nephroblastoma in one of monozygous twins and in another sibling. *Am J Hum Genet* 1975; **27**: 155–164.

101. Strom T. A Wilms tumour family. *Acta Paediatr* 1957; **46**: 601–604.

102. Fitzgerald WL, Hardin HC. Bilateral Wilms tumour in a Wilms tumour: case report. *J Urol* 1955; **73**: 468–474.

103. Knudson AG, Strong LC. Mutation and cancer: a model for Wilms tumour of the kidney. *J Natl Cancer Inst* 1972; **48**: 313–324.

104. Machin GA, McCaughey WTE. A new precursor of Wilms tumour (nephroblastoma): intralobular multifocal nephroblastomatosis. *Histopathology* 1984; **8**: 35–53.

Further reading

Barakat AY, der Kaloustian VM, Mufarris AA, Birbari AE. *Genetics in Medicine and Surgery Series. The Kidney in Genetic Disease*. Edinburgh: Churchill Livingstone, 1986.

Crawford M D'A. *Oxford Monographs on Medical Genetics*, No. 14. *The Genetics of Renal Tract Disorders*. Oxford: Oxford Medical Publications, 1988.

Wiedemann HR, Kunze, J, Crosse ER, Dibbern H. *An Atlas of Clinical Syndromes: a visual aid to diagnosis*, 3rd edn. London: Wolfe Publishing, 1992.

2

The embryological basis of urinary tract malformations

A.L. Freedman and E. Shapiro

The embryological development of the genitourinary (GU) tract exemplifies the complex choreography of events necessary in human embryogenesis. Precise synchronization in the movement and interaction of multiple cell types and tissue structures is required to produce these intricate organs. In many areas, the organization of tissues is in fact a result of induction by these cellular interactions. However, the general sequence of events is so graceful in its simplicity that an understanding of the normal course can provide convincing aetiologies for the many perplexing anomalies encountered clinically.

Disorders of the genitourinary system are quite common. Ten per cent of infants will be born with some GU abnormality [1]. Maternal fetal ultrasound can detect only a small percentage of these abnormalities, primarily hydronephrosis. GU abnormalities though account for 20% of the structural abnormalities that are found on prenatal ultrasound in 1% of normal pregnancies [2]. Mild hydronephrosis can be detected in up to 1/200 otherwise normal pregnancies [3]. Significant hydronephrosis, requiring postnatal intervention, can be detected in approximately 1 in 500 pregnancies [4]. Thus a relatively large number of children will be born with a diagnosis of a urinary tract abnormality which will require further evaluation and management. Therefore, a basic understanding of normal GU tract development is important for those who care for these children [5].

Renal development

Normal renal development is dependent on the sequential progression of tubular and ductal morphogenesis. Each new complex set of tubules and ducts leads to the next step in differentiation, with each set developing from the same mesenchymal primordia [6–8].

The process starts when the embryo begins its ventral folding and the **intermediate mesoderm**, lying along the entire length of the dorsal body wall, lateral to the somites, is brought ventrally, losing its connection to the somites. These bilateral bands of mesenchyme are called **nephrogenic cords**. The cords produce a longitudinal bulge which is referred to as the **urogenital ridge**. It is from successive areas of this ridge that the source of the tubules and ducts will develop. This ridge will also provide the supporting structures of the gonad following the migration of the primordial germ cells [6–8].

Pronephros
During the beginning of the fourth week, the cervical portion of the urogenital ridge (level of the second to sixth somite) organizes clusters of cells into the primitive straight pronephric tubules [9]. The tail of these tubules forms a descending duct. In humans, these tubules are not believed to function, although they are analogous to the excretory system in some primitive fishes. The importance of the pronephroi is the establishment of the duct

which, as it descends, induces the formation of the mesonephros and is thus called the **mesonephric duct** [10]. The tubular structures themselves will degenerate and disappear.

Mesonephros

Later in the fourth week, a portion of the nephrogenic cord just caudal to the pronephros begins to form clusters of cells in response to induction by the ampulla of the descending mesonephric duct [8]. These clusters develop lumen and become vesicles which extend into S-shaped tubules which connect to the mesonephric duct. The medial portion of the tubule becomes invaginated by a capillary arising from the aorta. The capillary is designated the **glomerulus**, while the invaginated portion of the tubule is called the **capsule**. Together the capsule and glomerulus form what is termed a **corpuscle**. As the tubule develops, it lengthens and becomees increasingly convoluted and segmented, developing a proximal, distal and collecting tubule in addition to the glomerulus. Progressive generations of tubules form in a caudally directed migration wave. The most cranial tubules degenerate at the same rate to keep a steady number of total tubules, approximately 40 on each side [11].

Metanephros

At about 28 days, a diverticulum forms on the mesonephric duct along the posteromedial aspect where the terminal portion joins the cloaca. This diverticulum, termed the **ureteric bud**, extends in a dorsal–cranial direction, penetrating the caudal portion of the nephrogenic cord [11]. This caudal area contains the metanephric mesoderm and is also known as the **metanephric blastema**. The contact of the ureteric bud and the metanephric blastema induces the blastema to form tubules which become the nephrons of the mature kidney and the ureteric bud to form successive branches which develop into the renal pelvis, calyces and collecting ducts.

Nephron development

The most complex step in renal development is the induction of nephrons by the advancing ureteric bud derivatives. As the bud arises from the mesonephric duct, it enters the metanephric blastema. The blastema condenses around the bulbous advancing portion known as the **ampulla**. The ampulla is the site of active cellular proliferation, division, linear advancement, and nephron induction and attachment. The portion of the bud following behind the advancing ampulla is called the **collecting tubule**. All tubule division and nephronic induction is mediated by the ampulla. Ampullary division is dichotomous and the ampullary substance is apportioned equally between each two new ampullas. As the ampulla advances, the enveloping blastema is carried forward. As renal development progresses, the ability of the ampulla to induce and attach nephrons changes. These changes can be categorized into four distinct periods of renal development [11].

The first period, which begins with the outgrowth of the ureteric bud at about 28 days (Figure 2.1(a)) and lasts until the fourteenth to fifteenth week, is characterized by each ampulla's ability to induce only one nephron and only when free of any other attached nephron. The bud is initially surrounded by the metanephric mesenchyme. Following the passage of the first 7–10 divisions, the collecting tubules begin to form. As the tubules form, the blastema begins to display its pluripotentiality, with those cells near the tubules developing into connective structures, while those cells near the ampulla initially remaining as blastema. As the ampulla progresses, those tissues adjacent to the ampulla develop along the nephrogenic path, while others around the tubules develop into connective tissue. Cells peripheral to the advancing tubule remain undifferentiated blastema.

The initial 7–10 divisions occur prior to the blastema obtaining the ability to differentiate. These early branches expand and coalesce in order to form the renal pelvis (four to six branches), and the major and minor calyces (three to five branches). Following these divisions, the ampulla become less bulbous and assumes a more narrow configuration.

At approximately 8 weeks, nephrons begin to develop throughout the blastema regardless of the degree of branching or number of generations of the collecting tubules. Tubules in the midpole are generally at the third generation of branching, while those in the polar regions are usually in the fifth generation.

(a)

(b)

(c)

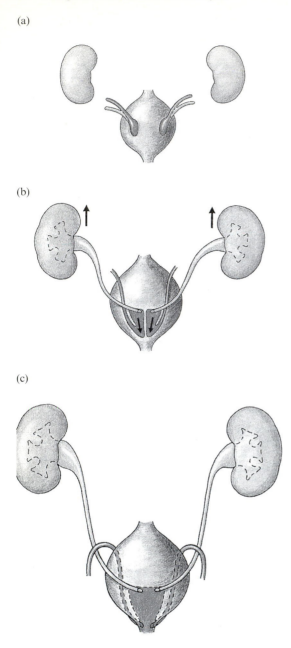

Figure 2.1 (a) 4–5 weeks. Primitive bladder. Ureteric buds arise from the mesonephric ducts. (b) 6–9 weeks. Penetration of the metanephric blastema by the ureteric buds at 5 weeks is followed by ascent of the primitive kidneys. The segment of mesonephric duct between the ureteral bud and urogenital sinus (UGS) is the trigone precursor. (c) 8–12 weeks. Branching of the calyces and differentiation of the intrarenal collecting system. The mesonephric ducts are incorporated into the prostatic urethra to give rise to the ejaculatory ducts and seminal vesicles.

Asynchronous branching maintains the reniform shape of the kidney [9]. The induction and attachment of the first generation of nephrons is a unique event. As no ampulla presently is attached to a nephron, following their division each new ampulla induces and attaches a first generation nephron. This is the only time when there is the simultaneous induction of two nephrons. Following this, at each division the ampulla with an attached nephron divides into two. The two ampullas formed extend in opposite directions, parallel to the renal surface and at a right angle to the original tubule. The ampullas penetrate the adjacent blastema pushing the majority of tissue into the angle between the ampulla and tubule, while the remaining cells are stretched into a single layer on the subcapsular surface.

Within the blastema, lying in the angle of the collecting duct, an ovoid mass of cells separates and develops a lumen. This vesicle elongates into an S-shaped structure which then attaches to the ampulla. This structure will differentiate into a mature nephron. After each division of the ampulla, the attached nephron will advance with one branch while the other will induce the development of a new nephron. Only ampulla without an attached nephron will induce a new nephron during this period of development. The new nephron will attach to the ampulla before the ampulla advances more than a short distance from the branch point. If the nephron attaches too slowly and meets below the ampulla, it may not be carried to the next division and will degenerate. This form of nephron development continues for seven to eight ampullary divisions [11].

The second period is characterized as the time of arcade formation and extends from weeks 14 to 15 until weeks 20 to 22. During this period, the ampulla are no longer actively dividing, yet they are capable of inducing the formation of new nephrons despite the attachment of a previous nephron. Arcade formation is accomplished when an ampulla with an attached nephron induces the formation of a second nephron from the blastema cells lying adjacent to the ampulla in the angle between it and its collecting tubule. The second nephron temporarily attaches to the ampulla. The connecting portions of the two nephrons merge at the site of attachment to the collecting tubule. The connecting segment of the new nephron elongates, carrying the distal segment of the older nephron such that it drains into it rather than the ampulla. A new nephron then is induced from the blastema near the ampulla and the cycle is repeated [11].

As the process proceeds, a series of nephrons is formed with each nephron attached by its most distal segment to the terminal segment of the succeeding generation and with the most recent attached directly to the ampulla. This series of nephrons, all draining into a single collecting tubule, is termed an **arcade**. The glomerulus of the oldest nephron lies closest to the medulla and has the longest loop of Henle, while the glomerulus of the youngest lies close to the capsule and has a shorter loop. The forward advancement of the ampulla is passive and due to the interstitial growth of the collecting tubule. Occasional divisions may occur, advancing the arcade and beginning a second arcade on the other ampulla. The usual number of nephrons in series on an arcade is four, though it can vary from four to eight depending on when branching of the ampulla ceased.

The third period of nephrogenesis commences at 20–22 weeks and continues until 23–36 weeks [11]. During this period, the ampulla begin to grow again by active cellular proliferation, though without branching. The ampulla advances past the attachment of the arcade and induces a new nephron. These nephrons attach along the collecting tubule behind the ampulla's zone of active growth. The ampulla continues to grow, leaving the nephron behind and inducing new nephrons. In this way, the collecting tubule attains a series of four to six separately attached nephrons. The final nephron becomes the terminal portion of the collecting tubule. The glomerulae of these nephrons lie in the outer half of the cortex.

The fourth and final period begins at 32–36 weeks when the ampulla disappears and extends to adulthood. No further nephron induction can occur. All further changes are the result of interstitial growth and differentiation. The nephrons and collecting tubules elongate and gain further convolution. Each terminal collecting tubules usually has 9–11 attached nephrons, of which between five and seven are individual nephrons and there is an arcade of three to five additional nephrons. Completion of growth and differentiation of the nephrons continues well into postnatal life.

Renal ascent

The kidney 'ascends' during development from its initiation at the level of the upper sacral segments to the level of the upper lumbar spinal segments by four mechanisms. The most important mechanism is believed to be the relative increased growth of the caudal portion of the embryo, thereby growing away from the developing kidney. Other factors include the elongation of the ureter, the moulding of the kidney as it hurdles the umbilical arteries and, lastly, the growth and elongation of the spine [12–14]. During this process, the kidney will also rotate almost 90° such that the ventral hilum will rest facing in an anteromedial direction. This migration and rotation are complete by the end of the ninth week of gestation [15,16] (Figure 2.1(b)).

As the kidney ascends, the origin of the vascular supply changes with the initial arterial supply from the middle sacral and common iliac arteries. With further ascent, the kidney is supplied by successive branches of the aorta [17]. Caudal branches degenerate as cranial branches develop, though the failure to do so completely is believed to account for the frequent finding of multiple renal arteries [18]. Persistent fetal caudal vessels may tether the rotation of the kidney. Non-rotated kidneys are, therefore, associated with aberrant arterial supply [19].

Between the fourth and sixth week, the kidney may not ascend completely and remain in an **ectopic** position. The most common ascent anomaly is a **horseshoe kidney** [16]. Since the lower poles of these kidneys have some degree of fusion, the inferior mesenteric artery prevents full ascent by obstructing the cranialward path of these units. These kidneys remain at the level of L1–L2 and, like other ectopic renal units, derive their blood supply from nearby vessels [17]. Therefore, multiple arteries are commonly associated with them. It is thought that a slight alteration in position of the umbilical or common iliac artery may change the orientation of the migrating kidneys, leading to contact and fusion [12]. Another theory is based on abnormal formation of the tail or other pelvic organ leading to fusion [20].

Renal anomalies

The majority of congenital renal lesions can be attributed to a disturbance in the ureteric bud formation, placement or interaction with the metanephric blastema. Although a full discussion of the many congenital anomalies associated with renal development is beyond the scope of this chapter, a discussion regarding the embryogenesis of renal dysplasia and cystic disease is of particular importance to those evaluating the fetus.

Renal dysplasia

The embryological origin of renal cystic changes and dysplasia remains one of the most controversial areas in urological embryology. Renal dysplasia is a histological diagnosis characterized by primitive collecting tubules which are dilated and have fibrous collars and by focal cartilaginous metaplasia of the blastema. Most dysplastic kidneys are also cystic. The dysplasia can be global or segmental and is observed when there is evidence of obstruction (UPJ, ureterocele, ureteral agenesis or bladder outlet obstruction) in 90% of cases [21]. The most common form of renal dysplasia in children is the multicystic kidney, though dysplasia can also be found in many less common genetic malformation syndromes such as VACTERL, Meckel–Gruber syndrome and the bracho-oto-renal syndrome [22].

The debate over the pathogenesis of renal dysplasia, and in particular the role of anatomical obstruction, has become entrenched among two broad schools of thought. One school, first proposed by Mackie and Stephens [23], holds that renal dysplasia is the result of a malposition of the ureteric bud causing an improper interface between the emerging bud and the metanephric blastema. This misconnection is responsible for the disordered induction leading to dysplasia, while the misplacement of the bud along the mesonephric duct is responsible for the frequency-associated obstruction (or reflux) found due to an abnormal or ectopic ureteral position. Thus obstruction and dysplasia are both consequences of the same underlying condition but are not related by cause and effect. A less popular modified theory holds that dysplasia is related to a common mesodermal development abnormality accounting for the renal changes and frequently associated anomalies.

The second broad school of thought holds that dysplasia is the result of obstruction during a vulnerable period of nephrogenesis. This theory, supported by the pathological observations of Bernstein [21], assumes that rising intraluminal pressures due to distal obstruction disturb the induction of nephrons by the ampulla, leading to dysplastic changes in the blastema and loss of nephron development. Although the majority of experimental evidence supporting either hypothesis is based on animal models, the debate has a significant impact on clinical treatment. If one believes that obstruction is not a significant cause of renal dysplasia, then *in utero* intervention loses much of its theoretical justification. Though if one believes that obstruction is the primary cause of subsequent dysplasia, then the impetus would be for the institution of *in utero* decompression as early as possible.

The primary support for the arguments against obstruction as the cause of dysplasia arises from two sources. The first source was the failure by numerous investigators to reproduce dysplasia by ureteral ligation in animal models. Tanagho ligated the ureter of fetal lambs at a gestational age of 70–75 days, which developed only hydronephrosis without dysplasia [24]. Likewise, Thomasson ligated the ureters of fetal rabbits at 23–27 days' gestation (normal term at 30 days) and failed to establish dysplasia [25]. Maizels, using a chick embryo model, was able to reproduce dysplasia by the depletion of the metanephric blastema [26] but not by ureteral ligation [27]. Secondly, *in vitro* evidence of the effects of altering the potassium concentration [28] or extracellular matrix environment [29] in causing dysplasia, suggests to some that dysplasia is more likely due to disturbances in the ampulla–blastema interaction than a mechanical effect.

On the other hand, other investigators have been able to produce renal dysplasia in animal models. Beck demonstrated renal dysplasia in the fetal lamb by establishing obstruction during the first half of gestation between 50 and 70 days [30]. The pioneering work by Harrison and his associates have clearly shown that the development of dysplasia is related to the time and duration of obstruction [31]. In fact, early relief of the obstruction was shown to prevent dysplasia [32].

Thus it has been demonstrated that early obstruction can lead to dysplasia while later obstruction leads to hydronephrosis. One explanation for this has been that in the immature kidney, the collecting ducts and nephrons are short, straight and distensible, allowing for the conduction of pressure and formation of cysts and dysplastic elements. In contrast, the more mature kidney has tubules that are longer and more tortuous, which are held in a tighter connective tissue, thus making the parenchyma less distensible than the renal pelvis and calyces. Therefore, it is critical in evaluating or designing experiments to consider the time of onset of the obstruction, the duration of obstruction and the completeness of obstruction.

Renal cystic changes

Renal cystic changes in the fetal kidney have been broadly divided into four groups based on their pathological appearance [33]. From an aetiological standpoint, the changes can be divided into those due to an heritable genetic syndrome or secondary to obstruction.

Type I cysts are defined by their generalized enlargement of the terminal collecting duct branches bilaterally. These cysts typically correspond to those found in autosomal recessive polycystic kidney disease.

Type II cysts display a profound defect in the ampulla such that functional nephrons are not formed. All or part of one or both kidneys may be affected. These cysts are typically seen in multicystic dysplastic kidneys but may occur with other types of obstruction.

Type III cysts may occur in any part of the collecting duct or nephron and are almost always bilateral. They are usually not clinically apparent until adulthood, though can be seen at any age as in autosomal dominant polycystic kidney disease.

Type IV cysts reveal distention of the distal portion of the S-shaped nephron and are classically described in association with urinary back pressure due to obstruction. In children with severe obstruction, the type of cyst formation, type II versus type IV, may relate to the time of onset of the obstruction, with type II cysts occurring in very early obstruction [34].

Development of the ureter

The development of the ureter can be characterized by three structural processes: **lumen formation**, **elongation** and **muscularization**. The ureter begins with the outgrowth of the ureteric bud early in the fourth week, which changes in patency during development [35]. As the bud migrates forward, the proximal tube is initially patent throughout. At approximately 37–40 days, the ureter is found to be patent only in its midportion. The obliteration of the majority of the lumen is thought to be due to the rapid elongation of the ureter. The ureter then undergoes a period of lumen re-expansion, starting in the midsection and progressing toward both ends, with completion after day 40.

Throughout this process, the ureter has likewise undergone rapid elongation to accommodate further renal ascent. In fact, the ureter elongates farther than the kidney ascends, leaving a redundancy that is compensated for by tortuosity and folds [36]. These folds will usually straighten in the postnatal period by the rapid growth of the infant, though on occasion they become fixed and may act as an obstructing valve [37].

Muscularization begins at 12 weeks, approximately 3 weeks following the initiation of urine production. Muscle first appears in the upper ureter and the superficial sheath of the uretero-vesical junction. Bundles in the upper ureter develop and display a spiral orientation by 16 weeks and throughout the ureter by the twenty-first week. Complete muscularization with well-developed layering of the distal ureter and trigone is complete by 40 weeks [38].

Ureteral bud anomalies can be explained by understanding the relationship between the ureteral bud and the mesonephric duct. As previously discussed, the ureteral bud develops as a diverticulum from the mesonephric duct at the end of the fourth week. The mesonephric ducts then drain into the urogenital sinus with fusion of its epithelium and the mesenchyme of the mesonephric duct. The segment of mesonephric duct between the ureteral bud and UGS dilates and is termed the **trigone precursor** or **common excretory duct** [39]. This trigone precursor is then partially absorbed into the UGS [9]. The orifice of the mesonephric duct

migrates caudally and is lateral to the mullerian ducts at the level of the UGS, while
the ureteral bud migrates cranially [40]. The
ureteral orifice migrates cephalad and laterally
and the mesonephric duct crosses over the
ureter (rotating in a clockwise direction, as
viewed extravesically) and migrates medially
and caudally. Once the primitive trigone develops with the ureteral orifices well separated,
muscularization of the bladder occurs.

When the ureteral bud forms from a more
caudal site on the mesonephric duct, the
common excretory duct is somewhat shorter in
length than normal. This duct is then absorbed
earlier and allows the ureter to migrate more
cranial and lateral than its normal position.
The ureteral orifice tends to be associated with
a wider trigone that is deficient in muscle.
There more laterally positioned ureteral orifices have a shorter submucosal tunnel, therefore having a propensity for the development
of the vesicoureteral reflux [8,23,40].

When the ureteral bud develops at a more
cranial position on the mesonephric duct, a
longer common excretory duct is present. The
ureteral bud will remain associated with the
mesonephric duct for a longer period, leaving
less time for the ureter to migrate cranially
once it has separated from the mesonephric
duct. The ureteral orifice will therefore be
located closer to the bladder neck or in association with structures derived from the mesonephric duct including the seminal vesicle,
epididymis or vas deferens [40,41]. In the
female, the ureter may end in the vestibule,
vesical neck or vagina as well as in the remnant
of the mesonephric duct or **Gartner's duct**.
When bilateral ureteral ectopia occurs, the
bladder is small and poorly formed. This
congenital anomaly may suggest that normal
bladder development depends upon both the
storage of urine to stimulate the muscularization of the bladder as well as the normal
sequence of events associated with the absorption of the common excretory duct in the
development of the trigone and bladder neck
regions [42,43].

Duplication anomalies of the ureter

Complete ureteral duplication occurs when two
ureteral buds arise close together at the normal
position on the mesonephric duct and the
development of these buds follow the **Weigert–**

Meyer Law [44,45]. This law states that the
ureteral bud closest to the urogenital sinus
migrates first and is associated with the lower
pole ureter. The more cephalad bud maintains
its contact with the mesonephric duct with
delayed separation and is associated with the
upper pole ureter. The lower pole orifice is
more laterally positioned on the trigone while
the upper pole orifice is more medial. At
7 weeks, the lower pole ureter opens into the
urogenital sinus and rotates in a clockwise
direction. At 8 weeks, the upper pole ureter
opens into the urogenital sinus, rotates and
migrates cranially. Ureteral duplication with
upper pole ectopy and lower pole reflux will
result when the lower pole ureter develops
closer to the urogenital sinus, with the development of a short common excretory duct.
Therefore, it is more rapidly absorbed into the
urogenital sinus by 6 weeks with subsequent
rotation. The ureter will then have additional
time for cranial ascent which will result in a
ureteral orifice in a more lateral position with
a shorter submucosal tunnel which will likely
reflux. The upper pole ureter originates higher
on the mesonephric duct and development proceeds as described with single ureteral ectopia
[40,46].

Development of the cloaca and bladder

The terminal end of the hindgut is termed the
cloaca, which is the Latin term for 'sewer'. The
cloacal membrane is a bilaminar layer located
at the caudal end of the germinal disc which
occupies the infraumbilical abdominal wall.
Formation of the lower abdominal wall musculature and bones results from the ingrowth
of mesenchyme between the cloacal membrane's bilaminar layers. After the mesenchymal ingrowth occurs, the cloaca undergoes
septation by the **urorectal septum** at about
28 days [41] (Figure 2.2). Distally, the septum
meets the posterior remnant of the bilaminar
membrane which eventually perforates, forming the anal and urogenital openings. These
regions are evident by the 44th day of development. Proliferation of the mesenchyme around
the cloacal membrane forms the genital tubercle and the labioscrotal swellings. The paired
genital tubercles migrate medially and fuse in

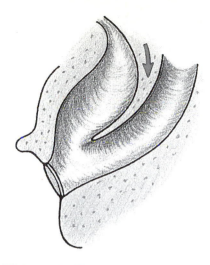

Figure 2.2 4–6 weeks. Formation and descent of the urorectal septum divides the primitive cloaca into the urogenital sinus anteriorly and the primitive rectum posteriorly.

the midline cephalad to the dorsal membrane before perforation.

The **exstrophy–epispadias complex** may occur due to failure of the cloacal membrane to be reinforced by mesenchymal ingrowth [47]. The cloacal membrane is also subject to premature rupture. Depending on the extent of the infra-umbilical defect and stage of development when rupture occurs, either bladder exstrophy or cloacal exstrophy results. Other theories of embryonic development suggest that the basic defect in exstrophy is an abnormal over-development of the cloacal membrane, pre-venting medial migration of the mesenchymal tissue and proper lower abdominal wall devel-opment [48]. Again, timing of the rupture of the cloacal defect determines the variant of the complex that results [47]. The bladder develops as a cylindrical tube lined by connective tissue at 10 weeks [49]. The apex of the vesico-allantoic canal narrows and becomes a thick fibrous cord, the **urachus** [10,50]. This thick cord persists in the adult as the **median umbili-cal ligament** [7]. There are several congenital anomalies of the urachus [51,52]. The urachal remnant may remain patent when it does not obliterate normally. This may persist in asso-ciation with the partially distended bladder or a vesicoumbilical fistula results due to failure of the bladder to descend normally. A urachal cyst may develop when the urachal lumen becomes filled with epithelium which has

undergone desquamation and degeneration. If the urachal apex remains patent, a blind external sinus may open at the umbilicus [52]. Finally, a blind internal sinus or diverticulum of the bladder apex may be seen on a cysto-gram. These are often associated with the prune belly syndrome [53].

The **epithelium of the bladder** is derived from the **urogenital sinus endoderm** [6–8]. Muscle layers develop from adjacent splanchnic mesenchyme. Muscularization of the bladder is noted by 13 weeks, with the development of circular, interlacing and longitudinal strands of smooth muscle [8]. The bladder wall is thickest at the level of the trigone. There is narrowing of the bladder lumen at the bladder neck or internal sphincter. The outer longitudinal layer is a complete coat extending from the bladder apex to the upper aspect of the prostate in males and the anterior wall of the vagina in girls [54]. At 20 weeks, the middle circular muscle layer is fine, but at the internal sphinc-ter it becomes closely packed and thick.

At the end of gestation, muscle bundles of the bladder are more coarse than those of the sphincter. The inner longitudinal layer is formed completely along the anterior wall of the bladder but posteriorly this layer is seen only in the region of the trigone. At this level, it extends distally to become contiguous with the longitudinal layer in the urethra [54]. At term, the fetal bladder has been seen with ultrasonography and noted to empty about 16 ml every 90 minutes [55]. The rate of fetal urine production is linearly related to gesta-tional age [55].

Gonadal development

The gonads of both sexes originate from three primary embryonic sources: the **coelomic epithelium**, the **intermediate mesenchyme** and the **primordial germ cells** [9,10]. As described with renal development, the intermediate mesenchyme dissociates from the somites to form the **urogenital ridge**. During the 5th week of gestation, an area of coelomic epithelium on the medial side of the urogenital ridge, adja-cent to the area of mesonephric development, begins to thicken and form the **gonadal ridge**. Finger-like projections of proliferating epi-thelial cells begin to expand into the underlying mesenchyme and form an outer **cortex** and inner **medulla**. These projections form the **primary sex cords**. During the 6th week, the primordial germ cells, which are found along the wall of the yolk sac near the allantois, migrate by ameboid movement along the dorsal mesentery of the hindgut and into the mesenchyme to become incorporated with the primary sex cords [56]. With the arrival of the germ cells, the indifferent gonad is formed.

Testicular development

The initiation of gonadal differentiation into a testis is believed to be in response to a **testis-determining factor (TDF)**. This factor is the product of the testis-determining factor in the **sex-determining region (SRY)** located on the short arm of the Y chromosome [57] which is expressed in the sex cord cells. The production of TDF causes the cells in the medullary sex cords [58] to differentiate into **Sertoli cells**. The sex cords will ultimately differentiate into mature **seminiferous tubules**. The cortical sex cords degenerate and are separated from the coelomic epithelium by a layer of connective tissue termed the **tunica albuginea** [6]. The Sertoli cells secrete **mullerian-inhibiting factor (MIF)**, which induces degeneration of the mullerian ducts between the eighth and tenth weeks [59,60]. Remnants of the mullerian duct persist in the male as the **appendix testis** at the cranial end and **prostatic utricle** at the caudal end. MIF may also induce the mesenchymal cells in the gonadal ridge to differentiate into **interstitial Leydig cells** in the ninth week. After this time, the Leydig cells will produce testosterone in response to chorionic gonadotropin from the placenta during this stage of gestation [61–63].

The deep portion of the seminiferous tubules of each sex cord narrows forming the **tubulus rectus**. These tubuli recti converge in the **rete testis**. The Sertoli cells, tubuli recti and rete testis all arise from the coelomic epithelium [64]. After 12 weeks, the rete testis becomes continuous with 15–20 mesonephric tubules, the **epigenitalis**, to form the **ductuli efferentes** [54]. With the onset of mullerian duct regression, the mesonephric duct differentiates under the influence of testosterone to become the **epididymis**, **vas deferens** and the **seminal vesicle** by the end of the 13th week. The seminal vesicles develop as buds from the caudal end of the mesonephric duct (Figure 2.1(c)). The

duct between the seminal vesicle and the urethra becomes the **ejaculatory duct** and **ampullae of the vas deferens**. The vas deferens becomes muscularized during the 28th week. Mesonephric tubules that are not incorporated into the ductus efferentes may remain as the vestigal **appendix epididymis** at the cranial end, while mesonephric tubules lying between the testis and epididymis that fail to degenerate remain as the **organ of Giraldes**.

Testicular descent

The testis enters a dormant state from the end of the first trimester until the seventh month of gestation when its descent will begin [65,66]. During this dormant period, the testis remains just inside the internal inguinal ring. The **gubernaculum** develops as a mesenchymal column running from its attachments to the gonad down to the scrotal swellings, through an opening in the anterior abdominal wall. Testicular descent begins with marked swelling of the gubernaculum, especially the scrotal portion. At the junction of the developing gubernaculum and the abdominal wall, a lip of peritoneum extends partially through the abdominal wall forming the **processus vaginalis** [67,68]. The **cremaster muscle** develops along the gubernaculum that is contained within the future inguinal canal. The cells of the gubernaculum begin to produce large amounts of intercellular matrix, which is rich in hyaluronic acid. The hyaluronic acid then increases the swelling by the uptake of substantial amounts of water until the gubernaculum resembles the consistency of the Wharton's jelly of the umbilical cord [69]. The swelling of the gubernaculum peaks at 28 weeks [66]. The distal gubernaculum separates from the dilated scrotal wall and forms a conical shape with the narrow apex attached to the testis and the swollen globular base lying in the scrotum. The cremaster and processus vaginalis also exhibit rapid growth, with the processus vaginalis developing a distal extension due to an active ingrowth of the peritoneal epithelium into the gubernacular mesenchyme [65]. The gubernaculum is thus divided into two concentric rings which are separated by the processus vaginalis: a central mesenchymal core and a peripheral ring containing the cremaster muscle. The intra-abdominal and inguinal portion of the central core involutes as the scrotal portion lengthens, until the scrotum is large enough to accept the gubernaculum and testis. The testicular vessels and vas deferens are rapidly growing, providing sufficient length to permit descent [70,71].

The testis descends rapidly through the inguinal canal, with the assistance of intra-abdominal pressure [72,73]. Once the testis descends, the inguinal canal no longer remains open by the gubernacular mesenchyme, and it closes behind the testis. The outer ring of gubernaculum differentiates into the internal and external cremasteric fasciae, and the processus vaginalis is obliterated except around the testis where it forms the **tunica vaginalis**.

Therefore, the three anatomical phases of testicular descent include:

1. Internal descent of the testis towards the internal inguinal ring due to the differential growth of the lumber region and pelvis.
2. Rapid passage of the testis through the very short inguinal canal as a result of gubernacular swelling.
3. Completion of descent through the external ring and into the scrotum after 26 weeks' gestation [66].

The chronological aspect of these events is supported by the prenatal ultrasound finding of testicular descent in 60% of male fetuses by 30 weeks and in 93% after 32 weeks [74].

Ovarian development

The development of the ovary is characterized as a delayed and slow process as compared to the testis [6,7]. The ovary is not identifiable until after the tenth week. The primary sex cords penetrate into the medulla to form a rudimentary **rete ovari**. This structure will then degenerate and disappear. The secondary sex cord, derived from the coelomic epithelium, will extend from the surface into the cortex of mesenchyme and become **cortical cords**. The primordial germ cells will become incorporated with these cortical cords and break up into isolated clusters called **primordial follicles**. The follicles consist of an **oogonium**, derived from the primordial germ cells, and a single layer of flat **follicular cells**, from the cortical cords. The oogonium will undergo active mitotic proliferation to form primary **oocytes**. Many degenerate, leaving approximately 2 million oocytes at birth. No further oocyte production

occurs postnatally. The primary oocytes become surrounded by follicular cells forming the **primary follicles**. The ovary descends to reach just inferior to the pelvic brim by the 12th week.

Development of the urogenital sinus

Indifferent stage

At about 6 weeks, after the cloaca has been divided by the urorectal septum, the anterior UGS is apparent. The UGS and genitalia will remain sexually indifferent until 10 weeks of development. The UGS is divided into three parts:

1. A superior portion or vesical part that is continuous with the allantois.
2. The second portion is the narrowed pelvic part.
3. Caudally, the portion which is closed externally by the urogenital membrane is termed the phallic portion [9].

The genital eminence forms between the umbilical cord and tail and is composed of a **genital tubercle** [75]. The genital eminence is surrounded by **genital swellings**. During gestational weeks 5–7, the opening of the UGS between the genital swellings (the primitive **urethral groove**) develops between paired **urethral folds** as a result of mesenchymal growth in the lateral margins of the phallic UGS. Once the urogenital membrane disintegrates at 7 weeks, the urethral groove is then lined by **endoderm** and proliferates to become the urethral plate which extends from the phallic portion of the UGS. The genital tubercle begins to elongate. The entire female urethra and the prostatic urethra in the male form from the urogenital sinus proximal to **mullerian** or **sinus tubercle** (the tubular uterovaginal primordium projects into the dorsal wall of the UGS producing this elevation). Longitudinal folds develop in the lateral aspect of the urethra which extend from the tubercle to the membranous urethra and are termed the plicae colliculi.

Posterior urethral valves are the most common cause of obstructive uropathy in males. Numerous theories have been proposed to explain the development of these obstructing leaflets. Tolmatschew proposed that valves may only represent an overdevelopment of the normal urethral wall folds and ridges [76]. Stephens suggested that the most common form, the type I valve, results from an abnormal anterior insertion and persistence of the distal aspect of the wolffian ducts, while type III may be explained by the persistence of the UG membrane [41].

Development of the urethra and external genitalia in the male

Masculinization of the indifferent external genitalia occurs following the elaboration of **testosterone** by the fetal testis at about 8–9 weeks of gestation [62]. Testosterone is then reduced to **dihydrotestosterone** (DHT) by the enzyme **5 alpha-reductase**, which is responsible for the virilization of the genitalia in the male [62].

At 10 weeks, the genital tubercle elongates pulling the urogenital folds ventrally. In the twelfth week, the endoderm of the urethral groove fuses forming the penile urethra and the ectodermal edges fuse forming the penile raphe [77]. The scrotal swellings enlarge and migrate caudally fusing to form the definitive scrotum. The process of fusion of the urethral folds is complete with formation of the glanular urethra during the fourth month. The **glanular urethra** forms by the process of both ventral fusion of the urethral folds with trapping of desquamated cells as well as primary canalization of a core of tissue by epithelial ingrowth of cells at the tip of the glans [78]. Failure or incomplete fusion of the endoderm of the urethral folds over the urethral groove results in varying degrees of **hypospadias** [79]. Anomalies of canalization of the glans result in the more common form of anterior hypospadias. During the twelfth week, the ectoderm at the level of the corona grows inward and breaks down forming the prepuce. The prepuce grows ventrally and covers the glans circumferentially. The development of a circumferential prepuce over the glans most always ensures normal positioning of the glanular meatus, except for the rare intact preputial variant of hypospadias associated with a megameatus and a deep glanular groove (MIP) [79]. The region of fusion of the preputial and urethral folds is termed the frenulum [80].

Development of the urogenital sinus, external genitalia and reproductive system in the female

The urethra and vagina are formed from the pelvic portion of the urogenital sinus. In the absence of circulating androgens, the external genitalia feminize during gestational weeks 12–28. The phallus is noted to curve ventrally and the labioscrotal swellings remain separate, except posteriorly where they form the **posterior commissure**. The urethral folds do not undergo the process of fusion and later form the **labia minora**. By the eighteenth week, the **labia majora** and the **clitoris** are apparent.

The female reproductive tract develops from the **mullerian ducts**. Mullerian duct development will not proceed in the absence of the mesonephric duct [13]. The mullerian ducts adhere to each other just before they project into the dorsal wall of the UGS, causing an elevation termed the **sinus tubercle**. When the fused tips contact the sinus tubercle, the ducts fuse cranially, forming a tube with a single lumen called the **uterovaginal primordium** or **canal** [81]. This tube will ultimately become the superior aspect of the **vagina** and **uterus** [6]. The cranial portion of the mullerian ducts which are unfused develop into the **fallopian tubes**. The original coelomic epithelial ostium remains as the abdominal opening of the fallopian tube. A septum initially divides the uterus into two cavities. This septum between the fused ducts disappears after 9 weeks, forming a single uterine cavity. The mesonephric ducts regress 1 week later, leaving a remnant in the female which is termed **Gartner's duct** [10]. Muscularization of the uterus is completed by 17 weeks' gestation and forms from the mesenchyme surrounding the mullerian ducts.

Vaginal development begins as early as 9 weeks with this Y-shaped solid mass of cells. The tissue of the sinus tubercle thickens, forming endodermal evaginations termed the **sinovaginal bulbs**. These sinovaginal bulbs give rise to the lower third of the vagina. The inferior portion of the uterovaginal canal becomes occluded by tissue termed the **vaginal plate**. The aetiology of this plate is unclear. It may form from the sinovaginal bulbs, the adjacent caudal end of the wolffian ducts, the mullerian ducts or a combination of these structures [13,82–84]. During the third to the fifth month of gestation, the plate elongates, and the central cells of the plate break down by a process of desquamation with the lower vaginal lumen appearing at 11 weeks. The lining of the vagina and cervix is derived from the endodermal epithelim of the definitive UGS [6]. By 20 weeks, canalization of the plate is complete [85]. Therefore, the vagina is of dual origin (the lower third is from the urogenital sinus while the upper two-thirds develops from the fused mullerian ducts).

Until late in fetal life, the vagina remains separated from the urogenital sinus by the **hymen**, which is a thin membrane of mesodermal tissue. The hymen represents the sinus tubercle and is invariably seen in females in which no anomalies of the urogenital tract are present. The male homologue of this structure is the **seminal colliculus**, which is a small elevation of the posterior wall of the prostatic urethra. As the vagina forms, the lower end of the vagina lengthens, and its junction with the UGS migrates caudally until it rests on the posterior wall of the definitive UGS. This thin hymenal membrane separates the lumen of the vagina from the cavity of the definitive UGS, which differentiates into the vaginal vestibule [6].

References

1. Vaughan Jr ED, Middleton GW. Pertinent genitourinary embryology. Review for the practicing urologist. *Urology* 1975; **6**: 139.
2. Woodard JR. The impact of fetal diagnosis on the management of obstructive uropathy. *Postgrad Med J* 1990; **66**: S37.
3. Chitty LS, Pembry ME, Chudleigh PM et al. Multicenter study of antenatal calyceal dilation by ultrasound. *Lancet* 1990; **336**: 875.
4. Thomas DFM. Fetal uropathy. *Br J Urol* 1990; **66**: 225.
5. Stephens FD. Embryopathy of malformations. *J Urol* 1982; **127**: 13 [guest editorial].
6. Larsen WJ. *Human Embryology*. New York: Churchill Livingstone.
7. Moore KL. *The Developing Human*, 4th edn. Philadelphia: WB Saunders.
8. Maizels M. Normal development of the urinary tract. In: *Campbell's Urology*, 6th edn. Philadelphia: WB Saunders, pp 1301–1343.
9. Hamilton WJ, Mossman HW. The urogenital system. In: *Human Embryology Prenatal Development of Form and Function*. New York: Macmillan Press, p 377.
10. Arey LB. *Developmental Anatomy*, 7th edn. Philadelphia: WB Saunders.
11. Potter EL. *Normal and Abnormal Development of the Kidney*. Chicago: Year Book Publishers, Chicago.
12. Boyden EA. Description of a horseshoe kidney associated with left inferior vena cava and disc-shaped suprarenal glands, together with a note on the occurrence of horseshoe kidneys in human embryos. *Anatom Rec* 1931; **51**: 187.
13. Gruenwald P. The normal changes in the position of the embryonic kidney. *Anat Rec* 1943; **85**: 163.
14. Maizels M, Stephens FD. The induction of urologic malformations: understanding the relationship of renal ectopia and congenital scoliosis. *Invest Urol* 1979; **17**: 209.
15. Weyrauch Jr HM. Anomalies of renal rotation. *Surg Gynecol Obstet* 1939; **69**: 183.
16. Bauer S, Perlmutter A, Retik A. Anomalies of the upper urinary tract. In: *Campbell's Urology*, 6th edn. Philadelphia: WB Saunders, pp 1357–1442.
17. Anson BJ, Riba LW. The anatomical and surgical features of ectopic kidney. *Surg Gynecol Obstet* 1939; **68**: 37.
18. Bremer JL. The origin of the renal artery in mammals and its anomalies. *Am J Anat* 1915; **18**: 179.
19. Nathan H, Glezer I. Right and left accessory renal arteries arising from a common trunk associated with unrotated kidneys. *J Urol* 1984; **132**: 7.
20. Cook WA, Stephens FD. Fused kidneys: morphologic study and theory of embryogenesis. In: Bergsma D, Duckett JW (eds) *Urinary Systems Malformations in Children*. Inc., Publishers, New York: Allen R Liss.
21. Bernstein J. Developmental abnormalities of the renal parenchyma: renal hypoplasia and dysplasia. In: Sommers SC (ed) *Pathology Annual*. New York: Appleton Century Croft, pp 213–247.
22. Jones KL. *Smith's Recognizable Patterns of Human Malformation*, 4th edn. Philadelphia: WB Saunders.
23. Mackie GG, Stephens FD. Duplex kidneys: a correlation of renal dysplasia with position of the ureteral orifice. *J Urol* 1975; **114**: 274.
24. Tanagho EA. Surgically induced partial urinary tract obstruction in the fetal lamb. III: Ureteral obstruction. *Invest Urol* 1972; **10**: 35.
25. Thomasson BM, Eassterly JR, Ravitch MM. Morphological changes in the fetal kidney after interuterine ureteral ligation. *Invest Urol* 1970; **8**: 261.
26. Maizels M, Simpson SB. Primitive ducts of renal dysplasia induced by culturing of ureteral buds denuded of condensed renal mesenchyme. *Science* 1983; **219**: 509.

27. Berman DJ, Maizels M. The role of urinary obstruction in the genesis of renal dysplasia. *J Urol* 1983; **128**: 1091.

28. Crocker JF. Human embryonic kidneys in organ culture: abnormalities of development induced by decreased potassium. *Science* 1973; **21**: 1178.

29. Spencer J, Maizels M. Inhibition of protein glycosylation causes renal dysplasia in the chick embryo. *J Urol* 1987; **138**: 984.

30. Beck AD. The effect of intrauterine urinary obstruction upon the development of the fetal kidney. *J Urol* 1971; **105**: 784.

31. Glick PL, Harrison MR, Noall RA et al. Correction of congenital hydronephrosis in utero. III: early mid-trimester ureteral obstruction produces renal dysplasia. *J Pediatr Surg* 1983; **18**: 681.

32. Glick PL, Harrison MR, Adzick NS et al. Correction of congenital hydronephrosis in utero IV: *in utero* decompression prevents renal dysplasia. *J Pediatr Surg* 1984; **19**: 649.

33. Osanthanondh V, Potter EL. Pathogenesis of polycystic kidneys. *Arch Pathol* 1964; **77**: 459.

34. Gasser B, Mauss Y, Ghnassia JP et al. A quantitative study of normal nephrogenesis in the human fetus: its implication in the natural history of kidney changes due to low obstructive uropathies. *Fetal Diagn Ther* 1993; **8**: 371.

35. Ruano-Gil D, Coca-Payeras A, Tejedo-Mateu A. Obstruction and normal recanalization of the ureter in the human embryo: its relation to congenital ureteric obstruction. *Eur Urol* 1975; **1**: 293.

36. Ostling K. The genesis of hydronephrosis: particularly with regard to the changes at the ureteropelvic junction. *Acta Chem Scand Suppl* 1942; **86**: 72.

37. Maizels M, Stephens FD. Valves of the ureter as a cause of primary obstruction of the ureter: anatomic, embryologic and clinical aspects. *J Urol* 1980; **123**: 742.

38. Matsuno T, Tokunaka S, Koyanagi T. Muscular development in the urinary tract. *J Urol* 1984; **132**: 148.

39. Alcaraz A, Vinaixa F, Tejedo-Mateu A et al. Congenital obstructive disease of the ureter. *Acta Urol Esp* 1989; **13**: 318.

40. Tanagho EA. Embryologic basis for lower ureteral anomalies: a hypothesis. *Urology* 1976; **7**: 451.

41. Stephens FD. *Congenital Malformations of the Urinary Tract*. New York: Praeger.

42. Williams DI, Lightwood RG. Bilateral single ectopic ureters. *J Urol* 1972; **44**: 267.

43. Noseworthy J, Persky L. Spectrum of bilateral ureteral ectopia. *Urology* 1982; **19**: 489.

44. Weigert C. Ueber einige Bildunsfehler der Ureteren. *Virchows Arch* (*Pathol Anat*) 1877; **70**: 490.

45. Meyer R. Normal and abnormal development of the ureter in the human embryo – a mechanistic consideration. *Anat Rec* 1946; **96**: 355.

46. Stephens FD. Anatomical vagaries of double ureters. *Aust N Z J Surg* 1958; **28**: 27.

47. Muecke EC. The role of the cloacal membrane in exstrophy: the first successful experimental study. *J Urol* 1964; **92**: 659.

48. Marshall VF, Muecke EC. Congenital abnormalities of the bladder. In: *Handbuch de Urolgie*. New York: Springer-Verlag, p 165.

49. Lowsley OS. The development of the human prostate gland with reference to the development of other structures at the neck of the urinary bladder. *Am J Anat* 1912; **13**: 299.

50. Hammond G, Yglesias L, David JE. The urachus: its anatomy and associated fasciae. *Anat Rec* 1941; **80**: 271.

51. Nix JT, Menville JG, Albert M, Wendt DL. Congenital patent urachus. *J Urol* 1958; **79**: 264.

52. Gearhart JP, Jeffs RD. Exstrophy of the bladder, epispadias, and other bladder anomalies. In Walsh, PC, Retik, AB, Stamey, TA et al. (eds) *Campbell's Urology* 1992, 6th edn. Philadelphia: WB Saunders, pp 1772–1821.

53. Lattimer JK. Congenital deficiency of the abdominal musculature and associated genitourinary anomalies: a report of 22 cases. *J Urol* 1958; **79**: 343.

54. Wood-Jones F. The musculature of the bladder and urethra. Anatomical Society, Great Britain and Ireland. *J Anat Physiol* 1901; **36**: 51.

55. Wladimiroff JW, Campbell S. Fetal urine production rates in normal and complicated pregnancy. *Lancet* 1974; **i**: 151.

56. Witschi E. Migration of the germ cells of human embryos from the yolk sac to the primitive gonadal folds. *Contrib Embryol Carnegie Instit* 1948; **32**: 67.

57. Berta P, Hawkins JR, Sinclair AH et al. Genetic evidence equating SRY and the testis-determining factor. *Nature* 1990; **348**: 448.

58. Fitzgerald M. Abdominal and pelvic organs. In: *Human Embryology*. New York: Harper & Row, p 106.

59. Guerrier DT, Tran, D, Vanderwinden, JM et al. The persistent mullerian duct syndrome: a molecular approach. *J Clin Endocrinol Metab* 1989; **68**: 46.

60. Josso N. Evolution of the mullerian-inhibiting activity of the human testis. *Biol Neonate* 1972; **20**: 368.

61. Payne AH, Jaffe RB. Androgen formation from pregnenolone sulfate by fetal neonatal adult human testis. *J Clin Endocrinol Metab* 1975; **40**: 102.

62. Siiteri PK, Wilson JD. Testosterone formation and metabolism during male sexual differentiation in the human embryo. *J Clin Endocrinol Metab* 1974; **38**: 113.

63. Clements KA, Reyes FI, Winter JSD, Faiman C. Studies on human sexual development. III. Fetal pituitary and amniotic fluid concentration of LH, CG and FSH. *J Clin Endocrinol Metab* 1976; **42**: 9.

64. Tuchmann-Duplessis H, Haegel P. Urinary system. In: *Illustrated Human Embryology*, vol. 2. New York: Springer-Verlag, pp 50–71.

65. Backhouse KM. Embryology of testicular descent and maldescent. *Urol Clin North Am* 1982; **9**: 315.

66. Heyns CF. The gubernaculum during testicular descent in the human fetus. *J Anat* 1987; **153**: 93–112.

67. Lemeh CN. A study of the development and structural relationships of the testis and gubernaculum. *Surg Gynecol Obstet* 1960; **110**: 164.

68. Wyndham NR. A morphological study of testicular descent. *J Anat* 1943; **77**: 179.

69. Fentener Van Vlissingen JM, Koch CAM, Delpech B et al. Growth and differentiation of the gubernaculum testis during testicular descent in the pig: changes in the extracellular matrix, DNA content and hyaluronidase, β-glucuronidase and β-N-acetylglucosaminidase activities. *J Urol* 1989; **142**: 837.

70. Backhouse KM. The gubernaculum testis in hunteri: testicular descent and maldescent. *Ann R Coll Surg (Engl)* 1964; **35**: 15.

71. Backhouse KM, Butler H. The gubernaculum testis of the pig. *J Anat* 1960; **94**: 107.

72. Geir HT, Marion GB. Development of the mammalian testis. In: Johnson AD, Gomes WR, Vandermark NL (eds) *The Testis*. New York: Academic Press, pp 1–45.

73. Frey HL, Peng S, Rajfer J. Synergy of abdominal pressure and androgens in testicular descent. *Biol Reprod* 1983; **29**: 1233.

74. Birnholz JD. Determination of fetal sex. *New Engl J Med* 1983; **309**: 942.

75. Spaulding MH. The development of the external genitalia in the human embryo. *Carnegie Contrib Embryol* 1921; **61**: 13, 67.

76. Tolmatschew N. Ein Fall von semilunaren Klappen der Harnrohre und von vergrosserter Vesicula Prostatica. *Arch Pathol Anat* 1870; **49**: 348.

77. Waterman, RE. Human embryo and fetus. In: Hafez ESE, Kenemans P (eds) *Atlas of Human Reproduction*. Hingham, MA: Kluwer Boston, Inc.

78. Rowsell AR, Morgan BDG. Hypospadias and the embryogenesis of the penile urethra. *Br J Plast Surg* 1987; **40**: 201.

79. Duckett JW. Hypospadias. In: Walsh, PC, Retik, AB, Stamey, TA et al. (eds) *Campbell's Urology* 1992, 6th edn. Philadelphia: WB Saunders, pp 1893–1919.

80. Hunter RH. Notes on development of prepuce. *J Anat* 1935; **70**: 68.

81. O'Rahilly R. The development of the vagina in the human. In: Blandau RJ, Bergsma D (eds) *Morphogenesis and Malformation of the Genital System. Birth Defects Original Article Series*, vol 13, pp 123–136.

82. Acien P, Arminana E, Garcia-Ontiveros E. Unilateral renal agenesis associated with ipsilateral blind vagina. *Arch Pathol* 1987; **240**: 1.

83. Bok G, Drews U. The role of the wolffian ducts in the formation of the sinus vagina: an organ culture study. *J Embryol Exp Morphol* 1983; **73**: 275.

84. Bulmer D. The development of the human vagina. *J Anat* 1957; **91**: 490.

85. Koff AK. Development of the vagina in the human fetus. *Carnegie Contrib Embryol* 1933; **140**: 24, 59.

3

Pathology of the kidney and urinary tract in infancy

C. Cullinane

Introduction

Disease of the kidneys and urinary tract in the fetus and infant are predominantly due to anomalous development and may be hereditary, genetic or sporadic [1]. Diagnosis requires a team approach [2]. The role of the pathologist is to confirm the clinical diagnostic findings, document associated or other anomalies, describe the pathological findings which may in some cases be definitive and contribute to our understanding of developmental pathology.

Anomalies of the kidney

Renal agenesis

Absence of the kidneys may be unilateral or bilateral. In bilateral renal agenesis both kidneys and ureters are absent and kidney tissue cannot be identified microscopically. The condition is not compatible with postnatal life and infants usually die shortly after birth from respiratory failure due to pulmonary hypoplasia rather than renal failure. In an autopsy review at British Columbia's Children's Hospital, bilateral renal agenesis represented 34% of serious renal system malformations with a male to female ratio of 3 : 1 [3]. The bladder is hypoplastic and may be absent. Genital anomalies are common with absence of testicular descent, failure of vas deferens and seminal vesicle development in males and abnormalities of fallopian tubes, uterine horns and upper vagina in females [4]. The adrenal glands are oval and flattened due to lack of moulding and lie against the posterior abdominal wall. Absence of urine leads to severe oligohydramnios which results in a constellation of dysmorphic features known as oligohydramnios Sequence. The features include abnormal facies with beaked nose, low-set posteriorly rotated ears, receding chin, bowing of legs with talipes, loose skin with large spade-like hands and pulmonary hypoplasia. The facial characteristics were originally described in association with bilateral renal agenesis [5] and became known as Potter's syndrome. However, it is recognized that similar features are seen in any condition with severe oligohydramnios. In a retrospective review of infants dying of Oligohydramnios Sequence, 34% had bilateral renal agenesis, 9% had unilateral agenesis with unilateral cystic dysplasia, 4% had a recessively inherited kidney disorder, 10% had minor urinary tract anomalies and 3% had normal urinary tracts [6]. Sirenomelia sequence, caudal regression sequence and MURCS association are often associated with bilateral renal agenesis [1]. Non-syndromal bilateral renal agenesis and unilateral agenesis with contralateral multicystic dysplasia originally thought to be sporadic, are often autosomal dominant with incomplete penetrance, a condition referred to as hereditary renal adysplasia [7,8]. The disease may recur in siblings with phenotypically normal parents [8]. Investigation of the family may reveal various renal anomalies [7]. It may also be associated with other malformations such as cleft palate, congenital heart defects, vertebral anomalies and with genital anomalies [8].

Unilateral renal agenesis is commoner and presents usually in adult life if the contralateral kidney is normal. When seen at autopsy in children it is usually an incidental finding, associated with contralateral renal dysplasia, or part of the spectrum of anomalies in syndromes where death has followed serious malformation in another system, e.g. cardiovascular. The ipsilateral ureter and hemitrigone are usually absent. Anomalies of ipsilateral genital tracts are common. The single kidney may show compensatory hypertrophy. Anomalies in other systems frequently encountered include oesophageal atresia, congenital heart disease, meningomyelocele and aplasia of the homolateral adrenal gland [9].

Supernumerary kidney(s)

This is a rare malformation with one or several ectopic kidneys in addition to the two normal ones. The supernumerary kidney is usually small, completely separate from and caudal to the ipsilateral normal kidney. The draining ureters may fuse or join the bladder separately [4].

Ectopic kidney

Caudal displacement of the kidney to the pelvis is the most common presentation. The displaced kidney is usually ovoid in shape and is often malrotated with pelvis anterior and distorted pelvicalyceal system. Kinking of the ureter predisposes the kidney to hydronephrosis and infection. Cystic dysplasia may be present. Genital anomalies such as hypospadias in males and vaginal abnormalities in females as well as anorectal anomalies may occur [4]. Cephalic displacement is very rare. The thoracic kidney is usually left sided and associated with diaphragmatic hernia or eventration [10].

Crossed renal ectopia is rare and characterized by location of both kidneys on the same side of the body. The kidneys may be fused and form unusual shapes [9]. The ureter of one kidney, usually the lower, crosses the midline to insert into the bladder on the opposite side. Hydronephrosis and dysplasia may be present.

Horseshoe kidney

Usually there is fusion of the lower poles of the kidneys which are displaced inferiorly. The isthmus of the fused kidney lies below the inferior mesenteric artery and the kidneys are malrotated with the pelvis and ureters lying anteriorly. Lack of moulding results in separate oval flat adrenals. Genital anomalies may be present. Association with trisomy 18 and Turner's syndrome is well recognized [1]. Doughnut kidney refers to fusion of the upper poles as well as the lower poles [9]. Dysplasia may be present if the ureter is obstructed.

Nephromegaly

Enlargement of the kidneys may be cystic or non-cystic, bilateral or unilateral. Bilateral cystic enlargement of the kidneys may be due to ureteropelvic obstruction with hydronephrosis, multicystic dysplasia, autosomal recessive polycystic kidney disease, Meckel's syndrome and, rarely, autosomal dominant polycystic kidney disease. The differential diagnosis for unilateral cystic nephromegaly includes multicystic dysplasia, hydronephrosis and multilocular cyst. Non-cystic nephromegaly is due to compensatory hypertrophy of normally differentiated renal parenchyma with increase in size of glomeruli, which also may be increased in number. Unilateral non-cystic nephromegaly is usually associated with contralateral renal agenesis or dysplasia. Rarely the enlarged kidney is due to the presence of tumour. Bilateral non-cystic nephromegaly is associated with maternal diabetes, Beckwith–Wiedemann syndrome, congenital diaphragmatic hernia and congenital nephrotic syndrome [11–13].

Renal hypoplasia

Most small kidneys show features of dysplasia and are best described as hypoplastic/dysplastic. True hypoplasia must be separated from small kidneys secondary to chronic infection and scarring. Bilateral hypoplasia refers to congenitally small kidneys which are less than 2 standard deviations below the expected mean and is divided into two types: simple hypoplasia and oligomeganephronia [14]. Simple hypoplasia shows decreased numbers of renal lobes and nephrons without hypertrophy or dysplasia and is extremely rare. Oligomeganephronia refers to congenitally small kidneys, usually bilateral, showing reduced numbers of lobules and nephrons with hypertrophy of glomeruli and tubules. Most cases are sporadic and are not associated with other anomalies. However, multiple malformations may be present [15] and the condition may be familial [16]. Renal insufficiency begins in infancy with chronic renal failure in the first decade, but those with severely affected kidneys may die in infancy [16]. It has been reported associated with right-sided renal agenesis in an 18-week fetus and 33-week preterm infant [17]. The cause of oligomeganephronia is unknown. Suggested aetiological factors include environmental and genetic abnormalities and deficient metanephric blastema [15–17].

Segmental hypoplasia (Ask–Upmark kidney)

This type of small kidney, unilateral or bilateral, is characterized by a transverse groove on the capsular surface with thinned underlying parenchyma showing deficient or absent glomeruli and atrophic tubules, due in most cases to reflux nephropathy [4].

Renal tubular dysgenesis

This is a rare autosomal recessive condition leading to oligohydramnios, oligohydramnios sequence, neonatal anuria and renal failure [18,19]. The kidneys are normal in shape and are usually slightly enlarged. The characteristic histological appearance is hypoplasia or absence of proximal tubules with crowding of glomeruli. Similar findings have been described in the kidneys in association with maternal use of ACE inhibitor for hypertension [20], donor twin in twin–twin transfusion [19] and haemosiderosis [21]. The onset of oligohydramnios before 20 weeks allows prenatal diagnosis. The pathological changes in the kidneys of two siblings (20 and 22 weeks' gestation) were less marked than in the kidney at term, with clearly recognizable proximal tubules which were reduced in number [22]. Ischaemia of renal parenchyma is a suggested pathogenetic mechanism [23].

Cystic disease of the kidney

Cysts in the kidney are a feature of a wide number of conditions, which may be sporadic, syndromic, genetic or familial. A team approach to diagnosis is necessary and frequently pathological features are specific.

Cystic dysplasia

This is the commonest cause of renal cysts in childhood. It is characterized by disorganized renal parenchyma resulting from anomalous metanephric differentiation and is part of a general anomaly of the whole urinary tract [24,25]. Studies of hereditary renal dysplasia support the primary defect in renal dysplasia being in the ureteral bud, with secondary effects varying from mild anomalies involving the ureter to severe anomalies such as agenesis and dysplasia [8,26]. The congenital anomalies of the urinary tract associated with renal dysplasia have an obstructive element. Generally the more severe the obstruction, the more severe the dysplasia. The dysplasia may be unilateral or bilateral, the former associated with ipsilateral ureteric anomalies and the latter with bilateral ureteric anomalies. Infravesical obstruction is associated with bilateral renal involvement. The kidney may show diffuse or segmental dysplasia. The latter accompanies ureteric stenosis, ectasia, duplication or urethrocele. Diffuse dysplasia shows a continuum from grossly enlarged multicystic kidney(s) to small hypoplastic kidney(s) and aplastic kidney(s), the latter consisting of a few small cysts [4].

Multicystic dysplasia is usually unilateral and presents as an abdominal mass in the neonate. The kidney is enlarged, often grossly, with loss of reniform shape and distortion by numerous cysts, the largest beneath the capsule (Figure 3.1). The pelvis and calyces are absent or poorly developed. The ureter is atretic throughout its length, or in its upper portion, and rarely is absent [27]. If bilateral, the prognosis is poor and oligohydramnios sequence with pulmonary hypoplasia leads to death from respiratory failure.

The diagnosis of renal dysplasia is based on the characteristic histological appearance (Figure 3.2). The microscopic appearance is variable, with disorganized parenchyma, cysts

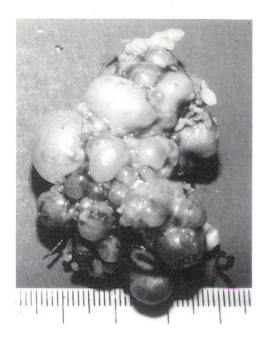

Figure 3.1 Cystic dysplasia with distortion of kidney by multiple cysts of varying size.

of varying size lined by cuboidal or flattened tubular epithelium, separated by fibrous stroma containing primitive tubules and glomeruli, foci of haemopoiesis, fat and often bars of cartilage. The histological hallmark is the primitive tubule lined by cuboidal or columnar epithelium, cuffed by concentric layers of mesenchymal cells. Nephrogenic rests

are occasionally present [28]. Rarely Wilms' tumour or renal carcinoma has developed in a multicystic kidney [29,30].

Infravesical anomalies or atresia, prune belly syndrome or megacystis–megaureter syndrome are associated with bilateral peripheral cortical dysplasia of variable degree accompanied by hydronephrosis. The extent and degree of renal involvement is dependent on the severity and duration of the obstruction.

Polycystic kidney disease

Polycystic kidney disease refers to two distinct forms of bilateral cystic renomegaly – autosomal recessive polycystic kidney disease (ARPKD) and autosomal dominant polycystic kidney disease (ADPKD). The genetic and familial nature of these diseases are discussed in Chapter 22.

Autosomal recessive polycystic kidney disease

This is the commonest hereditary renal disease in infancy and childhood [31]. The severity of renal involvement varies. Two clinical patterns of presentation are recognized. The infantile type is the most severe and is usually fatal in the neonatal period. The juvenile type presents as renal failure in later childhood and may be accompanied by portal hypertension. Differentiation from autosomal dominant polycystic

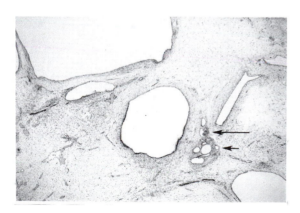

(a)

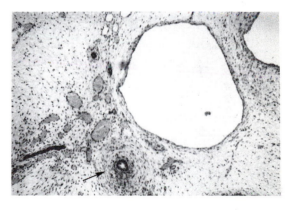

(b)

Figure 3.2 (a) Cystic dysplasia with cysts lined by flat epithelium separated by stroma containing cluster of tubules (short arrow) and glomerulus (long arrow) (H&E ×36). (b) Cystic dysplasia with tubule surrounded by concentric layers of mesenchymal cells (arrow) (H&E ×80).

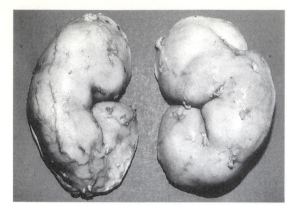

Figure 3.3 Smooth surfaced symmetrically enlarged kidneys of autosomal recessive polycystic kidney disease at term gestation.

kidney disease is based on family studies, radiology and histology, as laboratory investigations of renal function are not specific [32].

Infantile ARPKD is a rare disease characterized by bilateral symmetrical enlargement of the kidneys which retain their reniform shape (Figure 3.3). The capsular surface is smooth and typically the cut surface shows replacement of normal parenchyma by cylindrical radially orientated cysts, less than 2 mm in diameter (Figure 3.4). The pelvis, calyces and ureter are usually normal [4]. Microscopically the cysts, lined by cuboidal or flat epithelium, extend from the cortex to the medulla. Normal renal tubules and glomeruli are present between the cysts (Figure 3.5). Dysplastic-type tubules or glomerular cysts are not present.

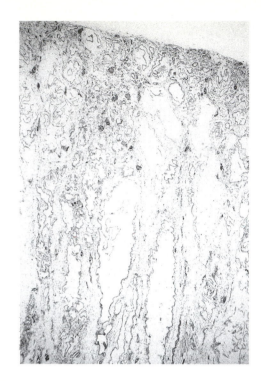

Figure 3.5 Autosomal recessive polycystic kidney disease, at term, showing cylindrical cysts extending from cortex to medulla with normal glomeruli and tubules between the cysts (H&E ×36).

The liver always shows expanded portal tracts with increased numbers of branching, angulated peripheral bile ducts and numerous blood vessels (Figure 3.6). This abnormality is known as biliary dysgenesis, or ductal plate malformation. In some patients, older children and

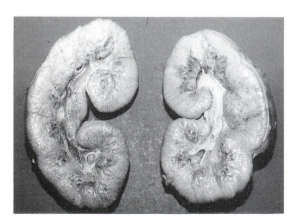

Figure 3.4 Cut surface of kidneys with autosomal recessive polycystic kidney disease at term showing radially orientated narrow cylindrical cysts.

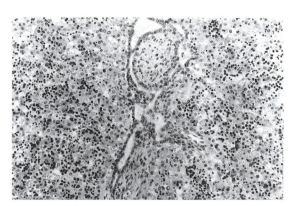

Figure 3.6 Biliary dysgenesis with branching bile duct in portal tract of liver (H&E ×204).

adults, the liver changes predominate and the presentation is with congenital hepatic fibrosis and portal hypertension. In infants with ARPKD oligohydramnios sequence is usually present with pulmonary hypoplasia. The oligo-hydramnios may only be detected in the third trimester of pregnancy. The massive kidneys also compress the chest contents contributing to the pulmonary hypoplasia and death results from respiratory failure.

Autosomal dominant polycystic kidney disease

This is usually a disease of adults and rarely presents in the fetus, neonate or child [32–34]. Death in early life is rarer in ADPKD than in ARPKD [32]. The kidneys are grossly enlarged and may be asymmetrical [35]. Microscopically cysts are present in both kidneys. They are lined by tubular epithelium, vary in size, are usually round and are present in cortex and medulla. Glomerular cysts may be present. The intervening parenchyma may be normal or show focal glomerulosclerosis. The liver is usually normal in the infant. Rarely cysts have been found in a liver biopsy taken in infancy [36].

Syndromes with renal cysts

Several syndromes are associated with cysts in the kidney. Cysts may be a minor or major component of these syndromes, and may be visible macroscopically or microscopically. Meckel–Gruber syndrome, an autosomal reces-sive condition, is characterized by posterior encephalocele, postaxial polydactyly and bilat-eral renomegaly [9]. The kidneys are greatly enlarged, smooth surfaced with retention of reniform shape, grossly resembling autosomal recessive polycystic kidney disease. However on cut surface there is no radial orientation of the cysts. The latter are round, involve cortex and medulla and are lined by flat or cuboidal tubular epithelium (Figure 3.7). The larger cysts are present towards the medulla. Between the cysts the tubules and glomeruli appear reduced in number and the interstitium is prominent. The ureters are atretic and the bladder is hypoplastic. Biliary dysgenesis simi-lar to that seen in ARPKD is another feature.

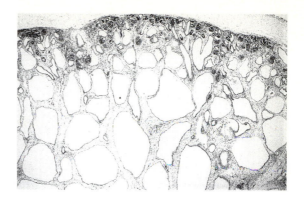

Figure 3.7 Meckel–Gruber syndrome at 18 weeks' gestation with round kidney cysts, larger towards the medulla (H&E ×36).

The disease is usually fatal in the neonate. Zell-weger's syndrome, an autosomal recessive con-dition, is often associated with persistent fetal lobulation and cortical cysts, usually micro-scopic, involving tubules and glomeruli with increased interstitial stroma containing small tubules [9]. In Jeune's syndrome, also auto-somal recessive, the extent and type of renal involvement varies from focal microcysts to extensive renal dysplasia [27]. All these syn-dromes are associated with biliary dysgenesis, similar to that seen in ARPKD.

Renal involvement in tuberous sclerosis consists of cysts and angiomyelolipomas [37]. The latter usually present in adolescence. In infancy the kidneys may be bilaterally enlarged with multiple cysts. Unilateral massive cystic enlargement in the neonate has been reported [38]. The histology of the renal cysts is dis-tinctive, consisting of a lining of hyperplastic eosinophilic tubular epithelium [39].

Glomerular cysts

Cystic dilation of Bowman's space may be associated with a variety of conditions. Renal cortical involvement may be focal or diffuse and is often referred to as glomerulocystic dis-ease. Diffuse cortical glomerular cystic change is rare, associated with a two-fold increase in kidney size and accentuation of lobulation [9]. Autosomal dominant polycystic kidney disease may present in the fetus as isolated renal glo-merulocystic disease [34]. An autosomal domi-nant condition with renal hypoplasia and glomerular cysts is described [40]. Cortical glomerular cysts have been found in trisomies, triploidy, monosomy X [3] and in multisystem syndromes [41]. The cysts are small and lined by flattened epithelium with a glomerular tuft in the lumen.

Medullary cysts

Juvenile nephronophthisis/medullary cystic disease is a spectrum of familial diseases causing renal failure in children and adults characterized histologically by interstitial fibrosis, tubular atrophy and cysts in the medulla. It is rare in infancy. Tubulo-interstitial nephritis with cortical microcysts associated with severe renal failure has been reported in infants [42].

Pathological changes in the liver

Portal tract fibrosis with bile duct enlargement or proliferation is seen with a variety of kidney diseases, including autosomal recessive polycystic disease, Meckel's syndrome and Jeune's syndrome and, rarely, in dominant glomerulocystic disease, tuberose sclerosis, autosomal dominant polycystic kidney disease and some types of juvenile nephronophthisis [43]. In the investigation of any cystic kidney disease a liver biopsy should routinely be taken in addition to the renal biopsy.

Anomalies of renal pelvis and ureter

Hydronephrosis

The hydronephrotic kidney shows dilatation of the pelvis, blunting of papillae and thinning of parenchyma. Microscopically, collecting ducts are dilated with tubular atrophy and interstitial fibrosis. Cortical atrophy, inflammation and scarring are associated with longstanding disease and secondary infection. Hydronephrosis is secondary to obstruction of the urinary tract and may be unilateral or bilateral. It may present in the fetus or neonate as an abdominal mass if unilateral or oligohydramnios sequence if there is severe bilateral kidney involvement.

Ureteropelvic junction obstruction

This is the usual cause of hydronephrosis. The junction of the ureter and pelvis is narrowed due to stenosis, hypoplasia or atresia. Dysplasia in the kidney is infrequent. It is an uncommon cause of non-dysplastic hydronephrosis in fetal and neonatal autopsies – only 9 of 21 cases in Taylor's series were due to ureteropelvic obstruction [3].

Duplication and ectopic ureter

Duplex kidney with duplication of the renal pelvis and ureter is a common abnormality of the urinary tract and is more frequent in females. It is usually asymptomatic unless complicated by infection. The upper portion of the duplex kidney is usually smaller, with a small pelvis and a few minor calyces. It may be complicated by hydronephrosis, chronic inflammation and reflux nephropathy and dysplasia. The draining ureter usually joins the ureter from the lower segment to form a single ureter. The ureters may remain separate, with the ureter draining the upper segment inserting ectopically into the bladder or occasionally into the vagina or urethra in females, prostatic urethra or ejaculatory ducts in males [4,9]. The upper segment ureter is prone to obstruction. Rarely a single ureter shows ectopic insertion.

Ureterocele

This is a cystic dilatation of the distal ureter at its insertion (normal or ectopic) into the bladder.

Anomalies of the bladder

Agenesis of the bladder is associated with major urinary tract anomalies and is very rare. Hypoplasia accompanies renal agenesis. Septation and duplication of the bladder are described [4]. Vesicorectal and vesicovaginal fistulas may occur. In the urorectal septum malformation sequence, which affects females, such fistulas are accompanied by pseudohermaphroditism and renal agenesis or dysplasia [44].

Exstrophy

This is due to failure or incomplete fusion of the lower anterior abdominal wall. The abnormality shows a spectrum from epispadias to the severest abnormality, cloacal exstrophy [45]. In bladder exstrophy the anterior bladder wall is absent, the pelvic bones are separated and the mucosa of the posterior bladder wall protrudes through the defect. The transitional bladder mucosa merges with skin at the margin of the defect. Prolonged exposure of the bladder mucosa results in infection, cystitis cystica and squamous metaplasia [4]. In cloacal exstrophy the exposed bladder mucosa is present laterally with intestinal mucosa centrally into which the ileum and blind-ending colon open. Anomalies of genitalia and kidneys, anal atresia and omphalocele are also present [46].

Anomalies of the urethra

Obstruction of the urethra may be due to valves, diaphragm or stenosis. The effect on the proximal urinary tract is dependent on the degree of obstruction, whether complete, partial or intermittent, and its duration.

Posterior urethral valves in males are the commonest cause of abnormal bladder outflow. Severe obstruction leads to prune belly syndrome.

Prune belly syndrome

This syndrome is characterized by the triad of absent abdominal wall muscle, undescended testes and urinary tract anomalies [47]. The aetiology is usually thought to be due to obstruction, although anatomical obstruction cannot be demonstrated in all cases. The obstructions identified in association with the syndrome include urethral valves or diaphragm, urethral stenosis, atresia or multiple lumens [48]. Pathological study of the lower urinary tract in prune belly syndrome showed abnormal prostatic growth and development [49]. More recently, it has been suggested that urethral obstruction distal to the prostate may be the underlying cause, with resultant increased pressure leading to dilated prostatic urethra and defective development of prostate [50].

Abdominal distension is due to dilated bladder (megacystis) and proximal urinary tract. The fetal bladder is thin walled with hypoplastic muscle fibres and may rupture. Fetal or neonatal ascites may be present [51]. In the neonate the bladder is trabeculated, with hypertrophy of the bladder neck. The proximal urethra, ureters and renal pelvises are dilated and the kidneys show peripheral cortical dysplasia. Urachus may be incorporated into the bladder [50]. In a review of 29 patients with prune belly syndrome (26 males, three females), associated anomalies included musculoskeletal anomalies secondary to oligohydramnios in 58%, gastrointestinal anomalies in 31% and genital anomalies in all females [52]. Severe renal involvement with extensive dysplasia and oligohydramnios is associated with a poor prognosis and death in the perinatal period, whereas in survivors renal dysplasia involves less than a third of the parenchyma [50].

Other diseases of the kidney

Nephrotic syndrome

The congenital nephrotic syndrome presents in the first 3 months of life and in the neonate is usually due to congenital nephrosis. The kidneys are large with stromal oedema and tubular microcystic change initially in the deep cortex. With disease progression the cortex becomes diffusely microcystic with interstitial fibrosis and chronic inflammation. The tubular dilation is probably secondary to heavy protein leakage from the glomeruli [9]. Pregnancy complications include premature delivery and mild intrauterine growth retardation. The placenta is characteristically large.

Other causes of nephrotic syndrome in the infant include congenital infection, usually syphilis, haemolytic-uremic syndrome, male pseudohermaphorditism and Wilms' tumour [53]. Acquired forms of nephrotic syndrome are rare in infancy [4].

Haemolytic uraemic syndrome

This disease presents usually in infants and young children with the triad of acute renal failure, microangiopathic haemolytic anaemia and thrombocytopenia. It is usually associated with verotoxin-producing *E. coli* infection and rarely with shigella, salmonella and viruses [54]. Histological features in the kidney include glomerular fibrin thrombi and fibrinoid necrosis, arterial and arteriolar thrombi with fibrinoid necrosis and intimal proliferation. Glomerular lesions are more marked in infants. The progressive occlusion of vessels may lead to diffuse cortical necrosis or widespread infarction [53].

Renal tubular transport abnormalities

Various hereditary disorders of renal transport are described. Symptoms may occur in infancy in some of these conditions. Histological features are not specific in the majority of cases [4].

Infection/inflammation

Systemic infections in the fetus and neonate may involve the kidney. Such infections may be congenital due to viruses and toxoplasmosis (TORCH), or fungi (candida, aspergillus, mucor and blastomyces) in the sick neonate on intravenous feeding and broad-spectrum antibiotics [53]. Microscopy of the kidney with viral infection, e.g. due to cytomegalovirus (CMV), shows typical owl's eye nuclear inclusions in tubular epithelium with chronic inflammation in the interstitium. Fungal infections usually result in multiple microabscesses in the parenchyma. Systemic bacterial infection due to *Staphylococcus aureus* causes acute pyelonephritis with swelling of the kidney due to interstitial oedema. Microscopy shows pus in the tubules, focal necrosis of tubular epithelium, acute inflammation in the interstitium and, in some cases, microabscess formation. Infants with congenital anomalies of the urinary tract are predisposed to recurrent ascending bacterial infections, usually due to *E. coli* and gram-negative bacilli. The changes of acute infection are similar to those noted above. However, in most cases because of longstanding recurrent inflammation the features are of chronic pyelonephritis. The kidney may be shrunken and scarred and histologically shows chronic inflammation in the interstitium and pelvic wall with lymphoid aggregates, tubular atrophy with thyroidization and interstitial fibrosis. Cortical involve-

ment with glomerular sclerosis, periglomerular fibrosis and atrophy occurs later in the disease.

Reflux nephropathy (chronic pyelonephritis) is usually due to vesicoureteric reflux complicated by recurrent infection. Intrarenal reflux with backflow in renal tubules due to increased pressure in the renal pelvis may be present [4,27,53].

Renal ischaemia/infarction

In the perinatal period renal necrosis due to asphyxia and hypoxia are the commonest cause of renal failure. Other causes of renal ischaemia in this age group include cyanotic congenital heart disease, hyaline membrane disease, infection, renal vein thrombosis and thrombosis secondary to umbilical artery catheter [9]. The extent of kidney necrosis is variable. Characteristically the necrosis in the neonate affects both the cortex and medulla, with sparing of peripheral cortex. Renal vein thrombosis is associated with large plum-coloured kidney(s) (Figure 3.8), which histologically show marked haemorrhage in association with necrosis. Renal vein thrombosis complicates renal hypoperfusion, and may be seen in infants of diabetic mothers [4,55]. Intrauterine onset may be associated with fetal hydrops. Renal artery occlusion by thromboemboli or rarely thrombosis due to polyarteritis nodosa may cause diffuse or segmental infarction of the infantile kidney [4].

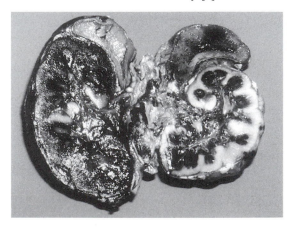

Figure 3.8 Thrombosis of inferior vena cava and renal veins, enlarged right kidney with diffuse haemorrhagic infarction, haemorrhage in medulla of left kidney with pale necrosis of cortex. Note haemorrhge also in left adrenal.

Tumours of kidney and urinary tract

An abdominal mass in childhood may be due to a number of kidney diseases, including dysplasia, polycystic renal diseases and neoplasia [56]. In a review of 226 tumours (abdominal, retroperitoneal and saccrococcygeal) in neonates and infants under 6 months of age, 54 kidney tumours were identified, the majority being mesoblastic nephroma [57]. Wilms' tumour, the commonest malignant renal tumour in childhood, has a peak incidence at approximately 2 years of age with approximately 15% of cases occurring in infants under 1 year of age in Western series, contrasting with East Asia where 25–40% of total incidence was in this age group [58]. Congenital Wilms' tumour is very rare [59]. A review of 32 neonates with solid malignant tumours over a 40-year period identified one case of Wilms' tumour [60]. Most nephroblastomatous lesions in the infant are benign or have low malignant potential. Wilms' tumour variants in the infant include monomorphous epithelial Wilms' tumour, cystic partially differentiated nephroblastoma and fetal rhabdomyomatous nephroblastoma and are associated with a good prognosis (see later). Three prognostic groups of renal tumours, based on histological features and survival, are recognized and have recently been termed low-, intermediate- and high-risk tumours [61].

Nephrogenic rests

The nephrogenic zone disappears from the fetal kidney at 34–36 weeks' gestational age. Foci of persistent nephrogenesis or nephrogenic rests may be found in less than 1% of perinatal autopsies but in up to 44% of kidneys with Wilms' tumour [62,63]. They are thought to represent precursor lesions of Wilms' tumour [62–64]. These rests are classified according to their position; perilobar rests are peripheral beneath the renal capsule, intralobar rests are found deeper within the cortex or medulla and by their histological appearance as dormant, maturing, hyperplastic or neoplastic [62]. Nephroblastomatosis refers to diffuse or multifocal rests which may be perilobar, intralobar or combined. When the entire kidney is involved the condition is referred to as universal or panlobar nephroblastomatosis. Intralobar rests are almost always identified in association with Wilms' tumour, which shows a predominance of stroma and heterologous differentiation, whereas perilobar rests are associated with peripheral triphasic Wilms' tumour with more epithelial and blastemal components. Intralobar rests occur with metachronous contralateral Wilms' tumour and in association with aniridia and Denys–Drash syndrome, whereas perilobar rests occur with synchronous bilateral Wilms' tumour and in association with hemihypertrophy and/or Beckwith–Wiedemann syndrome [62]. It has been suggested that the difference is due to timing of genetic events leading to Wilms' tumour, as intralobar rests occur chronologically earlier than perilobar nephrogenic rests [62,65]. Nephrogenic rests are very rarely associated with mesoblastic nephroma and have never been reported with clear-cell sarcoma or rhabdoid tumour [66]. Nephrogenic rests have also been described in association with congenital obstructive uropathy with or without dysplasia [28,67], trisomy 18 [68] and trisomy 13 [69,70].

Mesoblastic nephroma

This is a rare tumour accounting for approximately 3% of all childhood renal tumours [71]. However, it is the commonest solid kidney tumour presenting at birth or in early infancy [72]. Most cases present within the first 3 months of life. Its distinctive pathological and clinical features were recognized by Bolande [73]. Presentation is usually as an asymptomatic abdominal mass. Hypertension due to increased renin production by entrapped arterioles in the tumour has also been reported [74]. The tumour is typically unilateral and large, replacing most of the kidney. The gross appearance is of a solid lobulated whorled fleshy mass with no necrosis or haemorrhage. Rarely it is predominantly cystic [75]. The microscopic picture is characterized by nodules and fascicles of spindle cells with variable numbers of mitoses. Entrapped renal tubules are commonly found towards the margin (Figure 3.9). The tumour is not encapsulated and infiltrates the adjacent compressed renal parenchyma over a short distance. The tumour is confined to the kidney but may extend into the renal pelvis. Foci of rhabdomyoblastic

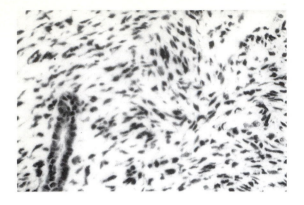

Figure 3.9 Mesoblastic nephroma with fascicles of spindle cells and entrapped renal tubule, lower left (H&E ×512).

differentiation, cartilage and myxoid stroma may be present [72]. Radical nephrectomy is the treatment of choice, with excellent prognosis. Incomplete excision is associated with local recurrence. Metastases have rarely been reported [76–78]. Recurrent or metastatic mesoblastic nephroma shows increased cellularity, necrosis, a high mitotic rate, haemorrhage and extension into adjacent structures [76,79]. The term atypical mesoblastic nephroma has been applied to these tumours [77]. However, the presence of these features has not correlated with the prognosis of mesoblastic nephroma in subsequent studies [78]. Adequacy of surgical excision is the most important prognostic factor. The patient's age must also be taken into account, as metastases have occurred in patients older than 3 months. Complete and repeated surgical excision without chemotherapy or radiotherapy is advised in children with atypical mesoblastic nephroma, recurrence or metastasis [78,80]. Karyotypic abnormalities in congenital mesoblastic nephroma include chromosome rearrangement at 11p15 region, hyperdiploidy and trisomy of chromosome 11 and hyperdiploidy in cellular variants [81–84].

Cystic partially differentiated Wilms' tumour and multilocular cyst

These are well-differentiated neoplasms which present as an abdominal mass in the neonate or infant. Nephrectomy is usually curative. The multilocular cyst or cystic nephroma is predominantly cystic with differentiated stroma between the cysts lacking blastema or other embryonic tissues, whereas cystic partially differentiated Wilms' tumour shows a predominance of blastema or other embryonic tissues in the septae [85]. Grossly the tumours are well circumscribed, vary in size and replace kidney parenchyma. The cysts are usually lined by tubular cuboidal or flattened epithelium, are discrete and do not communicate with the renal pelvis.

Metastases are not reported but cystic partially differentiated Wilms' tumour has recurred [85].

Wilms' tumour (nephroblastoma)

This is a malignant tumour of the kidney which may metastasize to lungs, liver, lymph nodes and rarely bone. Wilms' tumour may be unilateral or bilateral. Sporadic unilateral Wilms' tumour presents at a mean age of 45 months, with bilateral tumours presenting at a younger age [80]. The Wilms' tumour suppressor gene WT1 identified in 1990 at 11p13, codes a zinc finger protein which may act as a transcriptional represssor [86]. Wilms' tumour is associated with a number of clinical syndromes, including WAGR syndrome, Drash syndrome, hemihypertrophy, Beckwith–Wiedeman syndrome, Perlman syndrome and familial Wilms' tumour [72]. An interstitial deletion of chromosome 11 at p13 is found in WAGR syndrome and at p15 in Beckwith–Wiedeman syndrome. Nephrogenic rests are found in kidneys with Wilms' tumour and various associated syndromes as discussed earlier. The genetic events in Wilms' tumour development have recently been reviewed [87,88]. Multiple chromosomal anomalies are described [89,90].

Wilms' tumour usually presents as an abdominal mass. It is an embryonal tumour with disordered, aberrant nephrogenesis characterized histologically, in classic cases, by a triad of blastema, primitive tubules with occasional glomeruloid structures and stroma, the proportions of which vary (Figure 3.10). Mitoses, necrosis and focal haemorrhages are present. The tumour has a pushing margin and is well demarcated from adjacent renal parenchyma. Heterologous tissues such as striated muscle, cartilage, bone and primitive neural tissues may be found, more often in centrally located tumours, which tend to be associated with intralobar rests [62]. Variable expression

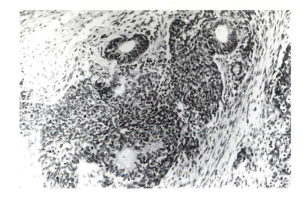

Figure 3.10 Wilms' tumour with blastema, primitive tubules and stroma (H&E ×204).

of Wilms' tumour genes correlates with these two phenotypes [65]. Postchemotherapy there is usually extensive scarring and necrosis and histologically the residual viable tumour may consist of more differentiated foci with tubules and glomeruli in a fibrous stroma or more undifferentiated tumour may persist. Rhabdomyoblastic differentiation in the stroma is more common in the Wilms' tumour post-treatment. Staging of the tumour is based histologically on adequacy of excision, presence or absence of capsular invasion and lymph node metastases. The presence of anaplasia is sought in biopsies and nephrectomy specimens. Anaplasia is characterized by large cells with atypical mitoses and large hyperchromatic nuclei, at least three times the size of those of adjacent cells [91]. It denotes unfavourable histology and is associated with a poorer prognosis. Anaplasia, however, is rare in children less than 2 years old [72]. The diagnosis of Wilms' tumour may be problematical when blastema only is present in a biopsy. The differential diagnosis then includes other small-celled tumours of childhood, including neuroblastoma, lymphoma, pPNET, rhabdomyosarcoma. Teratoid Wilms' tumour which has features of classical Wilms' tumour in association with teratoma-like tissues, is rare and has been reported in a 13-month-old child [92]. Extrarenal Wilms' tumour has occurred in infancy [93].

Monomorphous Wilms' tumour

This rare type of Wilms' tumour presents in infancy, and is characterized histologically by predominance of epithelial differentiation with closely packed primitive tubules. It is associated with a good prognosis and is usually confined to the kidney [94,95].

Fetal rhabdomyomatous Wilms' tumour

This type of Wilms' tumour occurs in children under 2 years of age. The tumour is large, polypoid and may project into the renal pelvis [96]. Histologically it consists mainly of well-differentiated striated muscle in a fibrous stroma with foci of blastema [72]. The tumour is bilateral in 30% of cases. The prognosis is usually good [72,94].

Sarcomatous tumours of the kidney

These are aggressive malignant renal neoplasms which may present in infancy and have a very poor prognosis.

Clear-cell sarcoma of the kidney

Clear-cell sarcoma or bone-metastasizing tumour usually presents between 1 and 2 years of age and is rare in infants less than 6 months old. It is characterized by its tendency to metastasize to bone and its histological appearance [97,98]. Grossly it resembles Wilms' tumour, forming a well-demarcated solid mass in the kidney. Histologically it differs from Wilms' tumour, with a diffuse cellular monotonous appearance of bland, round or spindle cells with clear cytoplasm and few mitoses. The vascular pattern is an important diagnostic feature, consisting of capillary rays with side branches forming arcades [72].

Malignant rhabdoid tumour of the kidney

This is a rare kidney tumour which frequently presents in infancy and rarely in the neonate [99]. Grossly the tumour is large, replaces the kidney and has a grey white cut surface with foci of necrosis and haemorrhage. Microscopically it consists of monotonous sheets or nests of large round cells with eccentric vesicular nuclei containing a prominent nucleolus and eosinophilic cytoplasm with hyaline inclusions. The latter consists of whorls of intermediate filaments ultrastructurally and is usually positive for vimentin and cytokeratin immunohistochemically. The tumour metastasizes widely to lung, liver, brain and bone [100]. It is associated with central nervous system tumours in approximately 15% of cases [101].

Ossifying renal tumour of infancy

This is a rare, benign tumour apparently arising from the papillary region of the medullary pyramids and forming a mass in the pelvis. It is characterized histologically by the presence of an osteoid core, osteoblasts and spindle cells [102]. Infants present with haematuria, and extension beyond the kidney has not been described.

Tumours of the lower urinary tract

Congenital rhabdomyosarcoma of the genitourinary tract is rare, second in frequency to head and neck tumours [103]. In a review of 95 cases of rhabdomyosarcoma, five occurred in the urinary tract of infants [104]. Tumours of the bladder or prostate are usually the botryoid subtype of embryonal rhabdomyosarcoma. In the bladder the tumour arises in the trigone and projects into the lumen as a polypoid pale oedematous mass resembling a bunch of grapes. Histologically it is characterized by a cambium layer of condensed primitive small hyperchromatic cells beneath the surface epithelium (Figure 3.11). The remainder of the mass consists of small dark stellate or spindle cells, which may be rather bland with infrequent mitoses, in a loose myxoid

stroma. Cells with eccentric eosinophilic cytoplasm or rhabdomyoblasts may be seen. Ultrastructurally Z-band material may be observed. Immunohistochemically the cells show positive cytoplasmic and nuclear staining with antibodies to desmin and MyoD1 respectively.

References

1. Jones KL (ed). *Smiths Recognisable Patterns of Human Malformation*, 4th edn. Philadelphia: WB Saunders, 1988.
2. Kaplan BS, Kaplan P, Ruchelli E. Inherited and congenital malformations of the kidney in the neonatal period. *Clin Perinatol* 1992; **19**: 197–211.
3. Taylor GP. Kidney and urinary tract. In: Dimmick JE, Kalousek DK (eds) *Developmental Pathology of the Embryo and Fetus*. Philadelphia: JB Lippincott, 1992; chap 19, pp 579–604.
4. Risdon RA (ed). Diseases of the kidney and lower urinary tract. In: Berry CL (ed) *Paediatric Pathology*, 2nd edn. Berlin: Springer-Verlag, chap 8, pp 409–466.
5. Potter EL. Facial characteristics of infants with bilateral renal agenesis. *Am J Obstet Gynecol* 1946; **51**: 885–888.
6. Newbould MJ, Lendon M, Barson AJ. Oligohydramnios sequence: the spectrum of renal malformations. *Br J Obstet Gynaecol* 1994; **101**: 598–604.
7. Roodhooft AM, Birnholz JC, Holmes LB. Familial nature of congenital absence and severe dysgenesis of both kidneys. *New Engl J Med* 1984; **310**: 1341–1345.
8. Moerman P, Fryns J-P, Sastrowijoto SH, Vandenberghe K, Lauweryns JM. Hereditary renal adysplasia: new observations and hypotheses. *Paediatr Pathol* 1994; **14**: 405–410.
9. Rapola J. The kidneys and urinary tract. In: Wigglesworth JS, Singer DB (eds) *Textbook of Fetal and Perinatal Pathology*, vol 2. Oxford: Blackwell Scientific Publications, 1991, pp 1109–1143.
10. Hawass ND, Kolawole TM, El Badawi MG, Patel PJ, Malabarey T. Intrathoracic kidney: report of 6 cases and a review of the literature. *Eur Urol* 1988; **14**: 83–87.
11. Sotelo-Avila C, Singer DB. Syndrome of hyperplastic fetal visceromegaly and neonatal hypoglycaemia (Beckwith's syndrome): a report of seven cases. *Pediatrics* 1970; **46**: 240–251.
12. Glick PL, Siebert JR, Benjamin DR. Pathophysiology of congenital diaphragmatic hernia: 1. Renal enlargement suggests feedback modulation by pulmonary derived renotropins – a unifying hypothesis to explain pulmonary hypoplasia, polyhydramnios and renal enlargement in fetus/newborn with congenital diaphragmatic hernia. *J Pediatr Surg* 1990; **25**: 492–495.

Figure 3.11 Botryoid rhabdomyosarcoma with small cells dispersed in a loose oedematous stroma and condensation of cells beneath surface epithelium (H&E ×80).

13. Tryggvasan K, Kouvalainen K. Number of nephrons in normal human kidneys and kidneys of patients with the congenital nephrotic syndrome. *Nephron* 1975; **15**: 62–68.

14. Boyd T, Rosen R, Redline RW, Genest DR. Non-dysplastic fetal renal hypoplasia associated with severe oligohydramnios. Clinical, pathologic and morphometric findings. *Paediatr Pathol Lab Med* 1995; **15**: 485–501.

15. Park SH, Chi JG. Oligomeganephronia associated with 4p deletion type chromosomal anomaly. *Pediatr Pathol* 1993; **13**: 731–740.

16. Moerman P, van Damme B, Proesmans W, Devlieger H, Goddeeris P, Lauweryns J. Oligomeganephronic renal hypoplasia in two siblings. *J Pediatr* 1984; **105**: 75–79.

17. Foster SV, Hawkins EP. Deficient metanephric blastema – a cause of oligomeganephronia? *Pediatr Pathol* 1994; **14**: 935–943.

18. Allanson JE, Pantzar JT, MacLeod PM. Possible new autosomal recessive syndrome with unusual renal histopathologic changes. *Am J Med Genet* 1983; **16**: 57–60.

19. Genest DR, Lage JM. Absence of normal-appearing proximal tubules in the fetal and neonatal kidney: prevalence and significance. *Human Pathol* 1991; **22**: 147–153.

20. Martin RA, Jones KL, Mendoza A, Barr M Jr, Benirschke K. Effect of ACE inhibition on the fetal kidney. Decreased renal blood flow. *Teratology* 1992; **46**: 317–321.

21. Bale PM, Kan AE, Dorney SFA. Renal proximal tubular dysgenesis associated with severe neonatal hemosiderotic liver disease. *Pediatr Pathol* 1994; **14**: 479–489.

22. Metzman RA, Hussan MA, Dellers EA. Renal tubular dysgenesis: a description of early renal maldevelopment in siblings. *Pediatr Pathol* 1993; **13**: 239–248.

23. Landing BH, Ang SM, Herta N, Larson EF, Turner M. Labelled lectin studies of renal tubular dysgenesis and renal tubular atrophy of post-natal ischaemia and end-stage kidney disease. *Pediatr Pathol* 1994; **14**: 87–99.

24. Risdon RA. Renal dysplasia: Part 1: A clinicopathological study of 76 cases. *J Clin Pathol* 1971; **24**: 57–71.

25. Risdon RA, Young LW, Chrispin AR. Renal hypoplasia and dysplasia. A radiological and pathological correlation. *Pediatr Radiol* 1975; **3**: 213–225.

26. Squiers EC, Morden RS, Bernstein J. Renal multicystic dysplasia: an occasional manifestation of the hereditary renal adysplasia syndrome. *Am J Med Genet (Suppl)* 1987; **3**: 279–284.

27. Risdon R. Cystic diseases of the kidney and reflux nephropathy. In: Anthony PP, MacSween RNM (eds) *Recent Advances in Histopathology*, vol 11. Edinburgh: Churchill Livingstone, chap 11, pp 163–184.

28. Dimmick JE, Johnson HW, Coleman GU, Carter M. Wilms tumorlet, nodular renal blastema and multicystic renal dysplasia. *J Urol* 1989; **142**: 484–485.

29. Oddone M, Marino C, Sergi C et al. Wilms' tumour arising in a multicystic kidney. *Pediatr Radiol* 1994; **24**: 236–238.

30. Birken G, King D, Vane D, Lloyd T. Renal cell carcinoma arising in a multicystic dysplastic kidney. *J Pediatr Surg* 1985; **20**: 619–621.

31. Kaplan BS, Kaplan P, Rosenberg HK, Lamothe E, Rosenblatt DS. Polycystic kidney diseases in childhood (Review). *J Pediatr* 1989; **115**: 867–880.

32. Kaariainen H, Koskimies O, Norio R. Dominant and recessive polycystic kidney disease in children: evaluation of clinical features and laboratory data. *Pediatr Nephrol* 1988; **2**: 296–302.

33. Edwards OP, Baldinger S. Prenatal onset of autosomal dominant polycystic kidney disease (Review). *Urology* 1989; **34**: 265–270.

34. Proesmans W, Van Damme B, Casaer P, Marchal G. Autosomal dominant polycystic kidney disease in the neonatal period: association with a cerebral arteriovenous malformation. *Pediatrics* 1982; **70**: 971–975.

35. Strand VVR, Rushton HG, Markle BM, Kapur S. Autosomal dominant polycystic kidney disease in infants: asymmetric disease mimicking a unilateral renal mass. *J Urol* 1989; **141**: 1151–1153.

36. Milutinovic J, Schabel SI, Ainsworth SK. Autosomal dominant polycystic kidney disease with liver and pancreatic involvement in early childhood. *Am J Kidney Dis* 1989; **13**: 340–344.

37. Zimmerhackl LB. Renal involvement in tuberous sclerosis complex: a retrospective survey. *Pediatr Nephrol* 1994; **8**: 451–457.

38. Miller ID, Gray ES, Lloyd DL. Unilateral cystic disease of the neonatal kidney: a rare presentation of tuberous sclerosis. *Histopathology* 1989; **14**: 529–532.

39. Bernstein J. Renal cystic disease in tuberous sclerosis (Review). *Pediatr Nephrol* 1993; **7**: 490–495.

40. Kaplan BS, Gordon I, Pincott J, Barratt TM. Familial hypoplastic glomerulocystic kidney disease: a definite entity with autosomal dominant inheritance. *Am J Med Genet* 1989; **34**: 569–573.

41. Bernstein J, Landing BH. Glomerulocystic kidney diseases [Review]. *Prog Clin Biol Res* 1989; **305**: 27–43.

42. Gagnadoux MF, Bacro JL, Broyer M, Habib R. Infantile chronic tubulo-interstitial nephritis with cortical microcysts: variant of nephronophthisis or new disease entity? *Pediatr Nephrol* 1989; **3**: 50–55.

43. Landing BH, Wells TR, Lipsey AI, Oyemade OA. Morphometric studies of cystic and tubulointerstitial kidney diseases with hepatic fibrosis in children. *Pediatr Pathol* 1990; **10**: 959–972.

44. Escobar LF, Weaver DD, Bixler D, Hodes ME, Mitchell M. Urorectal septum malformation sequence: report of cases and embryological analysis. *Am J Dis Child* 1987; **141**: 1021–1024.

45. Engel RM. Exstrophy of the bladder and associated anomalies. *Birth Defects* 1974; **10**: 146–149.

46. Johnston JH, Penn IA. Exstrophy of the cloaca. *Br J Urol* 1966; **38**: 302–307.

47. Eagle JF Jr, Barrett GS. Congenital deficiency of abdominal musculature and associated genitourinary abnormalities. A syndrome. *Pediatrics* 1950; **6**: 721–736.

48. Woodhouse CR, Ransley PG, Innes-Williams D. Prune belly syndrome – report of 47 cases. *Arch Dis Child* 1982; **57**: 856–859.

49. Popek EJ, Tyson RW, Miller GJ, Caldwell SA. Prostate development in Prune Belly Syndrome (PBS) and Posterior Urethral Valves (PUV): etiology of PBS – lower urinary tract obstruction or primary mesenchymal defect? *Pediatr Pathol* 1991; **11**: 1–29.

50. van Velden DJJ, de Jong G, van der Walt JJ. Fetal bilateral obstructive uropathy: a series of nine cases. *Pediatr Pathol Lab Med* 1995; **15**: 245–258.

51. Machin GA. Diseases causing fetal and neonatal ascites. *Pediatr Pathol* 1985; **4**: 195–211.

52. Manivel JC, Pettinato G, Reinberg Y, Gonzalez R, Burke B, Dehner LP. Prune belly syndrome: clinicopathological study of 29 cases. *Pediatr Pathol* 1989; **9**: 691–711.

53. Simonton SC, Dehner LP. The kidney and lower urinary tract. In: Stocker JT, Dehner LP (eds). *Pediatric Pathology*, vol 2. Philadelphia: JB Lippincott, chap 21, pp 825–871.

54. Drummond KN. Hemolytic uremic syndrome – then and now. *New Engl J Med* 1985; **312**: 116–118.

55. Katzman GH. Thrombosis and thomboembolism in an infant of a diabetic mother. *J Perinatol* 1989; **9**: 137–140.

56. Kissane JM, Dehner LP. Renal tumors and tumorlike lesions in pediatric patients [review]. *Pediatr Nephrol* 1992; **6**: 365–382.

57. Harms D, Schmidt D, Leuschner I. Abdominal, retroperitoneal and sacrococcygeal tumours of the newborn and very young infant. Report from the Kiel Paediatric Tumour Registry. *Eur J Pediatr* 1989; **148**: 720–728.

58. Stiller CA, Parkin DM. International variations in the incidence of childhood renal tumours. *Br J Cancer* 1990; **62**: 1026–1030.

59. Hrabovsky EE, Othersen HB, de Lorimier A, Kelalis P, Beckwith JB. Wilms' tumour in the neonate: a report from the National Wilms' Tumour Study. *J Pediatr Surg* 1986; **21**: 385–387.

60. Xue H, Horwitz JR, Smith MB et al. Malignant solid tumors in neonates: a 40 year review. *J Pediatr Surg* 1995; **30**: 543–545.

61. Delamarre JFM, Sandstedt B, Harms D, Bacon-Gibod L, Vujanic G. The new S10P (Stockholm) working classification of renal tumours of childhood. Letter to the editor. *Med Paediatr Oncol* 1996; **26**: 145–146.

62. Beckwith JB, Kiviat NB, Benadio JF. Nephrogenic rests, nephroblastomatosis and the pathogenesis of Wilms' tumor. *Pediatr Pathol* 1990; **10**: 1–36.

63. Bove KE, McAdam AJ. The nephroblastomatosis complex and its relationship to Wilms' tumour: a clinicopathologic treatise. *Perspect Pediatr Pathol* 1976; **3**: 185–223.

64. Machin GA. Persistent renal blastema (nephroblastomatosis) as a frequent precursor of Wilms' tumour. A pathological and clinical review. *Am J Pediatr Haematol Oncol* 1980; **2**: 253–261.

65. Yeger H, Cullinane C, Flenniken A et al. Coordinate expression of Wilms' tumor genes correlates with Wilms' tumor phenotypes. *Cell Growth Differ* 1992; **3**: 855–864.

66. Craver R, Dimmick J, Johnson H, Nigro M. Congenital obstructive uropathy and nodular renal blastema. *J Urol* 1986; **136**: 305–307.

67. Vujanic GM, Sandstedt B, Dijoud F, Harms D, Dellemarre JFM. Nephrogenic rest associated with mesoblastic nephroma – what does it tell us? *Pediatr Pathol Lab Med* 1995; 469–475.

68. Bove KE, Kofflet H, McAdams AJ. Nodular renal blastema. Definition and possible significance. *Cancer* 1969; **24**: 323–332.

69. Fujinaga M, Shepard TH, Fitzsimmons J. Trisomy 13 in the fetus. *Teratology* 1990; **41**: 223–228.

70. Keshgegian AA, Chatten J. Nodular renal blastema in Trisomy 13. *Arch Pathol Lab Med* 1979; **103**: 73–75.

71. Sanstedt B, Delemarre JFM, Krul EJ, Tournade MF. Mesoblastic nephromas: a study of 29 tumours from the SIOP nephroblastoma file. *Histopathology* 1985; **9**: 741–750.

72. Variend S (ed). Wilms' tumour and the nephroblastoma complex. In: *Paediatric Neoplasia. Current Histopathology*, vol 22. Dordrecht: Kluwer Academic, chap 2, pp 19–27.

73. Bolande RP, Brough AJ, Izant RH. Congenital mesoblastic nephroma of infancy. A report of eight cases and its relationship to Wilms' tumor. *Pediatrics* 1967; **40**: 272–278.

74. Cook HT, Taylor GM, Malone P, Risdon RA. Renin in mesoblastic nephroma. An immunohistochemical study. *Human Pathol* 1988; **19**: 1347–1351.

75. Ganick DJ, Gilbert EF, Beckwith JB, Kiviat N. Congenital cystic mesoblastic nephroma. *Human Pathol* 1981; **12**: 1039–1043.

76. Gonzalez Crussi F, Sotelo-Avila C, Kidd JM. Malignant mesenchymal nephroma of infancy. Report of a case with pulmonary metastases. *Am J Surg Pathol* 1981; **4**: 185–190.

77. Steinfeld AD, Crowley CA, O'Shea PA, Tefft M. Recurrent and metastatic mesoblastic nephroma in infancy. *J Clin Oncol* 1984; **2**: 956–960.

78. Vujanic GM, Delemarre JFM, Moeslichan S et al. Mesoblastic nephroma metastatic to lungs and heart – another face of this peculiar lesion: case report

and review of the literature. *Pediatr Pathol* 1993; **13**: 143–153.

79. Joshi VV, Kasznica J, Walters TR. Atypical mesoblastic nephroma. Pathological characterization of a potentially aggressive variant of conventional congenital mesoblastic nephroma. *Arch Pathol Lab Med* 1986; **110**: 100–106.

80. Beckwith JB. Wilms' tumour and other renal tumours in childhood: an update. *J Urol* 1986; **6**: 320–324.

81. Roberts P, Lockwood JR, Lewis IJ, Bailey CC, Batcup G, Williams J. Cytogenetic abnormalities in mesoblastic nephroma: a link to Wilms' tumor? *Med Pediatr Oncol* 1993; **21**: 416–420.

82. Carpenter PM, Mascarello JT, Krous HF, Kaplan GW. Congenital mesoblastic nephroma: cytogenetic comparison to leiomyoma. *Pediatr Pathol* 1993; **13**: 435–441.

83. Becroft DMO, Mauger DC, Skeen JE, Ogawa O, Reeve AE. Good prognosis of cellular mesoblastic nephroma with hyperdiploidy and relaxation of imprinting of the maternal IGF2 gene. *Pediatr Pathol Lab Med* 1995; **15**: 679–688.

84. Mascarello JT, Cajulis TR, Krous HF, Carpenter PM. Presence or absence of trisomy 11 is correlated with histological subtype in congenital mesoblastic nephroma. *Cancer Genet Cytogenet* 1994; **77**: 50–54.

85. Joshi VV, Beckwith JB. Multilocular cyst of the kidney (cystic nephroma) and cystic partially differentiated nephroblastoma. Terminology and criteria for diagnosis. *Cancer* 1989; **64**: 466–479.

86. Call K, Glasser T, Ito CY et al. Isolation and characterisation of a zinc finger polypeptide at the human chromosome 11 Wilms' tumor locus. *Cell* 1990; **60**: 509–520.

87. Re GG, Hazen-Nartin DJ, Sens DA, Garvin AJ. Nephroblastoma (Wilms' tumor): a model system of aberrant renal development [Review]. *Semin Diagn Pathol* 1994; **11**: 126–135.

88. Coppes MJ, Haber DA, Grundy PE. Genetic events in the development of Wilms' tumour [Review]. *New Engl J Med* 1994; **331**: 586–590.

89. Solis V, Pritchard J, Cowell JK. Cytogenetic changes in Wilms' tumors. *Cancer Genet Cytogenet* 1988; **34**: 223–234.

90. Wang-Wuu S, Soukup S, Bove K, Gotwals B, Lampkin B. Chromosome analysis of 31 Wilms' tumours. *J Cancer Res* 1990; **50**: 2786–2793.

91. Finegold M (ed). Wilm's tumour and other renal tumours of childhood. In: Beckwith JB (ed) *Pathology of Neoplasia in Children and Adolescents.*

Major Problems in Pathology, vol 18. Philadelphia: WB Saunders, 1986; chap 12, pp 319–320.

92. Vujanic GM. Teratoid Wilms' tumour: report of a unilateral case. *Pediatr Pathol* 1991; **11**: 303–309.

93. Wakely PE Jr, Sprague RI, Karnstein MJ. Extrarenal Wilms' tumour: an analysis of 4 cases. *Human Pathol* 1989; **20**: 691–695.

94. Ugarte N, Gonzalez-Crussi F, Hseuh W. Wilms' tumor, its morphology in patients under one year of age. *Cancer* 1981; **48**: 346–353.

95. Chatten J. Epithelial differentiation in Wilms' tumor: a clinico-pathological appraisal. *Perspect Pediatr Pathol* 1976; **3**: 225–251.

96. Wigger HJ. Fetal rhabdomyomatous nephroblastoma – a variant of Wilms' tumor. *Human Pathol* 1976; **7**: 613–623.

97. Marsden HB, Lawler W, Kumar PM. Bone metastasizing renal tumour of childhood. Morphological and clinical features, differences from Wilms' tumor. *Cancer* 1978; **42**: 1922–1928.

98. Sotelo-Avila C, Gonzalez-Crussi F, Sadowinski S, Gooch WM, Pena R. Clear cell sarcoma of the kidney: a clinopathologic study of 21 patients with long term follow up evaluation. *Human Pathol* 1986; **16**: 1219–1230.

99. Weeks DA, Beckwith JB, Mierau GW, Luckey DW. Rhabdoid tumour of the kidney. A report of 111 cases from the national Wilms' Tumor Study Pathology centre. *Am J Surg Pathol* 1989; **13**: 439–458.

100. Palmer NF, Sutton W. Clinical aspects of the rhabdoid tumour of the kidney: a report of the National Wilms' Tumor Study Group. *Med Pediatr Oncology* 1983; **11**: 242–245.

101. Fort DW, Tonk VS, Tomlinson GE, Timmons CF, Schneider NR. Rhabdoid tumor of the kidney with primitive neuroectodermal tumour of the central nervous system: associated tumors with different histologic, cytogenetic and molecular findings. *Genes Chromosomes Cancer* 1994; **11**: 146–152.

102. Sotelo-Avila C, Beckwith JB and Johnson JE. Ossifying renal tumor of infancy: a clinicopathologic study of nine cases. *Pediatr Pathol Lab Med* 1995; **15**: 745–762.

103. Kaufman SL, Start AP. Congenital mesenchymal tumours. *Cancer* 1965; **18**: 460–476.

104. Bale PM, Parsons ER, Stevens MM (eds). Pathology and behaviour of juvenile rhabdomyosarcoma. In: *Pathology of Neoplasia in Children and Adolescents*, vol 18. *Major Problems in Pathology*. Philadelphia: WB Saunders, chap 8, p 197.

4

Fetal renal function

S. Bewley and C.H. Rodeck

Introduction

The understanding of the pathophysiology of fetal renal function has been evaluated in animal studies, largely of the pregnant ewe. In the past 10 years, understanding of human fetal renal function has increased, due to the development of invasive techniques and treatments *in utero*.

Nephrogenesis

The development of the kidney is classically described in embryology as the formation of three successive organs, the pronephros, mesonephros and metanephros. The formation of nephrons occurs due to an inductive action of the branching ureteric bud on the surrounding mesenchyme [1]. There are 8–12 generations of nephrons in a human kidney [2], and new nephron formation occurs up to 36 weeks' gestation. Renal histology can provide a good index of fetal maturity. Human fetal urine production is thought to start once the first nephrons attain morphological maturity at 10 weeks of fetal life [3]. This is confirmed in the human by the observation that a fetal bladder can usually be seen at this gestation using transvaginal ultrasound scanning.

The kidney has little involvement in homeostasis which is largely performed by the placenta, although fetal urine is voided into the amniotic sac. In the second half of pregnancy amniotic fluid is largely derived from fetal urine, and is thus the simplest and traditional measure of function. Early fetal urine starts as a simple filtrate of blood, with high sodium loss. The control mechanisms mature throughout pregnancy. Only after birth, with a rapid rise in glomerular filtration rate (GFR), does the kidney behave as in the adult.

Animal studies

Renal blood flow

In fetal life the kidneys are a higher proportion of total weight than in the newborn, but renal blood flow (RBF) is much less; fetal kidneys receive 2–4% of cardiac output at the end of pregnancy compared to 15–18% in the newborn [4–6]. Despite differences in blood flow distribution between large mammals, fetal RBF per unit organ weight is similar [5,7,8]. RBF and filtration fraction are low and renal vascular resistance is high compared to the newborn [9–11]. RBF increases with gestation although so does renal mass, and RBF/unit mass remains constant prior to delivery [10].

Factors influencing renal blood flow

Factors that have been shown to control RBF include the renin–angiotensin (RA), renal sympathetic nervous system (SNS), prostaglandins, kallikrein–kinin (KK) and atrial natriuretic factor (ANF).

Renin has not been thought to cross the placenta as there is a fetal–maternal gradient [12] and no response to maternal nephrectomy. In addition, plasma renin cannot be stimulated after fetal nephrectomy [13] and maternal suppression with a high-salt diet does not affect the fetus [14]. However, renin can be detected in the maternal plasma of pregnant dogs following nephrectomy and it may cross the placenta to form angiotensin II and constrict stem villus arterioles [15]. The fetal renin–angiotensin system is very sensitive to acute haemorrhage [16,17] and hypoxia [18], and fetal responses are inhibited by the angiotensin I converting enzyme inhibitor, captopril [19]. Activation of the renin-angiotensin system raises fetal arterial pressure and decreases umbilical and renal blood flow [20–22]. The renin–angiotensin system may have an important role in haemorrhage, fetal survival and parturition.

Stimulation of renal sympathetic nerves leads to a fall in RBF and a rise in vascular resistance [23], whilst denervation inhibits hypoxia-induced vasoconstriction [24]. This is largely an α-adrenoceptor response, as activation of β-adrenoceptors causes vasodilatation [25]. It appears that maturation of the renal adrenergic system is associated with down-regulation of β-adrenoceptors in renal vessels [26].

Prostaglandins (PG) are released from fetal renal vessels and affect renal vascular tone and renin secretion [27]. High concentrations of PGE, PGF and PGFM are found in fetal urine [28]. Indomethacin causes an increase in vascular resistance and fall in RBF [29].

Kallikrein is associated with increased RBF, and its excretion increases during fetal maturation [30]. Intrarenal ANF leads to renal vasodilation [31], but systemic ANF produces a fall in RBF and a rise in renal vascular resistance, probably secondary to compensatory mechanisms [32]. ANF is found during fetal life in cardiocytes [33].

Glomerular filtration

GFR is low and increases during fetal life [34], but remains constant in relation to kidney weight [10]. After birth the GFR rises rapidly [35–37] via a recruitment of superficial cortical nephrons and an increase of the filtered load to the nephron [38].

Tubular function

There is a high rate of sodium excretion in the immature kidney and sodium reabsorption is relatively low, although it increases with gestational age [39,40]. This may be due to immaturity, the large extracellular volume, circulating naturietic factors and relative resistance to aldosterone [41,42]. Glucose reabsorption and renal plasma threshold for glucose is high (and increases with gestational age) [43]. Hyperglycaemia leads to glycosuria, diuresis and natriuresis [44], just as in the adult, providing an explanation for the osmotic diuresis and polyhydramnios seen in diabetic pregnancies.

Tubular secretion is immature although organic bases can be secreted by the fetal kidney [45]. Potassium secretion is low in early pregnancy, but increases with gestation [46]. The acid–base mechanisms mature with gestation. There is increasing excretion of acid and ammonium [47] and increasing bicarbonate and subsequent chloride resorption with age [47,48]. This is probably related to increasing carbonic anhydrase activity [49]. In severe acidosis, when placental regulation of acid–base balance is probably exceeded, there is an increase in hydrogen ion excretion by the fetal kidney [50]. An increase in the buffering capacity of the kidney can be provided by increased phosphate excretion which occurs with severe metabolic acidosis [50] and administration of cortisol [51]. Phosphate is the major urinary buffer and increased excretion allows increased excretion of protons and generation of new bicarbonate [52].

Factors affecting concentrating ability and tubular function

Fetal urine is hypo-osmotic, but can be concentrated or diluted by alterations in maternal hydration. The immature kidney does not concentrate urine well and the nephrons are relatively insensitive to the antidiuretic hormone arginine vasopressin (AVP). Fetal tubular function also responds to aldosterone (although sodium reabsorption is not accompanied by potassium excretion in fetal life), renin–angiotensin, kallikrein–kinin (which is inversely related to sodium excretion), prostaglandins, ANF (which increases sodium and

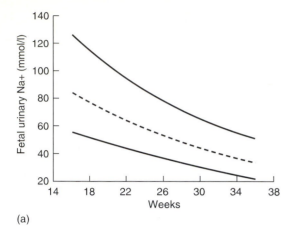

(a)

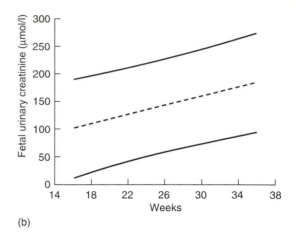

(b)

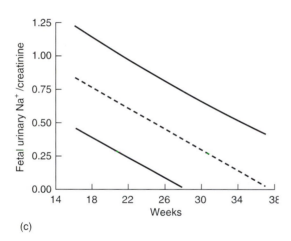

(c)

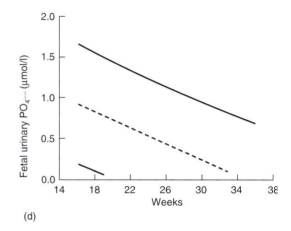

(d)

electrolyte excretion) and cortisol (which leads to a rise in GFR and phosphate reabsorption).

Changes during the transition from fetal to newborn life

In the sheep, delivery is associated with a rapid rise in GFR and decrease in urinary sodium excretion, accompanied by increases in plasma adrenaline and noradrenaline concentrations. There are no significant changes in renal blood flow velocity, renal vascular resistance or blood pressure. There are no significant changes in plasma renin activity, angiotensin II, aldosterone or arginine vasopressin [35]. The rise in GFR without increase in RBF may be due to intrarenal redistribution of blood

flow and recruitment of superficial glomeruli [38]. There are rapid changes in fractional sodium reabsorption which increases to adult levels within a day. This happens in term sheep fetuses and may be related to maturity, providing an explanation for the salt-losing condition of premature human infants.

Human studies

Much less is known about human fetal renal function as opposed to the large amount of animal data. There is great difficulty in the construction of normal ranges of blood and urinary constituents, let alone studies of func-

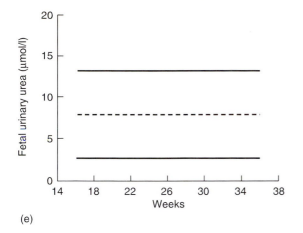

(e)

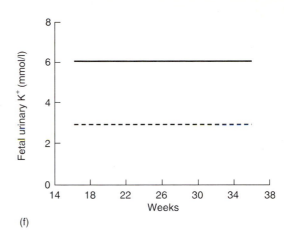

(f)

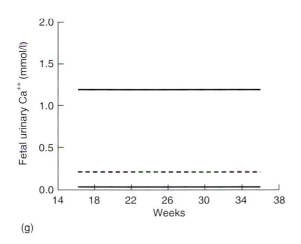

(g)

Figure 4.1 Normal ranges of fetal urinary sodium (a), creatinine (b), Na$^+$/creatinine ratio (c), phosphate (d), urea (e), potassium (f) and calcium (g). (Reproduced from reference [58] with permission.)

tion, due to the invasive nature of bladder or kidney sampling.

Renal blood flow

In the human, invasive measurements of renal blood flow are not possible, but indirect measurements of resistance, by Doppler ultrasound, confirm a high vascular resistance pattern in fetal life, that falls slightly towards term [53].

Urine production

Unlike the ovine urine circulation, which may be controlled by the urachus [54], human fetal urine normally flows only into the amniotic cavity, as the allantois degenerates early in gestation. Urine is produced at a rate of about 230–660 ml/day [55].

Normal human fetal plasma and urinary constituents

Sodium and potassium concentrations remain stable in fetal plasma, reflecting the efficiency of the feto-placental unit in maintaining constant electrolytes [56].

Lind collected fetal urine at termination hysterotomy and showed that the fetal kidney is capable of reabsorbing sodium and excreting urea from as early as 12 weeks [57].

Nicolini et al. [58] devised normal ranges of sodium, phosphate, creatinine and urea from a group of 26 fetuses with normal urinary tracts either undergoing elective termination of pregnancy (nine) or intraperitoneal transfusion (17). They found that sodium and phosphate decreased with increasing gestation, whereas creatinine increased and urea, calcium and potassium were unchanged (Figure 4.1).

Nicolaides et al. [59] devised normal ranges of sodium, total calcium, urea and creatinine from 20 fetuses with obstructive uropathy who subsequently were found to have normal renal function postnatally (13), or who were aborted (five) or had intrauterine death (one) without histological evidence of renal dysplasia. They too reported that sodium fell with gestation, whereas creatinine increased and urea concentrations did not change. Total calcium was unrelated to gestation.

In summary, the fall in urinary sodium and phosphate accompanied by an increase in creatinine with gestational age is consistent with increasing fetal GFR and tubular maturation, as seen in animal work.

Renal causes of oligohydramnios and polyhydramnios

Oligohydramnios and anhydramnios can be caused by abnormalities of the kidney such as renal agenesis and dysplasia, polycystic kidneys, bilateral multicystic kidneys and obstructive uropathy [60–63]. In severe early-onset growth retardation there is a redistribution of circulation to vital organs ('brain-sparing') and increased renal Doppler indices [53], suggesting a shift of blood flow away from the kidneys. This is associated with the development of oligohydramnios, and acute renal failure of the newborn.

Although classically caused by glucose osmotic diuresis, polyhydramnios is found in less than 10% of diabetic pregnancies [64]. Another cause of polyhydramnios with macrosomia is Beckwith–Weidemann syndrome [65,66]. Autosomal recessive disorders can lead to recurrent polyhydramnios via increased fetal voiding, such as Bartter's syndrome (juxtaglomerular hypertrophy, hyper-reninism and secondary hyperaldosteronism) [67] or Perlman's syndrome [68]. There can be a polyuric phase of renal damage and polyhydramnios is occasionally seen with fetal hydronephrosis.

The oligohydramnios/polyhydramnios sequence in monochorionic diamniotic twins,

thought to be due to twin–twin transfusion, is a dynamic process with wide and often unpredictable fluctuations in amniotic fluid volume [69].

Drugs affecting fetal renal function

Angiotensin-converting enzyme inhibitors, such as captopril and enalapril, have been reported to cause both animal and human fetal renal failure, antenatal and postnatal, and are associated with fetal and perinatal loss [70–75]. Indomethacin has been associated with human fetal renal failure [76,77] and has been used to treat polyhydramnios.

Assessment of renal function

The concept of *in utero* renal failure is slightly enigmatic as there is no direct need during *in utero* life for renal function, except to produce amniotic fluid, as the placenta performs all excretory functions. There are a variety of indirect and non-invasive ways to measure fetal renal function, including ultrasound scanning for liquor volume [78] and urine production rate [55], renal dimensions [79] and parenchymal echogenicity. However, even direct *in utero* sampling of kidney and bladder urine has limitations. The assessment of renal function is discussed in greater detail in Chapter 7.

References

1. Oliver J. *Nephrons and Kidneys: a quantitative study of development and evolutionary mammalian renal architectonics.*. New York: Harper & Row, 1968.
2. Potter EL. *Normal and Abnormal Development of the Kidney.* Chicago: Year Book Medical Publishers, 1972.
3. Gersh I. The correlation of structure and function in the developing mesonephros and metanephros. *Contrib Embryol Carnegie Inst Wash* 1937; **26**: 33–58.
4. Gilbert RD. Control of fetal cardiac output during changes in blood volume. *Am J Physiol* 1980 **238**: H80–86.
5. Paton JB, Fisher DE, Peterson EN, DeLannoy CW, Behrman RE. Cardiac output and organ blood flows in the baboon fetus. *Biol Neonate* 1973; **22**: 50–57.
6. Rudolph AM, Heymann MA. Fetal and neonatal circulation and respiration. *Ann Rev Physiol* 1974; **36**: 187–207.

7. Rudolph AM, Heymann MA. Circulatory changes during growth in the fetal lamb. *Circ Res* 1970; **26**: 289–299.

8. Behrman RE, Lees MH, Peterson EN, DeLannoy CW, Seeds AE. Distribution of the circulation in the normal and asphyxiated fetal primate. *Am J Obstet Gynaecol* 1970; **108**: 956–969.

9. Robillard JE, Weismann DN, Herin P. Ontogeny of single glomerular perfusion rate in fetal and newborn lambs. *Pediatr Res* 1981; **15**: 1248–1255.

10. Robillard JE, Kulvinskas C, Sessions C, Burmeister L, Smith FG. Maturational changes in the fetal glomerular filtration rate. *Am J Obstet Gynecol* 1975; **122**: 601–606.

11. Gruskin AB, Edelmann CM Jr, Yuan S. Maturational changes in renal blood flow in piglets. *Pediatr Res* 1970; **4**: 7–13.

12. Smith FG, Lupu AN, Barajas L, Bauer R, Bashore R. The renin angiotensin system in the fetal lamb. *Pediatr Res* 1974; **8**: 611–620.

13. Broughton-Pipkin F, Lumbers ER, Mo HJC. Factors influencing plasma renin and angiotensin II in the conscious pregnant ewe and its foetus. *J Physiol (Lond)* 1974; **243**: 619–636.

14. Stevens AD, Lumbers ER. Effect on maternal and fetal renal function and plasma renin activity of a high salt intake by the ewe. *J Dev Physiol* 1986; **8**: 267–275.

15. Glance DF, Elder MG, Bloxam DL, Myatt L. The effects of the components of the renin-angiotensin system on the isolated perfused human placental cotyledon. *Am J Obstet Gynecol* 1984; **149**: 450–454.

16. Robillard JE, Wietzman RE, Fisher DA, Smith FG. The dynamics of vasopressin release and blood volume regulation during fetal hemorrhage in the lamb fetus. *Pediatr Res* 1979; **13**: 606–610.

17. Brace RA, Cheung CY. Fetal cardiovascular and endocrine responses to prolonged fetal hemorrhage. *Am J Physiol* 1986; **251**: R417–R424.

18. Robillard JE, Weitzman RE, Burmeister L, Smith FG. Developmental aspects of the renal response to hypoxaemia in the lamb fetus. *Circ Res* 1981; **48**: 128–138.

19. Gomez RA, Robillard JE. Developmental aspects of the renal responses to hemorrhage during converting-enzyme inhibition in fetal lambs. *Circ Res* 1984; **54**: 301–312.

20. Iwamoto HS, Rudolph AM. Effects of endogenous angiotensin II on the fetal circulation. *J Dev Physiol* 1979; **1**: 283–293.

21. Ismay MJ, Lumbers ER, Stevens AD. The action of AII on the baroreflex response of the conscious ewe and its conscious fetus. *J Physiol* 1979; **288**: 467–476.

22. Berman W, Goodlin RC, Heymann MA, Rudolph AM. Effects of pharmocological agents on umbilical blood flow in fetal lambs in utero. *Biol Neonate* 1978; **33**: 225–235.

23. Robillard JE, Nakamura KT, Wilkin MK, McWeeny OJ, DiBona GF. Ontogeny of renal hemodynamic response to renal nerve stimulation in sheep. *Am J Physiol* 1987; **252**: F605–F612.

24. Robillard JE, Nakamura KT, Dibona GF. Effects of renal denervation on renal responses to hypoxaemia in fetal lambs. *Am J Physiol* 1986; **250**: F294–F301.

25. Nakamura KT, Matherne GP, Jose PA, Alden BM, Robillard JE. Ontogeny of renal β-adrenoceptor mediated vasodilation in sheep: comparison between endogenous catecholamines. *Pediatr Res* 1987; **22**: 465–470.

26. Robillard JE, Nakamura DT. Hormonal regulation of renal function during development. *Biol Neonate* 1988; **53**: 201-211.

27. Pace-Asciak DR. Prostaglandin biosynthesis and catabolism in the developing fetal sheep kidney. *Prostaglandins* 1977; **13**: 661.

28. Walker DW, Mitchell MD. Prostaglandins in urine of foetal lambs. *Nature* 1978; **271**: 161–162.

29. Matson JR, Stokes JB, Robillard JE. Effects of inhibition of prostaglandin synthesis on fetal renal function. *Kidney Int* 1981; **20**: 621–627.

30. Robillard JE, Lawton WJ, Weismann DN, Sessions C. Developmental aspects of the renal kallikrein-like activity in fetal and newborn lambs. *Kidney Int* 1982; **22**: 594–601.

31. Varille VA, Nakamura KT, McWeeny OJ, Matherne GP, Smith FG, Robillard JE. Renal hemodynamic response to atrial natriuretic factor in fetal and newborn sheep. *Pediatr Res* 1989; **25**: 291–294.

32. Robillard JE, Nakamura KT, Varille VA, Andresen AA, Matherne GP, VanOrden DE. Ontogeny of the renal response to natriuretic peptide in sheep. *Am J Physiol* 1988; **254**: F634–F641.

33. Wei Y, Rodi CP, Day ML et al. Developmental changes in the rat atriopeptin hormonal system. *J Clin Invest* 1987; **79**: 1325–1329.

34. Lumbers ER, Stevens AD. Factors influencing glomerular filtration rate in the fetal lamb. *J Physiol* 1980; **298**: 28P–29P.

35. Nakamura KT, Matherne GP, McWeeny OJ, Smith BA, Robillard JE. Renal hemodynamics and functional changes during the transition from fetal to newborn life in sheep. *Pediatr Res* 1987; **21**: 229–234.

36. Smith FG, Lumbers ER. Changes in renal function following delivery of the lamb by caesarian section. *J Dev Physiol* 1988; **10**: 145–148.

37. Smith FG, Lumbers ER. Comparison of renal function in term fetal sheep and newborn lambs. *Biol Neonate* 1989; **55**: 309–316.

38. Aperia A, Borberger O, Herin P, Joelsson I. Renal hemodynamics in the perinatal period: a study in lambs. *Acta Physiol Scand* 1977; **99**: 261–269.

39. Robillard JE, Ramberg E, Sessians C et al. Role of aldosterone on renal sodium and potassium excretion during fetal life and newborn period. *Dev Pharmacol Ther* 1980; **1**: 201.

40. Lumbers ER. A brief review of fetal renal function. *J Dev Physiol* 1983; **6**: 1–10.

41. Kleinman LI. Developmental renal physiology. *Physiologist* 1982; **25**: 103–110.

42. Spitzer A. The developing kidney and the process of growth. In: Seldin DW, Giebisch G (eds). *The Kidney: physiology and pathophysiology*. New York: Raven Press, 1985; pp 1979–2015.

43. Robillard JE, Sessions C, Kennedy RL, Smith FG. Maturation of the glucose transport process by the fetal kidney. *Pediatr Res* 1978; **12**: 680–684.

44. Smith FG, Lumbers ER. Effects of maternal hyperglycemia on fetal renal function in sheep. *Am J Physiol* 1988; **255**: F11–F14.

45. Elbourne I, Lumbers ER, Hill KJ. The secretion of organic acids and bases by the ovine fetal kidney. *Exp Physiol* 1990; **75**: 211–221.

46. Lumbers ER, Hill KJ, Bennett VJ. Proximal and distal tubular activity in chronically catheterised fetal sheep compared with the adult. *Can J Physiol Pharmacol* 1988; **66**: 697–702.

47. Kesby GJ, Lumbers ER. Factors affecting renal handling of sodium, hydrogen ions, and bicarbonate by the fetus. *Am J Physiol* 1986; **251**: F226.

48. Hill KJ, Lumbers ER. Renal function in adult and fetal sheep. *J Dev Physiol* 1988; **10**: 149–159.

49. Robillard JE, Sessions C, Smith FG. *In vivo* demonstration of renal carbonic anhydrase activity in the fetal lamb. *Biol Neonate* 1978; **34**: 253–258.

50. Kesby GJ, Lumbers ER. The effects of metabolic acidosis on renal function of fetal sheep. *J Physiol (Lond)* 1988; **396**: 65–74.

51. Hill KJ, Lumbers ER, Elbourne I. The actions of cortisol on fetal renal function. *J Dev Physiol* 1988; **10**: 85–96.

52. Pitts RF. *Physiology of the Kidney and Body Fluids*, 3rd edn. Chicago: Year Book Medical Publishers, 1974.

53. Vyas S, Nicolaides KH, Campbell S. Renal artery flow-velocity waveforms in normal and hypoxemic fetuses. *Am J Obstet Gynecol* 1989; **161**: 168–172.

54. Lye SJ, Freitag CL, Challis JRG. Ovine fetal urachus – physiological and hormonal control of its contractile activity. *Am J Physiol* 1988; **254**: F25–F31.

55. Campbell S, Wladimiroff JW, Dewhurst CJ. The antenatal measurement of fetal urine production. *J Obstet Gynaecol Br Cmwlth* 1973; **80**: 680–686.

56. Moniz CF, Nicolaides KH, Bamforth FJ, Rodeck CH. Normal reference ranges for biochemical substances relating to renal, hepatic, and bone function in fetal and maternal plasma throughout pregnancy. *J Clin Pathol* 1985; **38**: 468–472.

57. Lind T. The biochemistry of amniotic fluid. In: Sandler M (ed). *Amniotic Fluid and its Clinical Significance*. New York: Dekker, 1981; pp 1–25.

58. Nicolini U, Fisk NM, Rodeck CH, Beacham J. Fetal urine biochemistry: an index of renal maturation and dysfunction. *Br J Obstet Gynaecol* 1992; **99**: 46–50.

59. Nicolaides KH, Cheng HH, Snijders RJM, Moniz CR. Fetal urine biochemistry in the assessment of obstructive uropathy. *Am J Obstet Gynecol* 1992; **166**: 932–937.

60. Romero R, Cullen M, Grannum P et al. Antenatal diagnosis of renal anomalies with ultrasound. III. Bilateral renal agenesis. *Am J Obstet Gynecol* 1985; **151**: 38–43.

61. Romero R, Cullen M, Jeanty P et al. The diagnosis of congenital renal anomalies with ultrasound. II. Infantile polycystic kidney disease. *Am J Obstet Gynecol* 1984; **150**: 259–262.

62. Dungan JS, Fernandez MT, Abbitt PL, Thiagarajah S, Howards SS, Hogge WA. Multicystic dysplastic kidney: natural history of prenatally detected cases. *Prenat Diagn* 1990; **10**: 175–182.

63. D'Alton M, Romero R, Grannum P, DePalma L, Jeanty P, Hobbins JC. Antenatal diagnosis of renal anomalies with ultrasound. IV. Bilateral multicystic kidney disease. *Am J Obstet Gynecol* 1986; **154**: 532–537.

64. Lemons JA, Vargas P, Delaney JJ. Infant of the diabetic mother: review of 225 cases. *Obstet Gynecol* 1980; **57**: 187–192.

65. Weinstein L, Anderson C. *In utero* diagnosis of Beckwith–Wiedemann syndrome. *Radiology* 1980; **134**: 474.

66. Koontz KL, Shaw LA, Lavery JP. Antenatal appearance of Beckwith–Wiedemann syndrome. *J Clin Ultrasound* 1986; **14**: 57–59.

67. Sieck UV, Ohlsson A. Fetal polyuria and hydramnios associated with Bartter's syndrome. *Obstet Gynecol* 1984; **63**: 22S–24S.

68. Chitty LS, Griffin D, Johnson P, Neales K. The differential diagnosis of enlarged hyperechogenic kidneys with normal or increased liquor volume: report of five cases and review of the literature. *Ultrasound Obstet Gynecol* 1991; **1**: 115–121.

69. Bromley B, Frigoletto FD, Estroff JA, Benacerraf BR. The natural history of oligohydramnios/polyhydramnios sequence in monochorionic diamniotic twins. *Ultrasound Obstet Gynecol* 1992; **2**: 317–320.

70. Broughton Pipkin F, Turner SR, Symonds EM. Possible risk with captopril in pregnancy: some animal data. *Lancet* 1980; **i**: 1256.

71. Broughton Pipkin F, Wallace CP. The effect of enalapril (MK 421), an angiotensin converting enzyme inhibitor, on the conscious ewe and her fetus. *Br J Pharmacol* 1986; **87**: 533–542.

72. Kreft-Jeis C, Plouin P-F, Tchobroutsky C, Boutroy M-J. Angiotension-converting enzyme inhibitors during pregnancy: a survey of 22 patients given captopril and nine given enalapril. *Br J Obstet Gynaecol* 1988; **95**: 420–422.

73. Hulton SA, Thomson PD, Cooper PA, Rothberg AD. Angiotensin-converting enzyme inhibitors in pregnancy may result in neonatal renal failure. *S Afr Med J* 1990; **78**: 673–676.

74. Schubiger G, Flury G, Nussberger J. Enalapril for pregnancy-induced hypertension: acute renal

failure in a neonate. *Ann Intern Med* 1988; **108**: 215–216.

75. Thorpe-Beeston JG, Armar NA, Dancy M, Cochrane GW, Ryan G, Rodeck CH. Pregnancy and ACE inhibitors. *Br J Obstet Gynaecol* 1993; **100**: 692.

76. Itskovitz J, Abramovici H, Brandes JM. Oligohydramnion, meconium and perinatal death concurrent with indomethacin treatment in human pregnancy. *J Reprod Med* 1980; **24**: 137–140.

77. Veersema D, de Jong PA, van Wijck JAM. Indomethacin and the fetal renal nonfunction syndrome. *Eur J Obstet Gynecol Reprod Biol* 1983; **16**: 113–121.

78. Phelan JP, Smith CV, Broussard P, Small M. Amniotic fluid volume assessment with the four-quadrant technique at 36–42 weeks' gestation. *J Reprod Med* 1987; **32**: 540–542.

79. Grannum P, Bracken M, Silverman R, Hobbins JC. Assessment of fetal kidney size in normal gestation by comparison of ratio of kidney circumference to abdominal circumference. *Am J Obstet Gynecol* 1980; **136**: 249.

5

The kidney/lung loop

D. De Mello and L.M. Reid

Introduction

The association in the newborn of absent kidneys with lung hypoplasia is well recognized as Potter's syndrome and points to a critical effect of the kidney on lung development [1–3]. Evidence indicates that in some way or another the kidney influences lung growth at three stages:

1. Early during the embryonic and fetal periods.
2. Later, as organogenesis prevails.
3. In the final weeks before parturition.

The nature of kidney influence on human lung growth seems to be different at these different stages of development. Certain features of fetal kidney and lung development occur during the same phases of gestation (Figure 5.1).

In addition to similarity in timing, both lung and kidney are concerned with an epithelial mesenchymal dialogue that produces successive branches of hollow tubes. Furthermore, fusion of vascular and epithelial basement membrane produces a thin blood–gas barrier in the lung, in the kidney a thin layer between urine forming space and collecting duct. In both systems hollow tubes ultimately connect to the exterior. Whereas in lung the unit is the acinus, probably in kidney it is better considered as a collecting duct with the structures draining into it. The mesangial cell is reminiscent of the pericyte. Each organ is sensitive to hypoxia, the main response by the kidney being production of erythropoietin probably from the juxtacapillary apparatus: in the lung the main manifestation is vasoconstriction and vascular cell remodelling.

The nature of the growth modifications indicate metabolic or growth factor influences [4], although the usual theory emphasizes urine contribution to amniotic fluid as the way the kidney influences lung [1,2]. While this may be important in the late phase, in the early phase it is unlikely to be critical. The simple assumption is that the fetal kidney produces urine, that this contributes to amniotic fluid, that is inhaled into the fetal lung and so distends and stents the airspaces. This represents an uncritical and incomplete assessment of the available evidence on lung development and, more importantly, hampers development of new concepts to drive significant experiments. For example quantitative analysis of lung hypoplasia in Potter's syndrome shows that the airways have failed to branch normally. This happens early during intrauterine development, before urine production is significant, and points to a chemical not a mechanical influence. This chapter aims to present evidence on this wider role for the kidney in fetal lung development through metabolic and growth factor pathways and, finally, to present evidence for a contribution from the lung to kidney development, so closing a kidney/lung feedback loop. Tracheal ligation has recently been shown to produce significant correction of the lung hypoplasia associated with renal agenesis or damage.

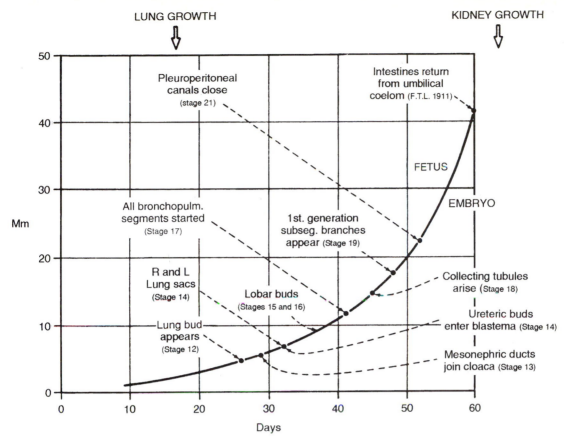

LUNG GROWTH   KIDNEY GROWTH

Figure 5.1 Curve illustrating stages in rate of growth of lungs (and kidneys) during embryonic period proper (first 52 days). (Reproduced from reference [76] with permission.)

Normal development

The following features of normal fetal lung development provide a framework for qualitative and quantitative assessment of lung growth and are key to the identification and interpretation of prenatal kidney influence on the lung. In lung, as in any other organ, development includes two aspects – *growth in size*, that includes mass of tissue as well as an increase in the number of its anatomical units, and *maturation or differentiation* of tissues.

The premature lung is not a miniature newborn, nor is the newborn a miniature adult [5,6]. At different ages the template or blueprint that determines lung development is different. Shifts in template often occur fast, although the new pattern may dominate for some time. These shifts in template represent windows in time, when the lung is especially susceptible both to injury and to experimental manipulation. Such times of 'shift' warrant special study. To use a communications metaphor, a switch is pulled and the programme changes, representing a change in biological signal. Questions to be asked are how the change in signal is induced and how the new signal is transduced to the given structural and functional pattern.

When the overall growth pattern is disturbed the resultant abnormal structure may be incompatible with life at birth. In other instances, the abnormality seems restricted in time and is followed by relatively normal development so that lung and patient are viable. Growth may be incomplete during the affected phase so that the lung is quantitatively abnormal, with a reduced number of units, or aberrant and so qualitatively abnormal. Certainly, an incomplete phase does not preclude a normal and timely switch to the next phase.

Normal appearance of an organ does not mean that all phases of development have been normal. An experiment reported by Clemmons [7] offers an example in the kidney. Administration of a nephrotoxin during the early phase of kidney development produced no apparent structural abnormality in the mature organ; normal later phases seemed able to correct the earlier aberration [7]. This implies that relatively late functional disorders could result from such early abnormality in structure. Clemmons' experiments imply that some cases of lung hypoplasia could result from abnormal kidney growth early in development, even if subsequent growth 'corrects' the kidney. Abnormal kidney growth could be 'occult', but the secondary effect on the lung apparent.

Stages of lung development

Microscopic cross-section reveals three different stages of lung development. During the first stage, the **pseudoglandular**, hollow tubes lined by continuous epithelium branch to produce future airways and alveoli. During the next stage, the *canalicular*, the distal airspaces differentiate into primitive air sacs with epithelial thinning and endothelium/epithelium fusion to form a blood–gas barrier. During the third, the *saccular* or *alveolar* stage, this differentiation continues, and further alveolar multiplication occurs until viability is achieved [5,6,8,9].

The Laws of Lung Development

The Laws of Lung Development describe the separate timing and nature of airway, alveolar and vascular growth, providing a timetable to interpret abnormal growth.

Law I deals with the airways. *The bronchi and bronchioli are present by the 16th week of intrauterine life.* Any reduction in airway number in the mature organ indicates abnormal growth during the first 16 weeks of gestation [8,10] (Figure 5.2).

Law II concerns alveolar growth. *At birth the alveolar spaces are more primitive than in the adult: they total about 20×10^6. After birth they multiply, until at about 8 years, the adult complement of 300×10^6 is reached* [5,11,12] (Figure 5.3).

Law III summarizes vascular growth: it reflects the first two laws. *The preacinar branches of the pulmonary arteries appear at the*

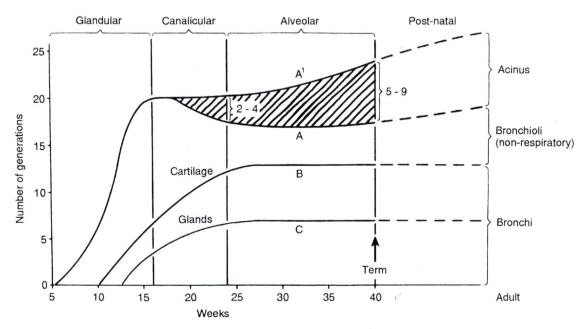

Figure 5.2 Development of the bronchial tree during gestation. Lobar bronchi appear at about 6 weeks' gestation, and by 16 weeks branching of future airways is complete. (Reproduced from reference [10] with permission.)

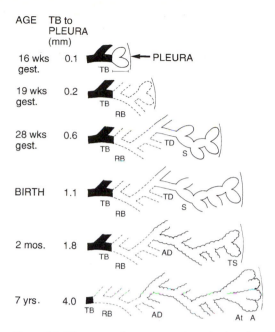

AGE | TB to PLEURA (mm)

16 wks gest. | 0.1

19 wks gest. | 0.2

28 wks gest. | 0.6

BIRTH | 1.1

2 mos. | 1.8

7 yrs. | 4.0

Figure 5.3 Diagrammatic representation of acinar length and intra-acinar air space growth during fetal life and childhood. AD = alveolar duct; AS = alveolar sac; At = atrium; RB = respiratory bronchiolus; S = saccule; TB = terminal bronchiolus; TD = terminal duct; TS = terminal sac. (Reproduced from reference [5] with permission.)

same time as the airways they accompany, whether bronchi or bronchioli; the intra-acinar arteries appear as alveoli grow [5,13–15] (Figure 5.4).

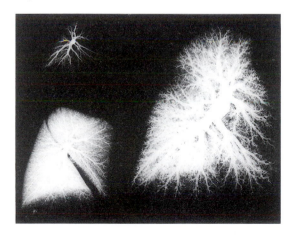

Figure 5.4 Arteriogram of the human lung at three ages: top left, newborn; bottom left, 18 months; right, adult. At birth, all preacinar arteries are present, but the background 'haze' representing intra-acinar arteries appears later. (Reproduced from reference [13] with permission.)

These Laws allow us to assess quantitatively the nature of an injury as well as to identify its timing and, in particular, to analyse hypoplasia.

A hypoplastic organ, here considered by reference to lung, may be structurally sound but miniature, that is small in weight or volume but with a normal number of units, or have a normal weight, mass or volume but a reduced number of units. Reduction can affect all or some of the systems (airways, alveoli or blood vessels) and with differential degrees of severity.

Species variation

The relative duration of these intrauterine stages varies in different species [16–18]. In the sheep, a species used for many fetal studies, a spurt of growth and differentiation occurs in the few weeks before birth [17,18]. The alveoli increase significantly in number, with corresponding augmentation of the vascular network. This spurt is probably typical of species that rapidly achieve independence at birth, as when the newborn learns quickly to run with the herd. In comparing prenatal experimental animal models of abnormal lung growth with human disease, allowance must be made for this species difference. The experimental studies described later in this chapter concern particularly the sheep, but the rabbit, rat and guinea-pig have also been used.

The opossum offers an intriguing variant. It is born after 12 days' gestation, migrates to the maternal pouch where oral fusion to the teat occurs; development continues for a further 48 days. While this demonstrates that lung development can occur in the absence of amniotic fluid, a mechanism very different from the human could be involved. A model of renal injury in the opossum has been established and is currently being used to investigate lung growth [19,20].

Evidence for kidney influence on lung development: a developmental kidney/lung loop

Evidence of a kidney/lung loop in development is provided by clinical and experimental findings that indicate that different mechanisms of modulation operate at each of three stages of gestation – early, middle and late.

Clinical

Clinically, influence at early or mid gestation is sometimes difficult to separate.

Early and middle phase

Historically, the evidence for a kidney to lung developmental loop came first in 1946 when Potter described the syndrome that bears her name [1–3]. It is characterized by renal agenesis, oligohydramnios, lung hypoplasia and an abnormal, rather characteristic, facies. At that time oligohydramnios was blamed for lung hypoplasia on the assumption that uterine wall pressure on the thoracic cage caused space restriction for the growing lung. This simple interpretation is put in doubt however, by exceptions: a normal lung can be found with oligohydramnios and a hypoplastic lung with polyhydramnios [21–25]. Of course findings at term are not necessarily those that operated during gestation.

More definitive are the results of a detailed study of hypoplastic lungs associated with renal agenesis or dysplasia, reported by Hislop et al. [4]. They found that in addition to a small lung, airway number is significantly reduced, sometimes to the equivalent of less than 12 weeks, indicating that lung development is disturbed during the phase of bronchial branching, before the sixteenth week of gestation, when the urine contributes little to amniotic fluid volume [26]. This study also showed reduced alveolar number and size (Figure 5.5), and an abnormal vascular bed with a reduced number of branches, but these were appropriate to the airways (Figure 5.6). Differences in detail were identified between cases of agenesis and cases of dysplasia. In the former dilatation of the arterial lumen and a thinner arterial wall point to greater abnormality.

Barth and colleagues [27] have recently analysed the vascular structure in a series of cases of renal agenesis and dysplasia. They confirmed the absence of muscular arteries within the acinus in the newborn, and established that in lung hypoplasia associated with renal dis-

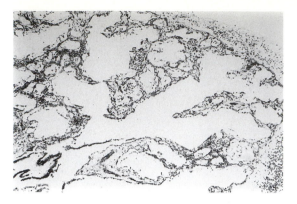

(a)

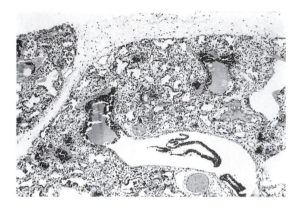

(b)

Figure 5.5 Photomicrographs of lung periphery from two infants born at term with congenital heart disease (as control) (a) and renal dysplasia (b), illustrating reduced acinar size and immature structure. (H&E × 80.)

ease, there is an increase in muscularity of the peripheral arteries.

Obstructive uropathy is also often associated with pulmonary hypoplasia. The way in which ureteral or urethral obstruction interferes with lung growth is not yet clear. It is likely that there are differences in nature and timing between the two levels of obstruction [28–31]. The analysis from Rotterdam of children with hypoplastic lungs and ureteral or urethral obstruction shows that the children in the two groups have a somewhat different prognosis, with the urethral being the worse [30,31]. The presence of lung hypoplasia, despite some functioning kidney, is not surprising if back pressure from accumulated urine has injured the kidney and interfered with renal function during early lung growth.

Obstruction early interferes with renal development [28]. The variety in nature and severity of the renal injury parallels variation in the degree of the associated lung effect. A middle-phase influence separate from that of the early phase is possible.

Late phase

Premature rupture of membranes (PROM) generally occurs relatively late in lung development [32–34]: the organ has already formed its airways and the future alveolar region is at the canalicular or saccular stage. While airways are complete the alveoli are still multiplying and differentiating. Premature rupture of membranes leading to amniotic fluid leak is likely to upset the two-way lung/amniotic fluid flow and balance (see below).

Because of a role in parturition, rupture of membranes is likely to shift the lung from a secretory to a fluid-absorbing organ. Normally this shift starts before birth and develops rapidly over a period of days [26,35,36]. Leakage of fluid from the lung at the beginning of parturition is the trigger that finally switches the lung from its intrauterine to extrauterine programme. Premature rupture of membranes perhaps leads to a premature change in programme, with a reduced production of lung liquid and so failure of the units to increase in number. At this late stage of intrauterine development, alveolar and vascular multiplication are arrested. In preparation for birth, it was thought that maturation of the surfactant system occurs, but the result of Franz et al. suggests that in the sheep, in the days before birth, rupture of membranes does not lead to premature maturation of the surfactant system [37].

In patients with premature rupture of the membranes and drainage of amniotic fluid, it can be said that amniotic fluid and lung development do interact and that the lungs are small, but the pathways and mechanisms by which these two are related is by no means clear.

It is known that the lung is small in infants with premature rupture of membranes and that alveolar number is reduced, but more detailed quantitation has not been carried out on these lungs [32,33]. This represents a late disturbance of amniotic fluid volume. It may

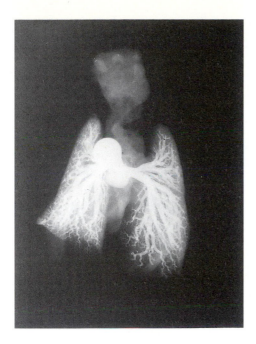

(a)

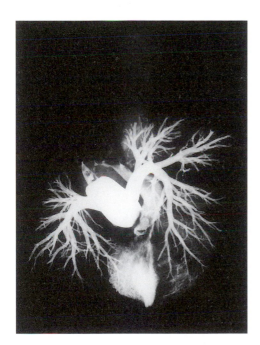

(b)

Figure 5.6 Arteriogram of the lung of: (a) renal agenesis and (b) renal dysplasia (×1). The arteries have been injected with a radio-opaque medium. (Reproduced from reference [4] with permission.)

be that it is the renal contribution to amniotic fluid that is critical at this stage, or it is possible that a metabolite or cytokine from the kidney is delivered to the lung in reduced amount. It could even be that reduced lung liquid production fails in its simple mechanical effect on stenting the lung, thus leading to reduced cell multiplication [25,38,39]. This effect could be relatively independent of kidney if it is seen because of an indirect outflow of lung liquid. But certainly in premature rupture of the membranes the interaction of amniotic fluid leak, and so reduced amniotic fluid volume, with lung hypoplasia, seems sequential [40].

A variety of anomalies of the urinary system is associated with lung hypoplasia, e.g. polycystic kidneys and prune belly associated with urinary outflow obstructive lesions like urethral atresia or posterior urethral valves [25]. In such cases of lung hypoplasia analysis of lung structure shows that not only is the lung small but also the airway number is reduced, indicating that lung development is disturbed during the phase of bronchial branching (authors' personal observation).

Experimental

Early damage to the kidney is exemplified by Clemmons' introduction of nephrotoxins to the chick kidney at various stages of development [7]. Nephrectomy is used as a way of introducing 'renal injury', but for technical reasons such surgery in the experimental animal is usually carried out later and so is not as relevant to human renal agenesis or dysplasia as to interference with renal function in the mid stages of gestation. Various forms of obstructive uropathy are also used, again usually in the mid phase of development. The late stage of amniotic fluid leak can be simulated in animals. The implication often made is that this serves as a model of early renal injury, but that is misleading. The numerous experimental examples of this are much more important as models of the various ways in which kidney function can influence lung development relatively late in gestation and of how lung liquid and amniotic fluid relate.

Early

Use of nephrotoxins

The use of nephrotoxins by Clemmons [7] to produce kidney injury in the chick has the advantage that it can be used in early stages of development. In 1977, Clemmons demonstrated that the kidney is an important site of proline synthesis for export 'use' by other organs, notably the lung. In the chick embryo he studied arginase activity in the developing kidney, since this enzyme influences the production of proline through the arginine–ornithine–proline cycle. Since active lung growth coincides with an increase in this enzyme, he included the lung in his examinations. By injecting nephrotoxins into the kidney during the mesonephric or metanephric stages and by radiolabelling, he was able to show reduced proline production by the kidney and reduced proline uptake and collagen synthesis in the lung. Histologically the lung was hypoplastic with sparse mesenchyme. This points to interaction of kidney with lung through biochemical or metabolic signals rather than by the volume of amniotic fluid, be it produced by lung or by kidney. It was of interest that injury to the mesonephros often left no sign in the newborn chick kidney, whereas injury to the metanephros was usually still apparent (J.J.W. Clemmons, personal communication).

In vitro experiments in mouse embryos demonstrate the importance of collagen in lung morphogenesis. A proline analogue azetidine-2-carboxylic acid depresses collagen accumulation to about 20% of the untreated controls. Even at low concentrations of the analogue the number of newly formed terminal buds is reduced and, with increasing dose, the overall growth of the epithelial tree is less [7,41–43] (Figure 5.7).

Injury to the fetal kidney reduces the supply of collagen, impairing fetal airway branching and growth in lung size.

Middle phase

Surgical – nephrectomy

Nephrectomy is usually carried out during the canalicular period and so is included with middle-stage interference.

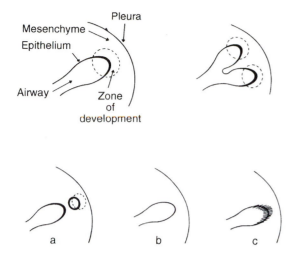

Figure 5.7 The lung arises as a ventral epithelial diverticulum from the foregut of the embryo: it is invested with mesenchyme. Interaction between epithelium and mesenchyme is essential to branching of airways and differentiation of lung. Abnormal organization at the zone of development produces congenital anomalies such as: (a) an extra focus, as seen in tracheal or bronchial cyst; (b) an absence of budding as in aplasia; or (c) abnormal interaction, as in various types of dysplasia. (Reproduced from reference [6] with permission.)

Bilateral kidney ablation does not precisely mimic human renal agenesis, since the timing is relatively later. In the nephrectomy model the earliest injury is usually produced during the pseudoglandular stage [44]. Bilateral nephrectomy is usually carried out during the canalicular stage after airway branching is complete. This results, although relatively late in gestation, in abnormal lung development and points to a continuing influence of kidney on lung. Thorburn in 1974 [45] reported that nephrectomy in fetal lambs interfered with subsequent growth without referring to its effect on lung.

In a recent study, Wilson and his colleagues [46] have carried out nephrectomy in sheep at 95 days' gestation, the fetus being delivered finally at 135 days. The second part of this experiment was of particular interest, in that in some animals tracheal ligation was combined with nephrectomy. This accelerates lung growth beyond the normal but the effect of the ligation was not as great in those animals in whom nephrectomy had been carried out as in those in whom kidney was present. This points to some lung independence from the kidney but also to a continuing influence from kidney

to lung, and favours a contribution mediated by a growth factor through the circulation.

Tracheal ligation before birth causes a big lung – in part at least because of lung liquid retention [17,47]. To test whether this could be produced after birth, these authors distended the right upper lobe of 5-week-old lambs with perfluorocarbon and ligated the lobar bronchus. The lobe increased greatly in size. Was this big lung a good 'quality' lung? Morphometric techniques that included estimates of alveolar density, alveolar surface area per unit lung volume, air space fraction as well as density of arteries of various sizes, established that the template to which this overgrown lung conforms is like the normal [48,49].

Perfluorocarbon was chosen as the distending agent because of its minimal absorption, and because it provided uniform distribution with minimal toxicity. It is virtually liquid Teflon, a hydrocarbon in which the hydrogen atoms have been replaced by fluorine, except for one bromine which confers radio-opacity. A radiograph demonstrates the established distension produced by the perfluorocarbon and the subsequent increase in volume of the distended lung can be assessed. The results of the experimental studies in the newborn lamb have already led to successful application of this procedure to human cases of diaphragmatic hernia [48].

Lung liquid from the experimental groups has been investigated for its mitogenic effect on W138 human lung fibroblasts, 3T3 murine fibroblasts and bovine capillary endothelial cells [50]. No sample of lung liquid affected the bovine cells. Normal liquid has a mitogenic effect on both the fibroblast lines, diaphragmatic hernia liquid has no effect on the human and minimal on the mouse, whereas diaphragmatic hernia and tracheal ligation liquid has a greater than baseline effect on both these cells. This mitogenic 'factor' is heat labile. From this and from the pattern of test cell response, the authors can conclude that this mitogenic 'factor', and presumably the effect on lung growth, is not mediated by platelet-derived growth factor (this is heat stable), or fibroblast growth or vascular endothelial growth factor (both the latter are mitogenic for bovine endothelium).

The stenting effect of the tracheal ligation is clearly important: increase in tracheal pressure as well as in volume of lung liquid occurs. The effect on growth could be achieved in a variety of ways by:

1. Increasing receptors or changing their receptivity.
2. Increasing retention of normal growth factors (this could include one derived from kidney).
3. Increasing the production of growth factors, autocrine and paracrine, by lung cells.

Of course, to varying degree these factors may all contribute. If there is a contribution from the kidney, then again this effect could be either by increased retention or by change in receptors.

Further experimental studies of the interaction between nephrectomy and tracheal ligation would be of significance. These should include morphometric analysis of the lung in the various experimental groups, both before and after correction, as well as analysis of the lung liquid in the nephrectomy and renal dysplasia groups. Even the possibility of perfluorocarbon distension as treatment for selected cases of lung hypoplasia with renal anomalies can be entertained.

Tracheal ligation in the adult does not have a similar effect. It seems necessary that the lung is in the programme stage of response to growth factor stimulus.

In the 6-month-old sheep, perfluorocarbon (PFC) was used to distend the right upper lobe with bronchus ligated, and pressure monitoring catheter within the bronchus. Age-matched controls underwent the same procedure but were sacrificed immediately after the initial installation of PFC. Upon retrieval, the PFC group showed no significant difference in lobar size based on lung segment volume to body weight ratio, total alveolar number or total alveolar surface area. Three weeks of PFC distension did not result in emphysematous changes based on histological appearance, air space fraction or alveolar numerical density. The capacity for postnatal lung growth seems lost in the adult lungs [49]. The histological results indicate that 3 weeks' exposure to the PFC appeared to be safe.

Surgical – obstructive uropathy and prenatal relief of obstruction

Surgical correction is often part of the experimental studies and, in some cases, has been carried out *in utero*. Improvement in lung growth after surgical correction of the renal lesion emphasizes the complex interaction between the kidney and lung.

Models of obstructive kidney damage are produced either by ligation of the urethra (with also, in the sheep, ligation of the urachus) [28,51,52] or bilateral ureteric ligation [53,54]. The ureteric injury, while it produces pelvic and renal changes, spares the bladder [28,29,55–58]. This is important when we come to consider 'effective' mechanisms. Urethral obstruction has the advantage that it can more easily be corrected *in utero*, by vesicostomy [59,60] (Figure 5.8).

In fetal lambs Adzick and Harrison [55] ligated both ureters, early in gestation, at 60 days, in the pseudoglandular phase. At term, lung volume to body weight is reduced, indicating hypoplasia, but microscopic morphometry showed that the total alveolar number relative to body weight was increased, as was the radial alveolar count. Thus the lung and its individual acini were polyalveolar. This represents an unusual dissociation between the size of lung and number of individual units. The stimulus to differentiation and alveolar multiplication seems to have been effective, although the lung did not achieve its normal size. It seems general nutritional requirements were not met or that some other required growth factor is needed.

It is intriguing that this seeming 'overgrowth' with ureteral obstruction parallels the clinical analysis in which it was shown that ureteral block seemed to have a better clinical outcome than urethral. This suggests that some contribution from the bladder is still available or that differences in the nature of kidney injury in the two types of obstruction are important [30,31].

Urethral obstruction has been done as early as the pseudoglandular phase but has more often been produced during the canalicular and alveolar phases. (In the sheep the pseudoglandular phase is up to 95 days.) Harrison et al. ligated the urethra, along with the urachus, in fetal lambs before 108 days of gestation to produce a model of urethral obstruction: this produced gross bilateral hydronephrosis and hydro-uretero-megacystis, with severe pulmonary hypoplasia associated with a high perinatal mortality [51,61]. In a second report, Harrison and colleagues pro-

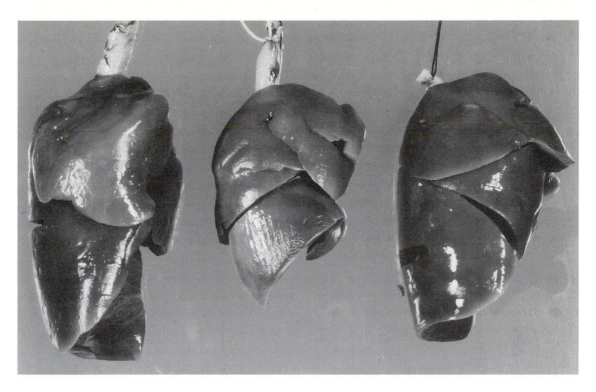

Normal   Obstructed   Reversed

Figure 5.8 Gross appearance of inflation-fixed fetal sheep lungs removed near term (135 days), showing relative size of right lungs (NORMAL), bladder obstruction with oligohydramnios (OBSTRUCTED) and bladder obstruction followed by *in utero* vesicostomy with restoration of lung volume (REVERSED). (Reproduced from reference [46] with permission.)

duced urethral and urachal obstruction in 17 fetal lambs between 93 and 107 days. In nine fetuses, the obstruction was relieved *in utero* by suprapubic cystostomy. The other eight fetuses proceeded to term with persisting obstruction: four of these fetuses were stillborn, and of the other four, all had respiratory insufficiency with only one survival; the lungs in all were severely hypoplastic. Of the decompressed, seven survived, and had less respiratory distress at birth with significantly increased lung weight and resolution of the hydronephrosis. The question arises, to what extent it is relief of lung compression from the hydronephrosis – the feature usually invoked – or how much the improved lung growth is because kidney function is better so kidney influence through a growth factor is restored. If so, does this reach the lung through urine or through the circulation?

Nakayama and colleagues [62] investigated bladder neck obstruction in the fetal rabbit. At 25 days, either bladder neck obstruction was produced or amniotic fluid was shunted into the maternal abdominal cavity. In this study the aim was to produce oligohydramnios. The newborns in both experiments had significantly decreased lung weight. In another experiment the 'correction' was attempted either through thoracic decompression by producing an abdominal hernia or by restoring the amniotic fluid volume by constant infusion of saline. Both procedures resulted in larger lungs in relation to body weight. This was taken as evidence that space limitation from the large bladder or that the constriction associated with oligohydramnios had interfered with lung growth. The results of these experiments do not indicate how lung growth had been impaired.

Peters et al. showed that after fetal bladder neck obstruction at 60 days the obstructed animals, at term, had a reduced lung volume to body weight ratio and a reduced air space fraction. Decompression of urethral obstruction at 112–124 days showed significant increase in lung weight, although it did not return to normal. Morphometric analysis of these lungs was not carried out. In experiments rather similar in design, bladder obstruction was produced at 60 days and *in utero* decompression at 195 days [52,59,60]. The corrective effect of decompression varied: in some, considerable improvement in lung maturation and amniotic fluid volume occurred; in others, renal dysplasia and lung hypoplasia persisted with little improvement. The authors concluded that the degree of renal damage from the original obstruction was the critical determinant of later recovery. The restoration of amniotic fluid seemed to parallel the improvement in lung structure. Whether this represents a marker of lung growth or its instigator needs additional analysis [51,53,61]. Production of growth factors, as from the amnion itself, also needs to be considered.

Most experimental models of 'renal injury' toward the end of gestation have been produced by amniotic fluid drainage. The assumption is often made that this corresponds with early renal injury but this model of oligohydramnios corresponds to the clinical condition of PROM (premature rupture of membranes) [34,38,62–67]. For example, Harding, Hooper and Dickson in 1990 [66], during the last third of gestation, by draining amniotic fluid produced 2–9 days of oligohydramnios in 20 sheep. This resulted in a reduction in lung liquid, increased tracheal pressure, increased pressure in the fetal pleural space and abdomen, and increased flexion of the fetal thoracolumbar spine. It was this last factor that they considered caused loss of fetal lung liquid.

Adzick and his colleagues [38] produced oligohydramnios in the fetal rabbit at 24 days (term 31 days) by shunting amniotic fluid into the maternal abdominal cavity. In another series of lambs, fetal breathing movements were impaired by high cervical cord section, and in a third group both procedures were performed [55]. This plan was to investigate the effect of amniotic fluid volume as well as of breathing movement, one suggestion being that reduced amniotic fluid volume produces an effect by interfering with breathing [38,55,66]. In each experimental group the lungs were smaller than in unoperated controls: the smallest lungs occurred when both procedures were combined. The effect of the amniotic fluid shunting was prevented by tracheal ligation. The question whether this results from internal stenting by lung liquid, as suggested by the authors, or because of the effect of growth factors present in the retained liquid has not been settled.

Moessinger and colleagues [40,64,68] carried out a series of experiments in which the guinea-pig fetus was exposed to oligohydramnios. They considered that it was the time of onset and, to a lesser extent, duration that were most important in determining the degree of impairment. Irrespective of duration, the greatest effect was during the canalicular period. Lung hypoplasia developed even in the absence of deformities, which themselves were directly correlated with the degree of oligohydramnios. This indicates that oligohydramnios itself is not the major feature. The effect of breathing movements was also investigated by these authors [40,64]. Again while major interference with breathing can produce a small lung, restricted breathing does not seem to be the critical feature for oligohydramnios. The presence of breathing movements was not a predictor of outcome in these cases.

In babies less than 34 weeks of age, renal agenesis does not influence body weight, but in older cases babies with agenesis tend to be lighter in weight. In the presence of hydramnios the babies tend to be bigger, again pointing to the fact that there is some other feature responsible for growth. It may be that the size of the infant reflects the better production of lung factors or that the amnion, known to be an important producer of fluid, is also a producer of growth factors.

Physiological features of amniotic fluid and lung liquid

The lung makes its own liquid that also contributes to amniotic fluid. The classic studies of Strang and his colleagues [26] have emphasized that although there is some exchange in each direction, the composition of lung liquid is so different from amniotic fluid that these systems do not equilibrate, indicating the relative independence of lung liquid. In recent years although many questions still remain, our understanding of the flux between lung liquid and the amnion has increased [35,67,69,70]. Is it the reduced contribution of lung liquid by the lung that causes the oligohydramnios rather than the oligohydramnios that causes lung hypoplasia [63]? A tracheal stenosis or tracheo-oesophageal fistula is often associated with oligohydramnios.

In a series of experiments it has been shown that drainage of lung liquid, notably through a tracheostomy, leads to small lungs. In early studies, Alcorn and her colleagues [47] showed that the lungs so produced were small in volume but that they showed morphological maturation as there was a greater density of Type II pneumocytes containing large numbers of lamellar bodies. The compliance of the lung was less than normal. Recently, Fewell and colleagues [69] have investigated the timing and effect of tracheostomy in fetal lambs. Seven ewes with twin fetuses were studied. Tracheostomy was performed on one fetus of each pair, and on the other sham operation. Lung liquid is produced as early as 94 days' gestation in the lamb and is steady until about 48 hours before birth.

The tracheostomy changes the pressure relations within the lung since the positive pressure within the trachea is no longer present to produce a distending force and presumably also, during attempted breathing, the negative phasic effect of diaphragm movement is removed. On the other hand, since distensibility of the lung increases near term, in the absence of the closed glottis, respiration will cause an increase in lung volume. Several studies have shown that cells respond to stretch by dividing and it may be that in the near-term lamb diaphragmatic breathing is important to produce stretch. Liggins for one considers this a significant factor in near-term lung maturation (G.C. Liggins, 1983 personal communication). Tracheostomy does not produce a change in the phosphatidyl choline content of lung or in air space stability [37].

In a clinical investigation, Moessinger and his colleagues [64] investigated fetal breathing patterns in PROM patients who survived and in a group associated with a number of renal anomalies. The patients with PROM, irrespec-

tive of outcome, spent the same or less time breathing as controls, while the fetuses with renal anomalies, oligohydramnios and lung hypoplasia spent more time. It seems that the fetal breathing does not help identify those infants at risk of lung hypoplasia. Furthermore, the weight, surface area and mean thickness of the diaphragm of patients with hypoplasia was similar to gestational age-matched controls. The mean fibre size was appropriate to gestational age. Carmel and colleagues [71] ligated the trachea in rabbits near term and showed that its presence for up to 5 days produced, on average, a 40% increase in lung to body weight ratio with thinning of alveolar walls and terminal bronchioli as well as dilatation. In the lamb, Alcorn and colleagues [47] produced the same effect near term, after 21–28 days' ligation. The increased lung volume was based on lung growth as well as accumulation of a greater liquid volume. This was in contrast to the tracheal drainage, which gave reduced lung to body weight ratio, thickened alveolar walls and a relative increase in density of Type II cells.

While the study of tracheal drainage or ligation is throwing light on pathophysiology and the role of lung liquid in lung growth, experimentally the urological surgeons are now exploiting the effect of tracheal ligation to help correct the hypoplasia that, for whatever reason, is associated with renal injury. Wilson and his colleagues [46] have shown that after nephrectomy combined with ligation of the trachea a striking increase in lung mass and weight occurs. This gives a degree of lung growth far above the normal. The normal stability and distensibility of these lungs suggest that they are functionally mature, but more detailed analysis, particularly of the vascular bed, is awaited.

A dramatic example of the expansive force of the growing lung is demonstrated by Wilson and his colleagues [72,73] who have combined tracheal ligation with a surgically produced diaphragmatic hernia. Here the lung has sufficient force to push the intestines, previously placed surgically within the thorax, to below the diaphragm, and the lung grows down into the abdominal cavity. The biological effect therefore of the retention of lung liquid, not in continuity with the amniotic cavity, is striking. (The animals with kidneys still present achieve an even greater response to tracheal ligation, which indicates that even in this rather dramatic model of lung independence from the kidney, the kidney still contributes.)

Clinical cases of lung hyperplasia and hypertrophy are seen in similar conditions, as with laryngeal atresia [24].

Lung to kidney loop

The discussion above emphasizes the influence of kidney on lung growth. Evidence from non-renal disease indicates that lung is also the source of growth factors influencing the kidney and other organs.

For example, Glick and his colleagues [74] developed the hypothesis that in congenital diaphragmatic hernia (CDH), due to compression, the lung cannot respond to pulmonary growth factors (PGF), notably one produced by the kidney: they postulated that this is modulated by a feedback signal from the lungs by what they called pulmonary-derived renotropin (PDR). They further postulated that if the lungs were not responding normally to PGFs, the pulmonary hypoplasia would stimulate the lung to overproduce PDR and that the excess would produce enlarged kidneys in newborns with CDH. In 30 autopsy cases of newborns with CDH they found that the kidney weight was greater than the control weight in 77%, in 57% by more than one standard deviation. Such feedback suggests that the kidney/lung loop is balanced by a lung/kidney loop. The interaction between the two organs comes full circle.

A similar endocrine function for the lung is apparent from its production of the so-called hepatocyte growth factor (HGF) [75]. Although named by reference to the hepatocyte, it is a potent growth factor for epithelial cells from various sites, including renal tubular cells. Within 12 hours of unilateral nephrectomy, HGF mRNA increased in the intact lung to about five times the normal level. *In situ* hybridization showed that after hepatectomy the mRNA signal for HGF was markedly increased in endothelial cells of lung. The lung/kidney loop is evidently only one of many interactions between lung and other organs.

Conclusions

From these data certain tentative conclusions and suggestions can be made:

1. That before the sixteenth week of intrauterine life, normal kidney development is necessary for normal lung growth.
2. That disturbed renal function at this period of gestation leads to reduced airway branching, reduced arterial branching (presumably venous as well) and abnormal development of the arterial wall.
3. That this reduced lung growth is at least in part mediated by failure of adequate proline production by the kidney: during its development the lung uses proline produced by the kidney for collagen production.
4. That the lung hypoplasia associated with the kidney deficiency can be modified (prevented partially, completely or even overcorrected) by the increased retention of lung liquid. This suggests that some renal-derived factor is relatively deficient when the kidney is abnormal but that if the smaller dose is in some way made more effective, growth can proceed.
5. That the difference in lung growth following ureteral or urethral blockage indicates that the effect of these abnormalities is not exclusively through kidney damage by back pressure of urine. It could be that in these two models, kidney injury is different in its timing, severity or rate of development, or that the kidney and bladder each independently produces growth factors so that urethral block produces greater injury than ureteral. This fits with the worse prognosis clinically of urethral obstruction. Alternatively, the same factor could be produced at both sites and the effect on lung growth reflects a dose reduction in growth factor.
6. That late leak of amniotic fluid, probably because of associated lung liquid leak, causes hypoplasia, of a different type from that occurring in early injury.
7. That a lung to kidney loop is also in place.

The techniques of molecular biology enable the induction of genes and their protein products – manipulations that have the potential to further elucidate the nature of the interactive control between kidney and lung. For the moment it is clear that a powerful kidney to lung loop normally exists as one of the intertwining loops forged between organs through the action of growth factors.

References

1. Potter EL. Bilateral renal agenesis. *J Pediatr* 1946; **29**: 68–76.
2. Potter EL. Facial characteristics of infants with bilateral renal agenesis. *Am J Obstet Gynecol* 1946; **51**: 885–888.
3. Potter EL. Bilateral absence of ureter and kidney. *Am J Obstet Gynecol* 1965; **25**: 3–12.
4. Hislop A, Hey E, Reid L. The lungs in congenital bilateral renal agenesis and dysplasia. *Arch Dis Child* 1979; **54**: 32–38.
5. Hislop A, Reid L. Growth and development of the respiratory system: anatomical development. In: Davis JA, Dobbing J (eds) *Scientific Foundations of Paediatrics*, 2nd edn. London: Heinemann Medical Publications, 1981; pp 390–431.
6. deMello DE, Davies P, Reid LM. Lung growth and development. In: Simmons D (ed) *Current Pulmonology*, vol 10. Chicago: Year Book Medical Publishers, pp 159–208.
7. Clemmons JJW. Embryonic renal injury: a possible factor in fetal malnutrition. *Pediatr Res* 1977; **11**: 404 (abstract).
8. Reid LM. The lung: its growth and remodeling in health and disease. Edward BD. Neuhauser Lecture. *AJR* 1977; **129**: 777–788.
9. Reid L. Lung growth in health and disease. (Tudor Edwards Lecture.) *Br J Dis Chest* 78: 113–134.
10. Bucher U, Reid L. Development of the intrasegmental bronchial tree: the pattern of branching and development of cartilage at various stages of intra-uterine life. *Thorax* 1961; **16**: 207–218.
11. Dunnill MS. Quantitative methods in the study of pulmonary pathology. *Thorax* 1962; **17**: 320–328.
12. Davies G, Reid L. Effect of scoliosis on growth of alveoli and pulmonary arteries and on right ventricle. *Arch Dis Child* 1971; **46**: 623–632.
13. Reid L. The pulmonary circulation: remodeling ingrowth and disease. The 1978: J Burns Amberson Lecture. *Am Rev Resp Dis* 1979; **119**: 531–546.
14. deMello D, Reid LM. Arteries and veins. In: Crystal RG, West JB, Barnes PH, Chernick NS, Weibel ER (eds) *The Lung: scientific foundations*, vol 1. New York: Raven Press, pp 767–777.
15. deMello DE, Reid LM. Pre and postnatal development of the pulmonary circulation. In: Chernick V, Mellins RB (eds) *Basic Mechanisms of Pediatric Respiratory Disease: cellular and integrative*. Philadelphia: BC Dekker, pp 36–54.
16. Rendas A, Lennox S, Reid L. Aorta–pulmonary shunts in growing pigs. Functional and structural assessment of the changes in the pulmonary circulation. *J Thor Cardiovasc Surg* 1979; **77**: 109–18.
17. Alcorn DG, Adamson TM, Maloney JE et al. A morphologic and morphometric analysis of fetal lung development in the sheep. *Anat Rec* 1981; **201**: 655–667.
18. Docimo SG, Crone RK, Davies P et al. Pulmonary development in the fetal lamb: morphometric study of the alveolar phase. *Anat Rec* **229**: 495–498.
19. Steinhardt GF, Vogler G, Salinas-Madrigal L, LaRegina M. Induced renal dysplasia in the young oppossum. *J Pediatr Surg* 1988; **23**: 1127–1130.
20. Steinhardt G, Salinas LM, Phillips R, deMello DE. Fetal nephrotoxicity. *J Urol* 1992; **148**: 760–763.
21. Jeffcoate TNA, Schoot JS. Polyhydramnios and oligohydramnios. *Can Med Assoc J* 1959; **80**: 77–86.
22. Kohler HG. An unusual case of sirenomelia. *Teratology* 1972; **6**: 295–302.
23. Bates HR. Hydramnios and the fetal lung: a selective review. *Am J Obstet Gynecol* 1979; **135**(1): 154–156.
24. Wigglesworth JS, Desai R, Hislop AA. Fetal lung growth in congenital laryngeal atresia. *Pediatr Pathol* 1987; **7**: 515–525.
25. Mandell J, Peters CA, Estroff JA, Benaceraf BR. Late onset of severe oligohydramnios associated with gento-urinary abnormalities. *J Urol* 1992; **148**: 515–518.
26. Strang LB. Growth and development of the lung: fetal and postnatal. *Annu Rev Physiol* 1977; **39**: 253–276.
27. Barth PJ, Ruschoff J. Morphometric study on pulmonary arterial thickness in pulmonary hypoplasia. *Pediatr Pathol* 1992; **12**: 653–663.
28. Beck DA. The effect of intra-uterine urinary obstruction upon the development of fetal kidney. *J Urol* 1971; **105**: 784–789.
29. Nakayama DK, Harrison MR, deLorimier AA. Prognosis of posterior urethral valves presenting at birth. *J Pediatr Surg* 1986; **21**: 43–45.
30. Reuss A, Wladimiroff JW, Scholtmeijer RJ et al. Prenatal evaluation and outcome of fetal obstructive uropathies. *Prenat Diagn* 1988; **8**: 93–102.
31. Reuss A, Wladimiroff JW, Stewart PA et al. Non-invasive management of fetal obstructive uropathy. *Lancet* 1988; 949–950.
32. Perlman M, Williams J, Hirsch M. Neonatal pulmonary hypoplasia after prolonged leakage of amniotic fluid. *Arch Dis Child* 1976; **51**: 349–353.
33. Thibeault DW, Beatty EC Jr, Hall RT, Bowen SK, O'Neill DH. Neonatal pulmonary hypoplasia with premature rupture of fetal membranes and oligohydramnios. *J Pediatr* 1985; **107**: 273–277.
34. Rotschild A, Ling EW, Puterman ML, Farquharson D. Neonatal outcome after prolonged preterm rupture of the membranes. *Am J Obstet Gynecol* 1990; **162**: 46–52.
35. Kitterman JA, Ballard PL, Clements JA et al. Tracheal fluid in fetal lambs: spontaneous decrease prior to birth. *J Appl Physiol* 1979; **47**: 985.

36. Maloney JE. Preparation of the respiratory system for the early neonatal period. *J Dev Physiol* 1984; **6**: 21–30.

37. Frantz ID III, Adler SM, Thach B et al. The effect of amniotic fluid removal on pulmonary maturation in sheep. *Pediatrics* 1975; **56**: 474–476.

38. Adzick NS, Harrison MR, Glick PL et al. Experimental pulmonary hypoplasia and oligohydramnios: relative contributions of lung fluid and fetal breathing movements. *J Pediatr Surg* 1984; **19**: 658–665.

39. Dickson KA, Harding R. Decline in lung liquid volume and secretion rate during oligohydramnios in fetal sheep. *J Appl Physiol* 1989; **67**: 2401–2407.

40. Moessinger AC, Singh M, Donnelly DF et al. The effect of prolonged oligohydramnios on fetal lung development, maturation and ventilatory patterns in the newborn guinea pig. *J Dev Physiol* 1987; **9**: 419–427.

41. Halme J. Development of protocollagen proline hydroxylase activity in the chick embryo. *Biochem Biophys Acta* 1969; **192**: 90–95.

42. Alescio T. Effect of a proline analogue, azetidine-2-carboxylic acid, on the morphogenesis *in vitro* of mouse embryonic lung. *J Embryol Exp Morphol* 1973; **29**: 439–451.

43. Schriver CR, McInnes RR, Mohyuddin F. Role of epithelial architecture and intracellular metabolism in proline uptake transtubular reclamation in PRO/Re Mouse kidney. *Proc Natl Acad Sci USA* 1975; **72**: 1431–1435.

44. Plopper CG, Kendall JZ, Saldana-Gautier LR et al. Lung development in the nephrectomized ovine fetus. *J Dev Physiol* 1984; **6**: 313–327.

45. Thorburn GD. The role of the thyroid gland and kidneys in fetal growth. In: Elliot KM, Knight J (eds) *Size at Birth. Proceedings of Ciba Foundation Symposium New Series No. 27, London, March 1974.* Elsevier: Amsterdam, 1974; pp 185–200.

46. Wilson JM, DiFiore JW, Peters CA. Experimental fetal tracheal ligation prevents the pulmonary hypoplasia associated with fetal nephrectomy: possible application for congenital diaphragmatic hernia. *J Pediatr Surg* 1993; **28**: 1433–1440.

47. Alcorn D, Adamson TM, Lambert TF et al. Morphological effects of chronic tracheal ligation and drainage in the fetal lamb lung. *J Anat* 1977; **123**: 649–660.

48. Fauza DO, DiFiore JW, Hines MH et al. Continuous intrapulmonary distention with perfluorocarbon accelerates postnatal lung growth: Possible application for congenital diaphragmatic hernia. *American College of Surgeons Surgical Forum* 1995; **46**: 666–669.

49. Nobuhara KK, Fauza DO, DiFiore JW. et al. Continuous intrapulmonary distention with perfluorocarbon accelerates neonatal but not adult lung growth. *J Pediatr Surg* (In Press).

50. DiFiore JW, Wilson JM. Lung liquid from fetal lambs with tracheal occlusion is mitogenic to pulmonary cells in vitro. *American College of Surgeons Surgical Forum*, 1994; **45**: 666–668.

51. Harrison MR, Nakayama DK, Noall R et al. Correction of congenital hydronephrosis *in utero* I. The model: fetal urethral obstruction produces hydronephrosis and pulmonary hypoplasia in fetal lambs. *J Pediatr Surg* 1983; **18**: 247–256.

52. Docimo SG, Luetic T, Crone RK et al. Pulmonary development in the fetal lamb with severe bladder outlet obstruction and oligohydramnios: a morphometric study. *J Urol* 1989; **142**: 657–660.

53. Glick PL, Harrison MR, Noall RA et al. Correction of congenital hydronephrosis *in utero* III. Early mid-trimester ureteral obstruction produces renal dysplasia. *J Pediatr Surg* 1983; **18**: 681–687.

54. Hu LM, Davies P, Adzick NS et al. Lung growth after intrauterine bilateral ureteral obstruction. *FASEB* 1987; (4865) 1151.

55. Adzick NS, Harrison MR, Glick PL et al. Fetal urinary tract obstruction: experimental pathophysiology. *Semin Perinatol* 1985; **9**: 79–90.

56. Pringle KC, Bonsib SM. Development of fetal lamb lung and kidney in obstructive uropathy: a preliminary report. *Fetal Ther* 1988; **3**: 118–128.

57. Peters C, Carr MC, Lais A et al. The response of the fetal kidney to obstruction. *J Urol* 1992; **148**: 503–509.

58. Peters CA, Vasavada S, Dato D et al. The effect of obstruction on the developing bladder. *J Urol* 1992; **148**: 491–496.

59. Peters CA, Docimo SG, Luetic T et al. Effect of *in utero* vesicostomy on pulmonary hypoplasia in the fetal lamb with bladder outlet obstruction and oligohydramnios: a morphometric analysis. *J Urol* 1991; **146**: 1178–1183.

60. Peters CA, Reid LM, Docimo S et al. The role of the kidney in lung growth and maturation in the setting of obstructive uropathy and oligohydramnios. *J Urol* 1991; **146**: 597–600.

61. Harrison MR, Nakayama DK, Noall R et al. Correction of congenital hydronephrosis *in utero* II. Decompression reverses the effects of obstruction on the fetal lung and urinary tract. *J Pediatr Surg* 1982; **17**: 965–974.

62. Nakayama DK, Glick PL, Harrison MR et al. Experimental pulmonary hypoplasia due to oligohydramnios and its reversal by relieving thoracic compression. *J Pediatr Surg* 1983; **18**: 347–353.

63. Barss VA, Benacerraf BR, Frigoletto FD Jr. Second trimester oligohydramnios, a predictor of poor fetal outcome. *Am J Obstet Gynecol* 1984; **64**: 608–610.

64. Moessinger AC, Fox HE, Higgins A, Rey HR, Al Haideri M. Fetal breathing movements are not a reliable predictor of continued lung development in pregnancies complicated by oligohydramnios. *Lancet* 1987; 1297–1299.

65. Nicolini U, Fisk NM, Rodeck CH et al. Low amniotic pressure in oligohydramnios – is this the cause of pulmonary hypoplasia? *Am J Obstet Gynecol* 1989; **161**: 1098.

66. Harding R, Hooper SB, Dickson KA. A mechanism leading to reduced lung expansion and lung hypoplasia in fetal sheep during oligohydramnios. *Am J Obstet Gynecol* 1990; **163**: 1904–1913.

67. Harding R, Dickson KA. Fetal breathing and pressures in the trachea and amniotic sac during oligohydramnios in sheep. *J Appl Physiol* 1991; **70**: 293–299.

68. Moessinger AC, Collins MH, Blanc WA et al. Oligohydramnio-induced lung hypoplasia: the influence of timing and duration in gestation. *Pediatr Res* 1986; **20**: 951–954.

69. Fewell JE, Hislop AA, Kitterman JA, Johnson P. Effect of tracheostomy on lung development in fetal lambs. *J Appl Physiol* 1983; **55**: 1103–1108.

70. Hill LM. Abnormalities of amniotic fluid. In: Nyberg DA, Mahony BS, Pretorius DH (eds) *Diagnostic Ultrasound of Fetal Anomalies – text and atlas*. Littleton, MA: Year Book Medical, pp 38–66.

71. Carmel AN, Friedman F, Adams FK. Fetal tracheal ligation and lung development. *Arch Dis Child* 1965; **109**: 452–456.

72. DiFore JW, Fauza DO, Slavin R, Wilson JM. Experimental fetal tracheal ligation and congenital diaphragmatic hernia: a pulmonary vascular morphometric analysis. *J Pediatr Surg* 1995; **30**: 917–924.

73. DiFore JW, Fauza DO, Slavin R, Peters CA, Fackler JC, Wilson JM. Experimental fetal tracheal ligation reverses the structural and physiological effects of pulmonary hypoplasia in congenital diaphragmatic hernia. *J Pediatr Surg* 1994; **29**: 248–257.

74. Glick PL, Siebert JR, Benjamin DR. Pathophysiology of congenital diaphragmatic hernia: I. Renal enlargement suggests feedback modulation by pulmonary derived renotropins – a unifying hypothesis to explain pulmonary hypoplasia, polyhydramnios, and renal enlargement in the fetus/new born with congenital diaphragmatic hernia. *J Pediatr Surg* 1990; **25**: 492–495.

75. Yanagita K, Nagaike M, Ishibashi H et al. Lung may have an endocrine function producing hepatocyte growth factor in response to injury of distal organs. *Biochem Biophys Res Commun* 1992; **182**: 802–809.

76. O'Rahilly R, Boyden EA. The timing and sequence of events in the development of the human respiratory system during the embryonic period proper. *Z Anat Entwicklungsgesch* 1973; **141**(3): 237–250.

6

Obstetric management of prenatally diagnosed uropathies

G.C. Mason, H. Irving and R.J. Lilford

Introduction

The availability of high-resolution ultrasound has allowed early evaluation of the fetal urinary tract. It is now possible to reliably visualize the fetal kidney, with transvaginal ultrasound, as early as the twelfth week of gestation [1]. The ultrasound appearance of the normal urinary tract (Figure 6.1) is well documented and this has led in turn to the description of the abnormal. Abnormality ranges from mild dilatation of the renal calyces to gross distension of the bladder and ureters or complete absence of the kidneys. Urinary tract anomalies are among the most frequently encountered abnormalities by ultrasound, with an incidence between 0.1 and 0.48% [2,3]. In Rosendahl's [3] series over two-thirds of the cases were identified in the third trimester. Abnormalities may not be apparent at the time of the routine 'dating' ultrasound performed between 16 and 20 weeks' gestation and therefore when ultrasound is performed in the third trimester it should include an assessment of the fetal renal tract. In addition to the above, mild pyelectasis occurs in a further 2–3% [4].

Prior to the introduction of ultrasound the majority of renal tract anomalies would remain

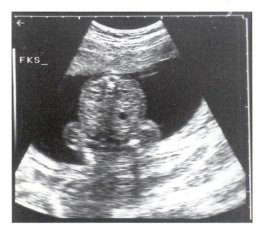

(a)

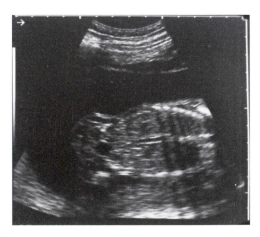

(b)

Figure 6.1 Normal fetal urinary tract at 18 weeks' gestation. (a) Transverse scan through fetal abdomen to show normal kidneys in cross-section, on each side of the fetal spine. (b) Coronal scan through fetal abdomen to show normal kidneys on either side of the fetal aorta, with normal fluid-containing fetal bladder in the pelvis.

silent both *in utero* and in the neonatal period. A proportion of these babies would have deteriorating renal function [2] and present in childhood with renal failure. It is likely that the appropriate follow up of a significant uropathy, diagnosed *in utero*, may prevent long-term renal damage [5–8], but it is difficult to measure the effect of routine scanning and follow-up on childhood and adult morbidity and mortality. Not all antenatally diagnosed anomalies will be significant, as a proportion will resolve *in utero* or neonatally, with approximately 50% of cases of 'fetal hydronephrosis' being normal at follow-up [9,10]. The increased anxiety generated in the parents must be considered whenever an apparent abnormality is demonstrated in the fetus.

Thus antenatal detection raises many obstetric dilemmas based on our inadequate knowledge of the natural history of these features. Faced with an abnormality of the renal tract the obstetrician has to answer a number of important questions. Is the abnormality likely to be of any significance? If so – What are the possible diagnoses? What is the probability of each of the various outcomes being associated with these ultrasound appearances? Is this abnormality likely to be associated with other abnormalities and/or a chromosomal disorder?

The finding of a renal anomaly should instigate a thorough sonographic investigation of the fetus to identify any other abnormalities. For example, the finding of a posterior encephlocele with bilateral renal cysts establishes the diagnosis of the autosomal recessive Meckel–Gruber syndrome. More often an absolute diagnosis cannot be achieved and when counselling the parents the prognosis is more important than the diagnosis. The prognosis will in part depend on the renal function, which can be assessed in a number of ways. Although Nolte et al. [11] have suggested a method to measure glomerular filtration in the fetus, most practitioners rely on indirect measures of fetal renal function. Estimation of liquor volume provides an important, albeit late, sign of renal function. Fetal bladder or ureteric sampling can be used for estimation of urinary electrolytes, in particular sodium and calcium which are the most useful markers of prognosis [12]. Although liquor is derived from a combination of fetal urine, fetal lung fluid, diffusion across membranes and, at early gestations, fetal skin, the majority is renal in origin. Oligohydramnios implies either a reduction in renal function, increased absorption or a leakage from spontaneous rupture of the membranes. Although the latter should become apparent from the history, a slow leak may go unnoticed or be masked by vaginal bleeding.

The prognosis for the fetus with oligohydramnios is poor, with the chances of survival being related not only to the underlying cause but also to the time of onset. The earlier the onset of oligohydramnios the more likely the fetus is to develop pulmonary hypoplasia. Attempts have been made to predict this condition by measuring chest diameters [13] and the presence [14] or absence of fetal breathing movements. Although it has been claimed that the presence of fetal breathing movements is associated with a normal outcome, this was not confirmed by others [15]. Amnioinfusion does not increase the incidence of fetal breathing movements, suggesting that the impairment of fetal breathing is not the cause of the pulmonary hypoplasia [16].

The management of oligohydramnios will depend on the likely underlying cause and gestation. Oligohydramnios secondary to renal agenesis, bilateral renal cystic dysplastic disease or a combination of dysplasia on one side and agenesis on the other will be universally fatal. The option of termination of pregnancy should be included in the counselling of such patients.

Fetal pyelectasis as a marker for Down syndrome

Recent reports have indicated a link between the finding of mild fetal pyelectasis and Down syndrome (Figure 6.2). The initial report from Benacerraf et al. [4] indicated that the normal anteroposterior diameter of the renal pelvis was less than 4 mm at 15–20 weeks, 5 mm between 20 and 30 weeks and 7 mm between 30 and 40 weeks. Abnormal findings were demonstrated retrospectively in 25% of Down cases. Two hundred and ten abnormal cases were demonstrated out of 7400 patients scanned, with seven being diagnosed as having Down syndrome. This gave a 3.3% incidence (predictive value positive) of Down syndrome in the presence of mild pyelectasis. More recent reports [17] have confirmed this

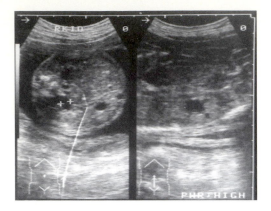

(a)

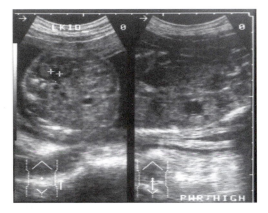

(b)

Figure 6.2 Bilateral mild fetal pyelectasis. Split images to show transverse and coronal scans through fetal kidneys. (a) Right kidney with anteroposterior (AP) diameter of renal pelvis = 5 mm. (b) Left kidney with (AP) diameter of renal pelvis = 6 mm.

association, indicating a predictive value of 1 in 90. However the predictive value in the absence of other markers fell to 1 in 340, which raises the question as to whether or not this should be an indication to offer invasive testing on its own.

Renal tract abnormalities and chromosomal abnormalities

One of the questions commonly asked on the finding of any ultrasound abnormality is could this be a marker for a chromosomal abnormality? We have seen that there is a weak asso-

ciation between pyelectasis and Down syndrome. Should therefore all renal anomalies require karotyping? Although many chromosomal anomalies have renal abnormalities as part of the syndrome, the association is weak in the presence of an isolated renal anomaly [18]. Therefore as a general rule karotyping should always be performed prior to *in utero* surgery, in particular for posterior urethral valves, and is recommended in bilateral renal agenesis (usually after delivery) and whenever the renal abnormality is found with one or more other anomalies.

Bilateral renal agenesis

The incidence of renal agenesis is between 1 in 3000 and 1 in 10 000 [19–21], with a male to female predominance of 2.5 to 1. Renal agenesis may occur as part of a syndrome or as an isolated finding. An accurate diagnosis will enable a precise recurrence risk to be given. Overall the recurrence rate is in the order of 3–5%. Syndromic causes of renal agenesis include autosomal recessive conditions such as Fraser syndrome [22], autosomal dominant for example branchio-oto-renal syndrome [23], X-linked recessive and as part of non-mendelian disorders such as the VATER syndrome [24]. Bilateral renal agenesis can also occur in association with chromosomal disorders, for instance trisomy 13 and 18, cat's eye syndrome and 4p syndrome.

Thirteen per cent of parents delivering a child with bilateral renal agenesis will themselves have silent unilateral renal agenesis. This rises to 30% after two affected children [25] and it is therefore worthwhile screening both parents with ultrasound.

The diagnosis is made by the inability to demonstrate fetal kidneys, absence of a bladder or no alteration in bladder size and oligohydramnios (Figure 6.3). Confirmation of renal agenesis can be assisted by the inability to demonstrate the renal artery with colour flow Doppler. In the past it has been suggested that bladder filling could be aided by maternal frusemide administration [26], however this has not been found to be of benefit.

The diagnosis has been highly accurate on ultrasound for some time, and with the increasing ultrasound resolution should become more so. *In utero* renal failure from other

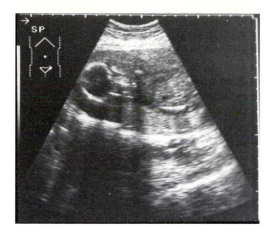

(a)

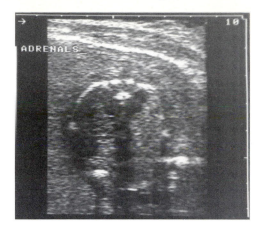

(a)

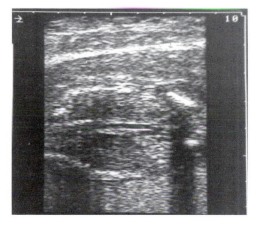

(b)

Figure 6.3 Bilateral renal agenesis. (a) Fetus in longitudinal section with severe oligohydramnios. (b) Coronal scan to show absence of kidneys on either side of fetal aorta.

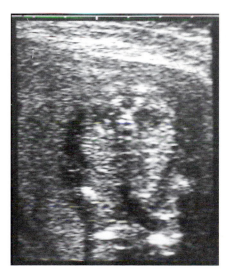

(b)

Figure 6.4 Bilateral renal agenesis with fetal adrenals. (a), (b) Transverse scans to show fetal adrenals on either side of fetal spine (note lack of pelvicaliceal systems).

causes may give a false-positive diagnosis [27]. Although the adrenal glands are of similar size, there is no evidence of adrenal hypertrophy in renal agenesis [28], and it should be possible to differentiate the characteristic discord appearance of the adrenal gland from the kidney with its demonstrable calyceal system (Figure 6.4). Even though the kidneys produce urine from about 10 weeks, they do not become the major contributor to amniotic fluid until 16 weeks. Oligohydramnios may be noticed as early as the fourteenth week, however normal liquor volumes at this stage do not exclude the diagnosis. The differential diagnosis must include any cause of profound oligohydramnios.

Babies born with bilateral renal agenesis show the classical appearance of Potter's syndrome. The typical findings are of absent kidneys and ureters, pulmonary hypoplasia and limb deformities. These babies have the characteristic facial features of low-set ears, a parrot beak nose, redundant skin, receding chin and a prominent fold arising at the inner canthus of the eye. The lungs weigh less than half the expected weight. The abnormal hand and foot positions, bowed legs and dislocated hips are probably a result of oligohydramnios [29]. The prognosis for such infants is invariably fatal. Between a quarter and a third will be stillborn, although the underlining mechanism of fetal demise is unknown. The remainder will die from pulmonary hypoplasia. Sixty per cent are born prematurely [30], with half of the cases demonstrating growth retardation.

Many of these fetuses have associated anomalies, with a 14% incidence of cardiovascular system (CVS) abnormality, 40% musculoskeletal malformation, 11% central nervous system (CNS) and 19% gastrointestinal abnormality [22]. Ten per cent of multicystic kidneys are associated with contralateral agenesis, in which case again the presentation will be of oligohydramnios. Unilateral renal agenesis occurs some 4–20 times [25,31] more often than bilateral renal agenesis. It occurs more commonly on the left and there is a male to female preponderance of 1.8 : 1. Providing the solitary kidney functions adequately, then the liquor volume will be normal and it may well go undetected *in utero*. There is evidence to suggest that this kidney will undergo compensatory hypertrophy *in utero* [32]. Associated genital anomalies are found in 25–50% of females and 10–15% of males. When agenesis is suspected care must be made to exclude an ectopic kidney prior to making the diagnosis. As usual a careful search for other anomalies should be made, as abnormalities of the cardiovascular system (30%), gastrointestinal tract (25%) and musculoskeletal system (14%) have been reported [33].

Ectopic kidney

The incidence is in the order of 1 in 500. Ectopic sites include the pelvis, abdomen, thorax and contralateral. The failure to demonstrate two kidneys in the usual site should instigate a search for one or more in an ectopic location.

Horseshoe kidney

The incidence is approximately 1 in 400, with a male preponderance of 2 : 1 [34]. The lower poles, which are joined, are usually displaced anteriorly. The diagnosis is not easy to make sonographically. A third of cases have associated anomalies in particular of the cardiovascular, skeletal and central nervous systems. There is an association with trisomy 18.

Renal cystic disease

Renal cysts are of four types: Infantile polycystic disease (Potter's type I); adult polycystic disease (Potter's type III): multicystic dysplastic kidney disease (Potter's type II), and isolated renal cysts. In infantile polycystic disease there is dilatation of the collecting tubules [35] (the distal portions of the ureteric buds), whereas in adult polycystic disease the cysts are visible in both the nephrons and the collecting tubules. In adult disease the number of nephrons involved is variable, which results in cysts interdispersed among normal renal tissue. Multicystic kidney disease is also characterized by cystic lesions, primarily as a result of dilated collecting tubules [36]. The underlying pathology in multicystic kidney disease is, in the majority of cases, obstruction with resultant increase in intraluminal pressure during nephrogenesis with resulting renal dysplasia. This explains why the condition is often associated with atresia of the upper ureter and/or renal pelvis. An obstruction occurring later in development can result in a hydronephrotic form of dysplastic kidney. It is not surprising therefore that bilateral obstruction, but of different degrees, will lead to cystic dysplasia on one side and apparent obstruction of the other.

All of these conditions are recognizable antenatally, although there are potential pitfalls with marked overlap in the ultrasound appearances between the conditions.

Infantile polycystic kidney disease

Infantile polycystic kidney disease is a rare autosomal recessive disorder with an incidence of 2 : 100 000 infants [37]. Both kidneys are symmetrically enlarged and contain numerous cysts which are typically 1–2 mm in diameter, although in some cases they can be larger and therefore resolvable on ultrasound. Sonographically the typical appearance is of an enlarged hyperechogenic kidney [38] (Figure 6.5) and this allows the antenatal diagnosis in

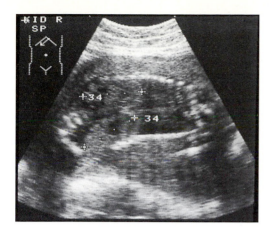

Figure 6.5 Infantile-type polycystic kidneys – large and echogenic with loss of normal intrarenal architecture.

the majority of cases [39]. In the presence of a family history the diagnosis can be made as early as 16 weeks' gestation, the diagnosis being based on the finding of bright kidneys, the absence of bladder filling and, in some cases, oligohydramnios. Renal enlargement as a sole finding is not sufficient to make the diagnosis, as this can be associated with a normal outcome [40]. The finding of enlarged bright kidneys, in the absence of a family history, is not necessarily the result of infantile polycystic kidneys and may be caused by the adult variety [41].

Four types of infantile polycystic kidney have been described; perinatal, neonatal, infantile and juvenile [42], the proportion of dilated renal tubules ranges from greater than 90% in the perinatal form to less than 10% in the juvenile form. The converse is found with periportal hepatic fibrosis with minimal in the perinatal group and gross fibrosis in the juvenile group. Recurrence within a family is usually of the same type [43]. As expected the greater the renal involvement, the more likely a diagnosis will be made *in utero*. The perinatal group is the most common [44] and can be diagnosed as early as the fourteenth week [45] and in the majority by the twenty-fourth week of gestation. However the finding of a normal renal appearance *in utero* does not exclude the possibility of one of the milder forms of infantile polycystic kidney disease. Bronshtein et al. [46] have suggested that the later onset forms may be diagnosable by long axis measurements but

this observation requires confirmation. In practice, in parents who have had an affected child, we would advise ultrasound at 16–18 weeks with a follow-up scan at 24 weeks, with a statement to the parents to the effect that a normal appearance is not a guarantee of a normal outcome.

Adult polycystic kidney disease

Adult polycystic kidney disease is an autosomal dominant disorder with approximately 1 in every 1000 people carrying the mutated gene. This is the third most prevalent cause of renal failure [47]. Although there appears to be virtually 100% penetrance of the gene, the expression varies, resulting in a wide range of ages for the onset and severity of the disease. Although some people remain entirely asymptomatic, the mean age of onset of symptoms is 35, with the mean age of diagnosis 43 [48]. Typical symptoms include loin pain, renal enlargement and renal failure. Hypertension is observed in the majority of patients, with 10–30% having demonstrable Berry aneurysms which are the cause of death in 10% of patients.

Although the disease affects both kidneys, one may be more severely affected than the other, giving the impression of unilateral disease *in utero*. The ultrasound appearance is of cystic echogenic kidneys with normal amniotic fluid (Figure 6.6). In this situation it is worth performing renal ultrasound on both parents, the finding of renal cystic disease in one of the parents would raise the prior probability considerably. However, failure to demonstrate abnormal kidneys in the parents does not exclude the diagnosis, which may arise from a new mutation or non paternity [49].

The diagnosis has been made prenatally by ultrasound as early as 14 weeks [50]. The syndrome can be associated with extrarenal cysts, in particular in the pancreas, spleen, lungs, testes and ovary. However these have not been diagnosed *in utero*. More accurate prenatal diagnosis can now be offered using a highly polymorphic probe linked to the locus of the mutant gene, which has been located on chromosome 16. Although rapid diagnosis has been described using the polymerase chain reaction [51], few parents seek prenatal diagnosis for this condition.

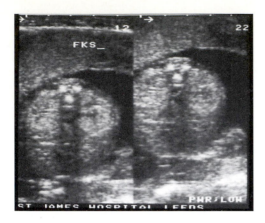

(a)

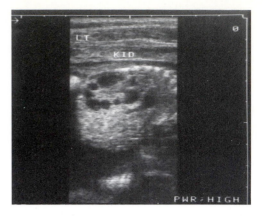

(a)

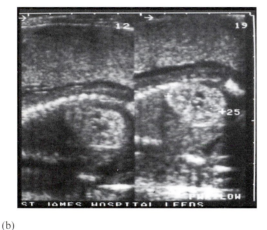

(b)

(b)

Figure 6.6 Adult-type polycystic kidneys – large and echogenic with visible cysts. (a) Transverse scans. (b) Sagittal scans.

Figure 6.7 Multicystic dysplastic kidney (MDK). (a) Sagittal scan through left MDK. (b) Transverse scan showing normal right kidney and left MDK.

Multicystic dysplastic kidney disease

Multicystic dysplastic kidney (MDK) disease is a sporadic condition with an incidence of approximately 1 in 10 000. There is a male/female preponderance of 2 to 1 in unilateral MDK. The disease can be unilateral, bilateral or segmental, with the cysts varying both in size and number. The classical appearance is of numerous cysts resembling a cluster of grapes involving the entire kidney with no normal renal parenchyma (Figure 6.7). The cysts themselves are of various sizes and *do not* communicate with each other. Occasionally a single large cyst may be seen which could be confused with a PUJ obstruction. The disease is bilateral in 20% of cases (Figure 6.8) and associated with contralateral renal agenesis in a further 10% of cases; in both situations oligohydramnios will be present and the bladder will not fill. In association with MDK the renal arteries are often very small or absent. In the remaining cases with unilateral MDK liquor would be normal. It is common to see a degree of mild renal pelvic distension on the contralateral side, but this lacks clinical significance [52]. In 10% of cases the contralateral kidney will demonstrate a PUJ obstruction (Figure 6.9). Provided there is a normally functioning kidney on the contralateral side, one

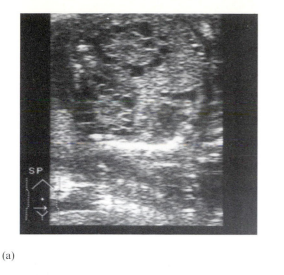

(a)

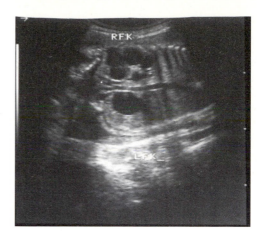

(a)

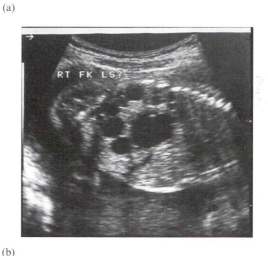

(b)

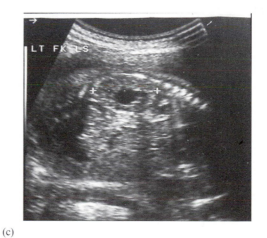

(b)

Figure 6.8 Bilateral multicystic dysplastic kidneys with absence of liquor. (a) Transverse scan. (b) Coronal scan.

(c)

Figure 6.9 Multicystic dysplastic kidney with contralateral PUJ obstruction. (a) Coronal scan. (b) Sagittal scan through right MDK. (c) Sagittal scan through right hydronephrosis due to PUJ obstruction (note normal renal parenchyma around the dilated collecting system).

would expect a normal liquor volume and a favourable prognosis for these children.

MDK ranges in size from massive enlargement (the most common cause of an abdominal mass in a neonate) to virtual agenesis. The finding of MDK disease warrants a detailed ultrasound evaluation to look for other anomalies, in particular cardiovascular abnormalities, hydrocephaly, microcephaly, spina bifida, diaphragmatic hernia, cleft palate, duodenal stenosis, imperforate anus, sirenomelia, tracheo-oesophageal fistula and bilateral absence of the radius and thumb [36]. Chromosomal anomalies have also been reported, but it is unusual for MDK to be the only abnormality. Unilateral multicystic kidneys are also associated with an increased frequency of congenital anomalies which are similar to those found in bilateral disease [29].

Unilateral MDK can be confused with a PUJ obstruction on ultrasound [6]. In MDK the cysts are usually multiple, peripheral, of variable size and are non-communicating. In the majority of cases the kidney will be enlarged. In PUJ obstruction the diagnosis is suggested by the presence of visible renal parenchyma, the fact that the cystic lesions are more central, non-spherical and communicating throughout the renal pelvis.

Isolated renal cysts

Renal abnormalities, in particular renal cystic disease, are found as part of many recognized syndromes. Certain syndromes, such as Zellweger's syndrome, asphyxiating thoracic dystrophy and Meckel's syndrome, nearly always have kidney involvement (Figure 6.10). In Meckel's syndrome 95% of cases demonstrate non-obstructive cystic renal dysplasia, with 80% having associated encephalocoele. Less common findings include polydactyly, cleft lip and palate. The identification of associated features may be difficult due to the oligohydramnios and one could argue for the need to instil normal saline by way of an amnioinfusion in order to obtain enhanced views of the fetus [56]. Conversely, this may not be necessary as the pregnancy is doomed to failure and such cases should be offered termination in view of the hopeless outcome. These cases do, however, typify the need to perform a very careful postnatal examination in order to make the correct diagnosis and adequately counsel the patients for the future. When a post-mortem is declined a careful external examination may in some cases allow the diagnosis to be made. If further information is required the parents will often agree to post-mortem ultrasound or radiology.

Renal cysts are found in various chromosomal abnormalities, in particular a third of fetuses with trisomy 13 (Figure 6.11) and 10% of fetuses with trisomy 18.

Renal tumours

Antenatally diagnosed fetal tumours are very rare. Most renal neoplasms are mesoblastic

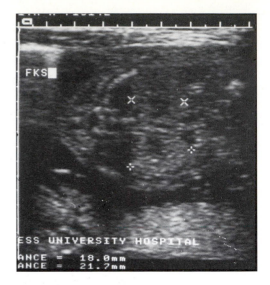

Figure 6.10 Dysplastic kidneys in thoracic asphyxiating dystrophy.

nephroma [53], which require postnatal surgical removal. Sonographic finding is of a large solitary, mainly solid, mass arising from the kidney. Polyhydramnios is frequently found in association [54,55], which may be due to pressure on the gastrointestinal tract from the tumour. The prognosis is good and there is no indication for obstetric interference.

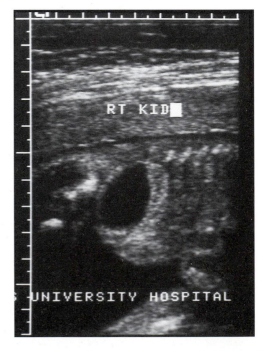

Figure 6.11 Isolated renal cyst in a fetus with trisomy 13.

Hydronephrosis

Hydronephrosis is the most commonly encountered fetal abnormality on ultrasound. It may be caused by either reflux, obstruction or low-pressure dilatation of the renal system. The obstruction can be at any level but typical sites include the ureteropelvic junction, the uterovesical junction and the urethra. We feel that postnatal follow-up should be mandatory whenever the renal pelvis exceeds 10 mm or if there is any calyceal dilatation.

Pelviureteric junction obstruction

Pelviureteric junction (PUJ) obstruction is the most common cause of fetal hydronephrosis [9] (Figure 6.12). The vast majority of cases are sporadic, although familial cases have been reported. The aetiology of the condition includes fibrous adhesions, bands, kinks, aberrant lower pole vessels and an unusual shape of the pyeloureteral outlet [57]. It is unusual to find any of the above and in the majority of cases the junction is patent and therefore

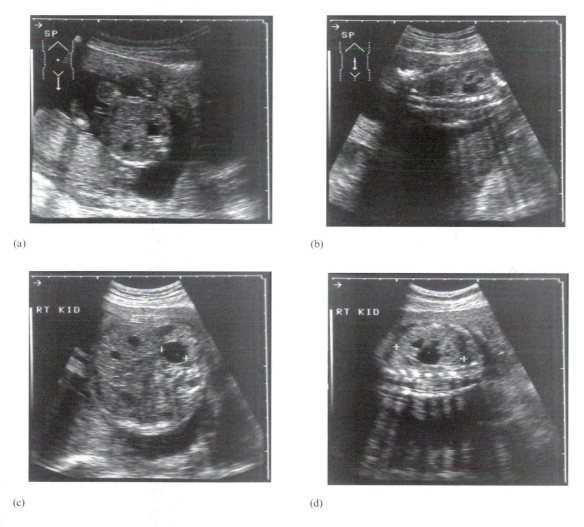

(a)　　　　　　　　　　　　　　　(b)

(c)　　　　　　　　　　　　　　　(d)

Figure 6.12 Progressive hydronephrosis due to PUJ obstruction. (a) Transverse scan at 18 weeks showing unilateral mild pelivicalyceal dilatation. (b) Coronal scan at 18 weeks. (c) Transverse scan at 30 weeks showing AP diameter of renal pelvis = 14 mm. (d) Coronal scan at 30 weeks showing dilated calyces.

pelvic dilatation would appear to be the result of a functional rather than an anatomical obstruction [58]. Thirty per cent of cases are bilateral and when unilateral are found more commonly on the left [59]. Extrarenal abnormalities are found in up to 19% of cases [60], but many are only diagnosed after birth. These include Hirschsprung's disease, cardiovascular abnormalities, neural tube defects, oesophageal atresia, imperforate anus, dislocated hips and the adrenogenital syndrome. Up to 27% of fetuses with PUJ obstruction will have associated anomalies of the urinary tract, including contralateral agenesis or cystic dysplastic kidney, vesicoureteric reflux, obstructive megaureter, meatal stenosis and hypospadias. The management depends on the degree of dilation.

There is no consensus of opinion as to what precise degree of dilation should be considered abnormal. At present we would only make the diagnosis of a PUJ obstruction based on finding a renal pelvis of greater than 10 mm in the anterior/posterior diameter with distension of the calyces. Even with this degree of dilation and more commonly with lesser degrees, it is possible for spontaneous resolution to take place prior to delivery (Figure 6.13). It is not unusual to find increased liquor in association with both unilateral and bilateral PUJ obstruction [61], although the underlying mechanism for this is unclear. The outlook for PUJ is extremely good and there is seldom a need for obstetric intervention. The most serious cases involve severe PUJ obstruction with contralateral renal agenesis or MDK. Such cases are rare, but when encountered may present with renal failure and oligohydramnios. In the remaining cases, serial ultrasound scans are recommended to check on fetal growth and liquor volume to ensure that oligohydramnios does not develop. However even with bilateral PUJ obstruction this rarely occurs. It is exceedingly important that such antenatally diagnosed fetuses are followed up by the paediatric urologists post delivery to confirm the diagnosis and plan future management.

Ureterocele

A ureterocele is a cystic dilation of the terminal end of the ureter. There is a female preponderance of 3 : 1. Between 10 and 15% of cases are bilateral [62]. When unilateral the left side is

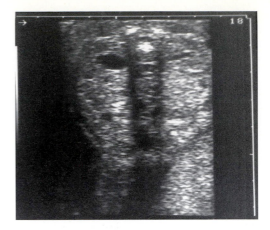

(a)

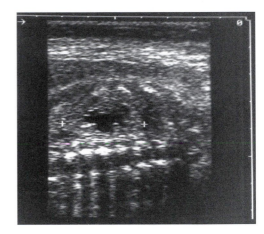

(b)

Figure 6.13 Transient pelvicalyceal dilatation at 24 weeks, with complete resolution by 36 weeks. (a) Transverse scan showing AP diameter of renal pelvis = 7 mm. (b) Coronal scan showing mildly dilated calyces.

the more common. The majority involve the upper pole of a duplex system (Figure 6.14). They can be observed by ultrasound when the fetal bladder is full. They are a cause of reflux (see below).

Megaureter with normal bladder

The normal ureter is approximately 1.5 mm wide. It is, therefore, not visible in the non-pathological state. Once it is dilated it is termed a megaureter. This is usually a sporadic condition more commonly found in males.

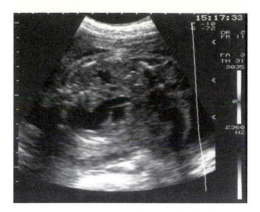

Figure 6.14 Duplex system with dilated upper pole moiety and ureter (lower pole moiety and contralateral single system show mild pyelectasis which later resolved).

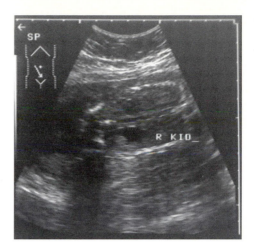

(a)

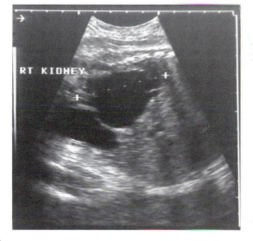

(b)

Figure 6.15 Megaureter due to ureterovesical junction obstruction. (a) Coronal scan at 18 weeks shows mild right pyelectasis. (b) Scan at 30 weeks shows gross hydronephrosis with a dilated tortous ureter.

Familial cases have been described, with vesicoureteric reflux being reported in 26–34% of asymptomatic siblings of affected individuals [63]. Causes can be divided into three groups depending on the precipitating factor, these being reflux, obstruction and an idiopathic group when the cause is neither due to reflux or obstruction but rather a functional abnormality of the ureteric wall. In obstetric practice it is usually impossible to differentiate these various causes of dilated ureters prior to birth.

The diagnosis is made sonographically by the finding of a tortuous fluid-filled structure that can be traced from the renal pelvis to the bladder (Figure 6.15). During its course it appears to touch the fetal spine. The differential diagnosis should include bowel obstruction and, in females, ovarian pathology. The former is usually associated with polyhydramnios, will be more anterior in the fetal abdomen and may demonstrate peristalsis, whereas the latter tends to be spherical in structure. In the absence of an enlarged fetal bladder, it is unlikely that this is secondary to a lower urinary tract obstruction, but it does not exclude it. Megaureter may be found in association with unilateral renal agenesis, incomplete duplex systems, ectopic kidney, contralateral cystic dysplastic kidney, horseshoe kidney and Hirschsprung's disease. In the vast majority of cases of both unilateral or bilateral megaureter the liquor volume will be normal, indicating relatively normal renal function and obstetric intervention is, therefore, not required. Occasionally renal damage may be underestimated when the liquor volume is increased due to a coexisting pathology such as bowel obstruction.

Megaureter and megacystis

With a distended bladder and bilateral megaureter, the most likely diagnosis is of urethral obstruction, secondary to posterior urethral valves or, less likely, urethral atresia. Other possible causes for such a finding include severe bilateral vesicoureteric reflux, the prune belly syndrome and the megacystis-micro-colon-intestinal hypoperistalsis syndrome.

Posterior urethral valves

Posterior urethral valves are sporadic in the majority of cases. The obstruction to urinary flow leads to hypertrophy of the detrusor muscle and gradual enlargement of the bladder. This eventually leads to reflux with resulting megaureter and hydronephrosis. Often one kidney and ureter are more severely affected than the other. It is possible on ultrasound, therefore, to appear to have unilateral renal pathology. The earlier the gestation at which the back pressure occurs on the kidney, the more likely this is to result in cystic dysplasia of that kidney. This has, therefore, led a number of workers to propose and to perform *in utero* bladder drainage. Other genitourinary system anomalies are found in 20–25% of fetuses with posterior urethral valves. These include duplication of the urethra, cryptorchidism and hypospadias. Some 20% of these fetuses are found to have chromosomal anomalies [64], including trisomy 18, 13, DEL2q and 69 XXY. Extrarenal anomalies include patent ductus arteriosus, microstenosis, tracheal hypoplasia, total anomalous pulmonary venus drainage, scoliosis and imperforate anus.

The findings on ultrasound are of a large thick-walled bladder, often with the characteristic keyhole shape, bilateral megaureter and hydronephrosis (Figure 6.16). The liquor volume will either be reduced or normal. With such a finding the fetal sex should be determined, as posterior urethral valves occur in males (Figure 6.17). The high incidence of chromosomal anomalies warrants a rapid karyotype analysis, at which time the bladder can be aspirated to assess renal function. The most reliable predictors of fetal outcome are the level of urinary sodium and calcium [12,65]. The presence of oligohydramnios and cystic dysplastic kidneys carries an extremely bad prognosis (Figure 6.18). Such a finding and/or a demonstration of an abnormal karyotype warrants the offer of a termination of pregnancy. Conversely, the finding of normal liquor volumes with low fetal urinary sodium and calcium levels indicates a good prognosis

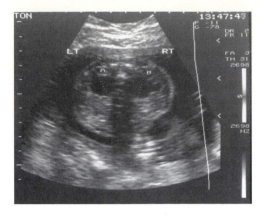

(a)

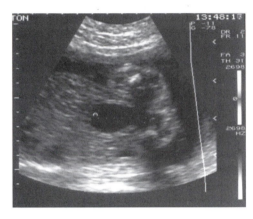

(b)

Figure 6.16 Urethral valves at 18 weeks. (a) Transverse scan showing bilateral hydronephroses. (b) Coronal scan showing distended 'keyhole-shaped' bladder.

(Figure 6.19). Having made the diagnosis, such cases should be followed with serial ultrasound scan to check liquor volume.

Prune belly syndrome

The prune belly syndrome is a combination of low-pressure dilation of the urinary tract, abdominal wall distension and cryptorchidism. The incidence is between 1 in 35 000 and 1 in 50 000, the majority of cases being male [66]. A genetic mode of inheritance has not been described, but recurrence in siblings have been reported. Cases have been described in association with trisomies 18 and

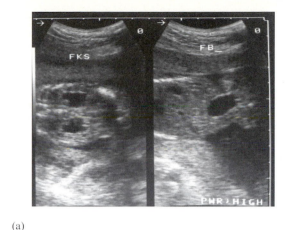

(a)

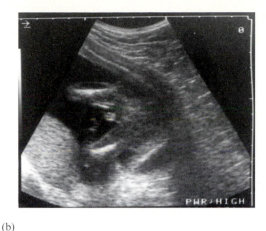

(b)

Figure 6.17 Urethral valves at 18 weeks. (a) Split image showing bilateral hydronephroses and distended bladder. (b) External genitalia confirm male gender.

13, and Turner's syndrome. An increased incidence has been found among twin pregnancies, with the incidence of twinning in prune belly syndrome being reported as 1 in 23 [67].

Fetuses with this condition are born with markedly deficient abdominal wall muscles. In 10% of cases there is an associated cardiovascular system abnormality. Other common abnormalities include talipes equinovarus, presumably secondary to oligohydramnios. Occasionally more severe limb abnormalities may be encountered, such as amputation and intestinal malrotation. The abdomen may be sufficiently enlarged as to cause dystocia at the time of delivery (Figure 6.20). The outlook is very variable and ranges from death in the neonatal period from pulmonary hypoplasia to a reasonable outlook although in the vast majority of cases abdominal wall surgery will be required, as will surgery to the urinary tract.

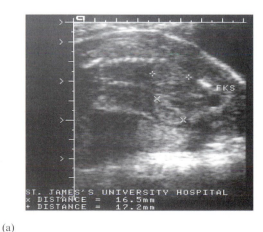

(a)

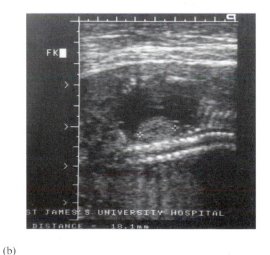

(b)

Figure 6.18 Dysplastic kidneys due to urethral valves with irreversible renal damage. (a) Small 'bright' kidneys and complete lack of liquor. (b) Small 'bright' kidney with surrounding urinary ascites.

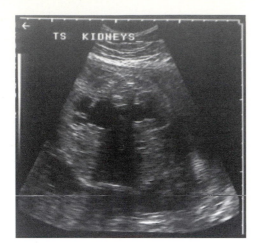

(a)

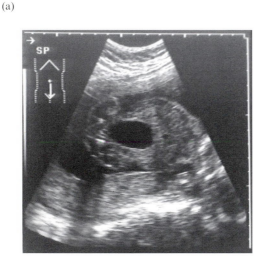

(b)

Figure 6.19 Urethral valves at 24 weeks with good prognosis confirmed by serial scans and urinary sampling. (a) Transverse scan showing bilateral hydronephrosis. (b) Distended bladder, but note presence of liquor.

Megacystis-microcolon-intestinal hypoperistalsis syndrome

This is a lethal autosomal recessive condition [68] and consists of a distended unobstructed bladder with a dilated small bowel and a microcolon. The condition should be considered, on finding an infant with a distended bladder, normal to increased amniotic fluid and dilated loops of small bowel (Figure 6.21). The probability is increased if the fetus is

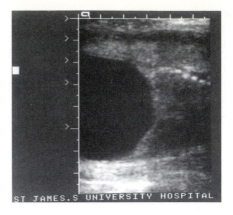

(a)

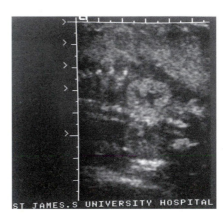

(b)

Figure 6.20 Prune belly syndrome. (a) Hugely distended urinary bladder extends up to diaphragm. (b) Dysplastic kidney with abnormal 'bright' renal parenchyma.

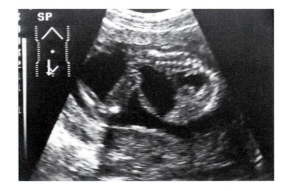

Figure 6.21 Megacystis-microcolon-intestinal hypoperistalsis syndrome: distended bladder, dilated ureter and hydronephrosis with normal liquor volume, but other scans revealed dilated fetal stomach and dilated loops of intestine.

female, since bladder outflow obstruction is rare in the female. The diagnosis can probably be made with certainty in the presence of a family history, however caution is needed in its absence. Being a lethal condition no obstetric intervention is required. However one case of dystocia at the time of delivery has been reported [69] secondary to the massively distended bladder. If this were anticipated it would be a simple matter to tap the bladder prior to attempting a vaginal delivery.

References

1. Bronshtein M, Yoffe N, Brandes JM, Blumenfeld Z. First and early second trimester diagnosis of fetal urinary tract anomalies using transvaginal sonography. *Prenat Diagn* 1990; **10**: 653–666.
2. Thomas DFM, Irving HC, Arthur RJ. Pre-natal diagnosis: how useful is it? *Br J Urol* 1985; **57**: 748–787.
3. Rosendahl H. Ultrasound screening for fetal urinary tract malformations: a prospective study in general population. *Eur J Obstet Gynecol Reprod Biol* 1990; **36**: 27–33.
4. Benacerraf BR, Mandell J, Estroff JA, Harlow BL, Frigoletto FD. Fetal pyelectasis: a possible association with Down's syndrome *Obstet Gynecol* 1990; **76**: 58–60.
5. Arthur RJ, Irving HC, Thomas DFM, Watters JK. Bilateral fetal uropathy. What is the outlook? *Br Med J* 1989; **298**: 1419–1420.
6. Greig AC, Raine PAM, Young DG et al. Value of antenatal diagnosis of abnormalities of the urinary tract. *Br Med J* 1989; **298**: 1417–1419.
7. White RHR. Fetal uropathy. *Br Med J* 1989; **298**: 1408–1409.
8. Gordon AC, Thomas DF, Arthur RJ, Irving HC, Smith SE. Prenatally diagnosed reflux: a follow-up study. *Br J Urol* 1990; **65**: 407–412.
9. Mandell J, Blyth BR, Peters CA, Retik AB, Estroff JA, Benacerraf BR. Structural genitourinary defects detected in utero. *Radiology* 1991; **178**: 193–196.
10. Gruenewald SM, Cohen RC, Antico VF, Farlow DC, Cass DT. Diagnosis and treatment of antenatal uropathies. *J Paed Child Health* 1990; **26**: 142–247.
11. Nolte S, Mueller B, Pringsheim W. Serum alpha 1-microglobin and beta 2-microglobulin for the estimation of fetal glomerular renal function. *Pediatr Nephrol* 1991; **5**: 573–577.
12. Nicolini U, Fisk NM, Rodeck CH. Fetal urine biochemistry: an index of renal maturation and dysfunction. *Br J Obstet Gynecol* 1992; **99**: 46–50.
13. Nimrod C, Nichollson S, Davies D, Harder J, Dodds G, Scuve R. Pulmonary hypoplasia testing in clinical obstetrics. *Am J Obstet Gynecol* 1988; **158**: 277–280.
14. Blott M, Greenough A, Nicolaides KH, Moscoso G, Gibb D, Campbell S. Fetal breathing movements as predictor of favourable pregnancy outcome after oligohydramnios due to membrane rupture in second trimester. *Lancet* 1987; **ii**: 129–131.
15. Moessinger AC, Fox HE, Higgins A, Rey HR, Al Haideri M. Fetal breathing movements are not a reliable predictor of continued lung development in pregnancies complicated by oligohydramnios. *Lancet* 1987; **ii**: 1297–1300.
16. Fisk NM, Talbert B, Nicolini U, Vaughan J, Rodeck CH. Fetal breathing movements in oligohydramnios are not increased by amnioinfusion. *Br J Obstet Gynaecol* 1992; **99**: 464–468.
17. Cortville JE, Dickie JM, Crane JP. Fetal pyelectasis and Down syndrome: is genetic amniocentesis warranted? *Obstet Gynecol* 1992; **79**: 770–772.
18. Edoux P, Choiset A, Leporrier N et al. Chromosomal prenatal diagnosis: study of 936 cases of intrauterine abnormalities after ultrasound assessment. *Prenat Diagn* 1989; **9**: 255–268.
19. Potter EL. Bilateral absence of ureters and kidneys. A report of 50 cases. *Obstet Gynecol* 1965; **25**: 3–12.
20. Carter CO, Evans K. Birth frequency of bilateral renal agenesis. *J Med Genet* 1981; **18**: 158.
21. Wilson RD, Baird PA. Renal agenesis in British Columbia. *Am J Med Genet* 1985; **21**: 153–169.
22. Burn J, Marwood RP. Fraser syndrome presenting as bilateral renal agenesis in three sibs. *J Med Genet* 1982; **19**: 360.
23. Carmi R, Binshtock M, Abeliovich D et al. The branchio-oto-renal (BOR) syndrome: report of bilateral renal agenesis in three sibs. *Am J Med Genet* 1983; **14**: 625.
24. Uehling DT, Gilbert E, Chesney R. Urologic implications of the VATER association. *J Urol* 1983; **129**: 352.
25. Roodhooft AM, Birnholz JC, Holmes LB. Familial nature of congenital absence and severe dysplasia of both kidneys. *N Engl J Med* 1984; **310**: 1341–1345.
26. Waldimiroff JW. Effect of furosemide on fetal urine production. *Br J Obstet Gynaecol* 1975; **82**: 221–224.
27. Romero R, Cullen M, Grannum P et al. Antenatal diagnosis of renal anomalies with ultrasound. III. Bilateral renal agenesis. *Am J Obstet Gynecol* 1985; **151**: 38.
28. Droste S, Fitzsimmons J, Pascoe-Mason J, Shepard TH, Mack LA. Size of the fetal adrenal in bilateral renal agenesis. *Obstet Gynecol* 1990; **76**: 206–209.
29. Bearman DB, Hine PL, Sanders RC. Multicystic kidney: a sonographic pattern. *Radiology* 1976; **118**: 685–688.
30. Ratten GJ, Beischer NA, Fortune DW. Obstetric complications when the fetus has Potter's syndrome. I. Clinical considerations. *Am J Obstet Gynecol* 1973; **115**: 890.
31. Austin CW, Brown JM, Friday RO. Unilateral renal agenesis presenting as a pseudo mass in utero *J Ultrasound Med* 1984; **3**: 177–179.

32. Hartshorne N, Shepard T, Barr M Jr. Compensatory renal growth in human fetuses with unilateral renal agenesis. *Teratology* 1991; **44**: 7–10.

33. Emmanuel B, Nachman R, Aronson N et al. Congenital solitary kidney. A review of 74 cases. *Am J Dis Child* 1974; **127**: 17.

34. Campbell MF. Anomalies of the kidney. In: Campbell MF, Harrison JH (eds) *Urology*. Philadelphia: WB Saunders, 1970; pp 1447–1452.

35. Fong KW, Rahmani MR, Rose TH, Skidmore MB, Connor TP. Fetal renal cystic disease: sonographic–pathologic correlation. *Am J Roentgenol* 1986; **146**: 767–773.

36. D'Alton M, Romero R, Grannum P et al. Antenatal diagnosis of renal anomalies with ultrasound, IV: Bilateral multicystic kidney disease. *Am J Obstet Gynecol* 1986; **54**: 532–537.

37. Potter EL. Type I cystic kidney: tubular gigantism. In: *Normal and Abnormal Development of the Kidney*. Chicago: Year Book 1972; pp 141–153.

38. Boal DK, Teel RL. Sonography of infantile polycystic disease. *Am J Radiol* 1980; **135**: 575–580.

39. Luthy DA, Hirsh JH. Infantile polycystic kidney disease. Observations from attempts at prenatal diagnosis. *Am J Med Genet* 1985; **20**: 505–517.

40. Romero R, Cullen M, Jeanty P et al. The diagnosis of congenital renal anomalies with ultrasound. II. Infantile polycystic kidney disease. *Am J Obstet Gynecol* 1984; **150**: 259–262.

41. Lilford RJ, Irving HC, Allibone EB. A tale of two prior probabilities – avoiding the false positive antenatal diagnosis of autosomal recessive polycystic kidney disease. *Br J Obstet Gynecol* 1992; **99**: 216–219.

42. Blyth H, Ockenden BG. Polycystic disease of kidneys and liver presenting in childhood. *J Med Genet* 1971; **8**: 257–284.

43. Sabbagha BE. *Diagnostic Ultrasound in Obstetrics and Gynaecology*. Philadelphia: JB Lippincott 1987; pp 387–388.

44. Romero R, Pilu G, Jeanty P, Ghidini A, Hobbins JC. Adult polycystic kidney disease. In: *Prenatal Diagnosis of Congenital Abnormalities*. Norwalk, Connecticut, California: Appleton & Lange, 1988; pp 268–270.

45. Bronshtein M, Kushnir O, Ben-Rafeal Z et al. Transvaginal sonographic measurement of fetal kidneys in the first trimester of pregnancy. *J Clin Ultrasound* 1990; **18**: 299–301.

46. Bronshtein M, Bar-Hava I, Blumenfeld Z. Clues and pitfalls in the early prenatal diagnosis of 'late onset' infantile polycystic kidney. *Prenat Diagn* 1992; **12**: 293–298.

47. Milutinovic J, Failkow PJ, Phillips LA et al. Autosomal dominant polycystic kidney disease. Early diagnosis and data for genetic counselling. *Lancet* 1980; **i**: 1203.

48. Zerres K, Volpel MC, Weiss H. Cystic kidneys. Genetics, pathologic anatomy, clinical picture and prenatal diagnosis. *Hum Genet* **68**: 104–135.

49. Journel H, Guyot C, Barc RM, Belbeoch P, Quemener A, Jouan H. Unexpected ultrasonographic prenatal diagnosis of autosomal dominant polycystic kidney disease. *Prenat Diagn* 1989; **9**: 663–671.

50. Ceccherini I, Lituania M, Cordone MS et al. Autosomal dominant polycystic kidney disease: prenatal diagnosis by DNA analysis and sonography at 14 weeks. *Prenat Diagn* 1989; **11**: 751–758.

51. Turco A, Peissel B, Quaia P, Morandi R, Bovicelli L, Pignatti PF. Prenatal diagnosis of autosomal dominant polycystic kidney disease using flanking DNA markers and the polymerase chain reaction. *Prenat Diagn* 1992; **12**: 513–524.

52. Kleiner B, Filly RA, Mack I et al. Multicystic dysplastic kidney: observations of contralateral disease in the fetal population. *Radiology* 1986; **161**: 27–29.

53. Guilian BB. Prenatal ultrasonographic diagnosis of fetal renal tumors. *Radiology* 1984; **152**: 69–70.

54. Blank E, Neerhout RC, Burry KA. Congenital mesoblastic nephroma and polyhydramnios. *JAMA* 1978; **240**: 1504.

55. Geirron RT, Ricketts NEM, Taylor DJ et al. Prenatal appearance of a mesoblastic nephroma associated with polyhydramnios. *J Clin Ultrasound* 1985; **13**: 488–490.

56. Fisk NM, Ronderos-Dumit D, Soliani A, Nicolini U, Vaughan J, Rodeck CH. Diagnostic and therapeutic transabdominal amnioinfusion in oligohydramnios. *Obstet Gynecol* 1991; **78**: 270–278.

57. Hanna MK, Jeffs RD, Sturgess JM et al. Ureteral structure and ultrastructure. Part II: Congenital ureteropelvic junction obstruction and primary obstructive megaureter. *J Urol* 1976; **116**: 725–730.

58. Antonakopoulos GN, Fuggle WJ, Newman J et al. Idiopathic hydronephrosis. *Arch Pathol Lab Med* 1985; **109**: 1097–1101.

59. Drake DP, Stevens PS, Eckstein HB. Hydronephrosis secondary to ureteropelvic obstruction in children. A review of 14 years of experience. *J Urol* 1978; **119**: 649.

60. Johannessen JV, Haneberg B, Moe PJ. Bilateral multicystic dysplasia of the kidneys. *Beitr Pathol Bd* 1973; **148**: 290.

61. Bosman G, Reuss A, Nijman JM, Wladimiroff JW. Prenatal diagnosis, management and outcome of fetal uretero-pelvic junction obstruction. *Ultrasound Med Biol* 1991; **17**: 117–120.

62. Mandell J, Colodny AH, Lebowitz R et al. Ureteroceles in infants and children. *J Urol* 1980; **123**: 921.

63. Dwoskin JY. Siblings uropathology. *J Urol* 1976; **115**: 726–727.

64. Nicolaides KH, Rodeck CH, Gosden CM. Rapid karyotyping in non-lethal fetal malformations. *Lancet* 1986; **i**: 283.

65. Crombleholme TM, Harrison MR, Golbus MS et al. Fetal intervention in obstructive uropathy: prognostic indicators and efficacy of intervention. *Am J Obstet Gynecol* 1990; **162**: 1239–1224.

66. Garlinger P, Ott J. Prune-belly syndrome. Possible genetic implications. *Birth Defects* 1974; **10**: 173.

67. Ives EJ. The abdominal muscle deficiency triad syndrome. Experience with 10 cases. *Birth Defects* 1974; **10**: 127.

68. Lilford RJ, Penman DG. The megacystis-microcolon-intestinal hypoperistalsis syndrome. A fetal auto-somal recessive condition. *J Med Ethics* 1987; **26**: 66–67.

69. Puri P, Lake BD, Gorman F et al. Megacystic-microcolon-intestinal hypoperistalsis syndrome. A visceral myopathy. *J Pediatr Surg* 1983; **18**: 64.

7

Fetal intervention

S. Bewley and C.H. Rodeck

Introduction

As perinatal mortality rates continue to fall, deaths due to fetal abnormality are proportionally increasing [1]. Renal problems, especially dilatation of the renal pelvis, are the commonest ultrasound abnormalities detected during pregnancy (Figure 7.1). Urinary tract abnormalities are found in 0.3% of the general population [2] and almost 1% of babies have a congenital uropathy of some kind [3], although rates as high as 1.8% have been quoted in the first trimester [4]. Malformations of the urinary tract are common, causing morbidity and mortality. Perinatal deaths due to renal abnormalities make up about 4% of those due to congenital abnormality [5].

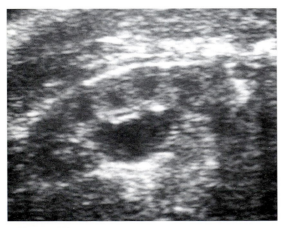

Figure 7.1 Ultrasound showing mild renal pelvic dilatation

There is a wide spectrum of severity, the poor outcome in obstructive uropathy being related to its secondary effects, rather than the disease itself which is surgically correctable. This is of especial importance because these effects may be preventable. Other renal diseases, such as multicystic kidney disease or polycystic kidneys, are easier to diagnose but the management options are very limited. Intervention can be diagnostic or therapeutic, and it is important both to obtain a prognosis for the parents and to help guide management. There are three main management options during fetal life: ultrasound follow-up, termination of pregnancy and *in utero* treatment to bypass the obstruction.

Definition and classification

Abnormalities of the fetal urinary tract fall into two groups:

1. *The collecting system* – dilatation of all or part of the urinary tract.
2. *The renal parenchyma* – cystic changes, bright echogenicity or reduced parenchyma.

Obstructive uropathy is considered when dilatation of all or part of the urinary tract is seen on ultrasound. Not all dilatation is due to obstruction however; it may be due to reflux or to a previous obstruction. For example, in the prune belly syndrome, megacystis and megaureter can be present without obstruction (Figure 7.2). If there is a dilated urinary tract

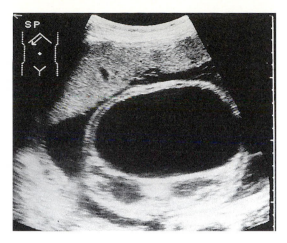

Figure 7.2 Megacystis and bilateral megaureter at 18 weeks with normal amniotic fluid.

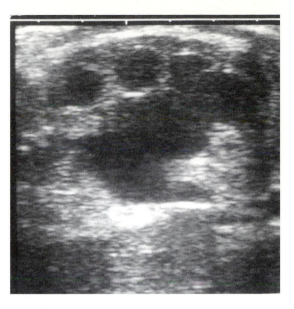

Figure 7.3 Moderate hydronephrosis with intra- and extrarenal pelvic dilation. Dilated calyces can be differentiated from cortical cysts by the demonstration of continuity with the renal pelvis.

with oligohydramnios, obstruction can be confidently diagnosed. Dilatation in the presence of normal amniotic fluid is likely to be functional, although there might be a partial or intermittent obstruction. Lax and tortuous ureters are another feature of non-obstructive distension. The minor degrees of hydronephrosis overlap with normal pelvic ureteric junctions (PUJ). There may be faulty innervation of the PUJ as there is no anatomical evidence of obstruction, and only a slight diminution of pelvic emptying will lead to distension.

The definition of severity of hydronephrosis is arbitrary and can be made subjectively (mild, moderate or severe) or objectively (using measurements of the pelvis and parenchymal thickness). Measurement of the anteroposterior diameter of the pelvis is made on transverse scan, and a cut-off of ≤5 mm is considered normal in the second trimester. The cut-offs for mild, moderate and severe hydronephrosis are 5–9 mm, 10–14 mm and ≥15 mm respectively (Figure 7.3).

Dilatation can be described in several ways:

1. Upper or lower urinary tract.
2. Unilateral or bilateral.
3. By precise site.

Upper tract dilatation can be caused by PUJ obstruction or functional dilatation, uretero-vesical obstruction, ureterocele and vesico-ureteric reflux and may be unilateral or bilateral. Lower tract obstruction is associated with bilateral disease, although the two sides may not be affected equally, and urethral obstruction is more serious as both kidneys are threatened.

There is a wide spectrum of severity of distension which can be broadly classified into three main clinical pictures:

1. *Upper tract dilatation* can be difficult to distinguish from reflux, and is probably largely functional. Even when bilateral, oligohydramnios is rare and there is a better prognosis than with lower tract obstruction [6]. No action usually needs to be taken, apart from karyotyping.
2. *Posterior urethral valves (PUV)* are associated with varying degrees of distension, dysplasia and oligohydramnios. Although there is dispute about the value of ultrasound screening for urinary tract abnormalities [3,7,8], the main objective is to identify these cases, as intervention during pregnancy may be of benefit.
3. *Urethral atresia* is the most severe form of obstructive uropathy associated with early-onset oligohydramnios. The kidneys are usually severely dysplastic, shrunken and echogenic. Urinary distension is variable, but can be enormous. No therapeutic action is presently possible.

Posterior urethral valves

Posterior urethral valves (PUV) or urethral atresia are suspected when megacystis accompanies dilated ureters. The birth of a male fetus with PUV is not common (1–2/10 000 male births [9,10]). There is an overlap of the severe end of PUV with urethral atresia, and also with prune belly (where no evidence of obstruction is seen at birth, although some features suggest *in utero* obstruction). There may or may not be oligohydramnios as the obstruction may be partial, or intermittent, or start at different gestational ages. The purpose of prenatal intervention is to halt or ameliorate the effects of obstruction, and is largely confined to cases of PUV.

The differential diagnosis of PUV includes other abdominal cystic lesions such as multicystic kidney, mesenteric cyst, ovarian cyst and bowel dilatation, amongst others (Figure 7.4). Megacystis-microcolon-intestinal-hypoperistalsis (MMIH) usually presents initially as megacystis alone, the gut dilatation appearing later in the third trimester. The prognosis is very poor with 80% mortality in infancy.

Prune belly syndrome

Prune belly syndrome is rare, occurring in approximately 1 in 30–50 000 births [11], and has been thought to be due to longstanding megacystis or gross urinary ascites that has resolved (Figure 7.5). It has been hypothesized that there could be a primary mesodermal defect affecting muscularization of both the abdominal and urinary tracts, which explains the lack of evidence for infravesical obstruction, particularly in females [12]. Alternatively, a temporary obstruction leads to dilatation of the urinary tract, secondary cryptorchidism and the development of urinary ascites. Occasionally, prune belly is found with PUV, and the finding of megalourethra also supports the concept of a distal (if transient) obstruction at the junction of the glandular and penile urethra [13,14]. This has been diagnosed antenatally [15]. Once there is massive, low pressure distension of the urinary tract it becomes difficult to treat. First, there is no vesicoamniotic pressure difference and thus no outward flow and, secondly, the abdominal wall is so flaccid that shunts, if inserted, fall out easily (C.H. Rodeck, unpublished observation, 1995).

Natural history of untreated obstructive uropathy

Knowledge of the natural history is essential to assess prognosis and the efficacy of therapeutic interventions. The poor perinatal outcome is associated with renal dysplasia and pulmonary

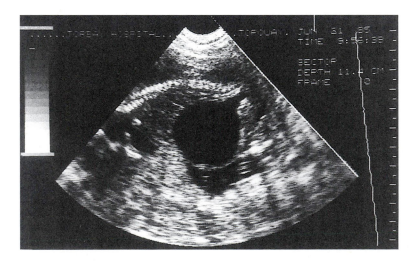

Figure 7.4 Dilated posterior urethra, with characteristic 'retort' shape and enlarged bladder in fetus with PUV at 20 weeks. Oligohydramnios adversely affects the quality of ultrasound visualization.

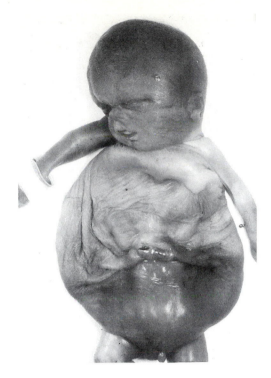

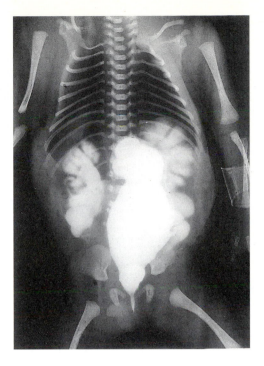

Figure 7.5 Fetus with massive prune belly syndrome secondary to urinary ascites, following termination of pregnancy at 24 weeks. Antenatal decompression of the abdomen was required to ensure vaginal delivery. (By courtesy of Virginia Sams.)

Figure 7.6 Post-mortem contrast study of a 36-week stillborn baby with Potter's syndrome demonstrating megacystis, megaureters and urethral atresia. (By courtesy of Virginia Sams.)

hypoplasia [16–18]. Potter's sequence of pulmonary hypoplasia, low-set ears, talipes and contractures is caused by longstanding oligohydramnios. Back pressure from obstruction can lead to reflux (Figure 7.6), extravasation of urine, bladder rupture, urinary ascites and urinomas [19–21].

To determine the natural history of untreated obstructive uropathy, Reuss et al. [22] examined a series of 43 consecutive cases of obstructive uropathy that were given no treatment. They found that 31 died (72%) and only 12 (28%) survived. The majority of those that died (23/31, 74%) had renal dysplasia and pulmonary hypoplasia (13/31, 42%). However, the outcome was heavily influenced by the 18 (42%) found to have other renal or extrarenal anomalies, including five abnormal karyotypes. Survival was related to the type of obstruction, with 8/9 survivors of PUV (89%) and 0/27 survivors with urethral atresia. When 76 consecutive cases of obstructive uropathy were divided into high- and low-level obstructions, the sur-

vival rates were 86% and 12% respectively [23]. In a series of infants presenting postnatally with PUV, Nakayama found that 5/21 (24%) died of pulmonary hypoplasia [17].

The discrepancy in survival figures may be due both to the bias in selecting pre- or postnatally and to the small numbers involved. However, this means that the results of *in utero* treatment compared to no treatment are difficult to assess.

There is also a discrepancy in the effect of sex on outcome. Reuss found the survival rate for females was better (4/6, 67%) than males (8/37, 22%) [22], although the International Registry reported the opposite, with lower survival amongst female fetuses (1/5, 20%) than males (29/57, 51%) [24]. Again, differences in case selection may be responsible.

The long-term prognosis of untreated PUV diagnosed *in utero* is unclear, and awaits follow-up studies. However, it probably includes reflux, recurrent urinary tract infection, chronic pyelonephritis, hypertension, renal failure, chronic dialysis and transplantation.

Assessment of prognosis in obstructive uropathy

Prognosis is determined by:

1. *The diagnosis* (and its severity and extent).
2. *Renal and lung function.*
3. The presence or absence of *other abnormalities.*

As outcome is strongly related to the presence or absence of other structural or chromosomal anomalies, diagnosis is initially concerned with confirming the abnormality and excluding other problems.

There are three ultrasound-guided invasive procedures relating to accurate diagnosis and assessment of renal function: amnioinfusion, karyotyping and urine sampling.

Diagnosis of associated abnormalities

Amnioinfusion in oligohydramnios

Amnioinfusion of 100–200 ml of normal saline using a 20G needle can be used to improve the ultrasound picture in cases of severe oligohydramnios (deepest pool of amniotic fluid <1 cm). Care has to be taken to avoid extra-amniotic instillation of fluid. This may be complemented by instillation of 10–20 ml of intraperitoneal saline to obtain a clearer view of the fetal kidneys, or lack of them [25]. In obstructive uropathy with oligohydramnios, amniotic fluid instillation is helpful in delineating talipes and other anomalies, especially subtle markers of chromosome defects. It is also used immediately before insertion of a shunt, as delineation of the fetal abdomen allows correct placement of the outer part of the catheter in the amniotic cavity and reduces the risk of trauma to the umbilical cord.

The prognosis for fetuses with anhydramnios without renal tract dilatation in the second trimester is very poor, as the differential diagnosis is renal agenesis, renal dysplasia, preterm premature rupture of the membranes or early-onset intrauterine growth retardation. The use of amnioinfusion can change the prenatal diagnosis in up to 13% of cases [26].

Karyotyping

The incidence of chromosomal anomaly varies both with gestational age of testing and with the renal pathology and is summarized in Table 7.1. The rate of karyotype abnormality is slightly higher when disease is bilateral, and very high when other abnormalities are present. Karyotyping can be performed on amniotic fluid, or more rapidly, using fetal blood or chorionic villi. It can also be performed on amniotic cavity washings after amnioinfusion and occasionally on urine samples.

Post-mortem

Good post-mortem follow-up is essential, ideally performed by a perinatal pathologist. Some anomalies are not, or cannot be, diagnosed antenatally and are only found at post-mortem (whether after termination, intrauterine or infant death). They may change the diagnosis, or have important implications for counselling regarding future pregnancies.

Table 7.1 Abnormal fetal karyotype in 682 fetuses with unilateral or bilateral renal abnormalities, divided into those with isolated problems or associated with additional malformations

Renal defect	Isolated		With other defects	
	Unilateral	Bilateral	Unilateral	Bilateral
Mild hydronephrosis	0% (0/10)	3% (5/163)	25% (2/8)	32% (30/95)
Moderate hydronephrosis		6% (5/81)		26% (10/38)
Severe hydronephrosis	1% (1/76)		64% (7/11)	
Multicystic kidney	2% (1/48)	4% (3/79)	44% (7/16)	33% (10/30)
Renal agenesis	0% (0/0)	5% (1/79)	33% (1/3)	40% (2/9)

Adapted from Cheng and Nicholaides [27].

Ultrasound assessment of the urinary tract

Ultrasound scanning is the mainstay of diagnosis although the presence of oligohydramnios, which removes the 'acoustic window', can lead to inaccuracies [28], which may be minimized with amnioinfusion [29,30].

Amniotic fluid volume

The simplest measure of renal function is the assessment of amniotic fluid volume. A normal amount implies that urine is being produced by the kidneys and that there is no, or at most partial, obstruction. Decreased amniotic fluid might be due to renal failure or a lack of micturition. This can be a subjective assessment, or objective, using the depth of the deepest pool, or amniotic fluid index [31] (AFI), from the four quadrants of the uterus, but all measures have poor reproducibility [32]. Oligohydramnios is defined as a deepest pool <2 cm, or AFI <8 cm.

Urine does not contribute significantly to the amniotic fluid until the second trimester [33]. Diagnosis of renal agenesis with oligohydramnios can be made at about 15–16 weeks, at the earliest.

Even in the second trimester, oligohydramnios is not a reliable indicator of renal failure. Nicolaides has reported that it may be seen in cases of obstructive uropathy with good prognosis (5/20, 25%), and not be present in many cases with renal dysplasia (15/40, 38%) [34].

Renal parenchyma

Ultrasound can be helpful in identifying some cases of dysplasia, but, again, it is not definitive. Hyperechogenicity of the renal parenchyma (brighter than the fetal lung fields) is suggestive of renal dysplasia, although the prediction is inaccurate with a sensitivity and specificity of only 73% and 80% [35]. Not all echogenic kidneys are dysplastic and vice versa. There is special difficulty in assessing echogenicity in those cases with severe hydronephrosis causing parenchymal compression, with oligohydramnios or with urinary ascites. In addition, appearances can change on serial scanning, or following urinary drainage or shunt insertion.

Renal cortical cysts

Mahoney et al. [35] independently compared antenatal ultrasound findings with histopathology of 49 kidneys from 33 fetuses with obstructive uropathy. Dysplasia was present in all 15 cases with renal cortical cysts (100% specificity), but the absence of cysts did not exclude it (19/34, 44% sensitivity). It can be difficult distinguishing between renal cysts and dilated calyces [36]. It is helpful when diagnosing the latter to demonstrate a communication with the pelvicalyceal system.

Hydronephrosis

The degree of hydronephrosis is the least reliable predictor of dysplasia. Calyceal blunting and parenchymal thinning predicts dysplasia with a sensitivity and specificity of only 41% and 73% [35]. It is understandable that dysplasia might occur without severe hydronephrosis, as urine production may decrease after dysplasia occurs and the dilatation subsides [37,38]. The urinary tract may also decompress after bladder rupture [19]. Urethral obstruction may lead to pronounced dilatation of the bladder and ureters and minimal pelvicalyceal dilation and still be associated with dysplasia [37,39].

Assessment of renal function

There are several non-invasive measures of renal function. The purpose of urine sampling is to gauge accurate information for prognosis, if a mother would proceed to termination or if an invasive procedure were contemplated. The major problem with the management of the prenatally diagnosed obstructive uropathies is the difficulty in obtaining predictive information about which fetus has adequate renal function now and which fetus, although having adequate function now, will not have in the future, and thus might benefit from relief of the obstruction. In addition to the lack of a predictive test, there is little known about long-term follow-up and renal function over years.

Indirect measures of function

Indirect measures of the functional potential of obstructed kidneys include bladder filling and emptying [40] and frusemide stimulation of urine production [41], but these measures have found little favour [42].

Fetal blood tests

Although fetal blood samples have provided normal ranges for substances of renal origin, most of these cross the placenta and therefore do not accumulate in renal failure. $\beta 2$-microglobulin, in contrast to urea and creatinine, does not cross the placenta, and might thus predict fetal glomerular function independently of maternal renal function. $\beta 2$-microglobulin has been found to be raised in fetal serum in fetuses with urinary tract anomalies, but as this may be so even with unilateral damage it is not yet a usual test [43]. Cord blood levels taken at birth in babies with antenatally diagnosed renal anomalies predict severe renal disease [44], although they are not used in practice.

Urine sampling

Urine can be obtained from either a distended bladder or the renal pelvis, or both (Figure 7.7). Normal ranges have been devised for a variety of compounds (see Chapter 4). Urine aspiration has several functions:

1. Urinary electrolytes can be evaluated.
2. Intravesical pressure can be measured.

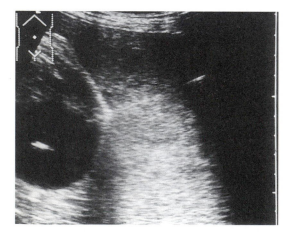

Figure 7.7 Ultrasound-guided placement of needle (entering from the right) into dilated bladder for urine sampling.

3. Refilling can be observed.
4. A comparison can be made between samples taken on different occasions or from different sites (bladder and both kidneys).

1. Urinary electrolytes

Urinary electrolyte composition changes as gestational age advances. Sodium and phosphate show a fall, whilst creatinine rises [45] (see Chapter 4). However, confusion has arisen in the literature because fixed levels have been used as criteria for selecting cases for shunting. For example, the cut-offs advised by Glick et al. [46] of urinary $Na^+ > 100\,mEq/l$, $Cl^- > 90\,mEq/l$ and osmolality $>210\,mosmol/l$ do not take account of the normal changes in urine electrolytes with gestation [47], and have proved unreliable [48,49].

Nicolini et al. [45] divided a group of 25 fetuses with obstructive uropathy into those with (15) and without (10) dysplasia. All fetuses had significantly decreased urea and increased calcium concentrations, whereas sodium, potassium and phosphate were significantly increased only in cases of dysplasia. Calcium was the most sensitive for the detection of renal dysplasia, and sodium the most specific.

Nicolaides et al. [34] showed that the fetuses with renal dysplasia (35) or infantile chronic renal failure (5) had significantly raised sodium and calcium, and significantly lower urea and creatinine, compared to fetuses with obstructive uropathy without dysplasia (20). All fetuses with multicystic kidneys had renal dysplasia. A combination of mildly hydronephrotic, hyperechogenic kidneys or moderate-to-severe hydronephrosis with either high calcium or high sodium was the best predictor of poor outcome.

The predictive properties of raised sodium and calcium were confirmed by Lipitz et al. [50] in a group of 25 fetuses with PUV. They also assessed $\beta 2$-microglobulin and N-acetyl-β-D-glucosaminidase, and noted that a raised $\beta 2$-microglobulin was found in many survivors with impaired renal function, suggesting that this was an early sign of renal damage, though not predictive of a fatal outcome.

A confounding factor in assessing renal function is the mixing of urine in the bladder from two differentially affected kidneys. To clarify this, it may be necessary to sample the bladder and kidneys separately. This has been shown by a case of successful shunting in a fetus with severely abnormal electrolytes from the bladder and one severely hydronephrotic kidney, but preservation of good function in the other [51].

2. Intravesical pressure

Although renal damage occurs when urinary pressure exceeds glomerular pressure and high urinary tract pressures have been reported in some children with obstructive uropathy, by contrast, low intravesical pressures are found in fetuses with low obstructive uropathies, even when high urinary sodium suggests renal damage [52]. End-stage failure would be expected to lead to absent renal function and urine production, low pressure and high sodium.

3. Reaccumulation of urine

Although the return of urine to the urinary tract after drainage is reassuring, as is the re-accumulation of amniotic fluid after shunting, these observations can occur in the presence of renal dysplasia [53] and thus do not provide conclusive evidence of good renal function. If reaccumulation is only noted in the bladder, it may be due to influx of old urine from tortuous ureters rather than new production.

4. Second sample

The extent of renal damage is not assessed by the speed of reaccumulation of urine in the urinary tract (although failure to reaccumulate is very sinister), but by the change in electrolytes. If the bladder is emptied, reaccumulation of urine enables a second sample to be taken the next day which may show an improvement, i.e. more physiological electrolytes, although such an observation can occur with dysplastic and normal kidneys alike [54]. In cases presenting early, when sodium is normally high, it is reassuring if a fall in sodium is demonstrated on a second urine sample.

Several workers have suggested serial sampling to assess function [54,55], reasoning that the first urine sample represents 'old' renal function, whereas the second represents 'current' function. However, there is a difference between 'freshly produced' first-day sampling, when electrolytes all tend to improve, and serial sampling which assesses maturation and the effect of the renal pathology on that maturation.

Weekly serial sampling

Sampling of the kidneys and bladder can immediately relieve the back pressure on the urinary tract, and may have a therapeutic value in itself. However, this would have to be continually repeated, and the time interval for reaccumulation is not clear. Serial decompression does not correct oligohydramnios and thus cannot protect the lungs and extremities, although it may have a place later in the third trimester.

Weekly serial sampling can be an essential part of management, particularly in cases presenting early in the second trimester, when it is both too early for shunting, and the physiological levels of sodium are too high to make the test of diagnostic value. Serial sampling should show a fall in sodium levels (indicating continued maturation of renal function) despite continuing ultrasound evidence of obstruction [45].

Nuclear magnetic resonance spectroscopy

High resolution nuclear magnetic resonance (NMR) spectroscopy can investigate the total biochemical composition of fetal urine, and the patterns of spectra in disease [56,57]. It has the advantage of tremendous complexity of information with preservation of the urine sample, but requires large capital costs, and is therefore only a research tool at present. There has been little work yet in fetal life, but it has the potential both for early recognition of a failing kidney and assessment of recovery.

The potential of *in utero* therapy

There are a range of management options in obstructive uropathy:

1. *Conservative* management (or masterly in-activity).
2. *Termination* of pregnancy.
3. *Monitoring* with the possibility of *in utero* intervention, or termination, depending on the results of serial scanning and samplings.
4. Early *delivery* (if mature enough).

Consideration of termination as an option is inversely related to the gestation at diagnosis. This is partly related to the worse prognosis, with early detection of the more severe abnormalities, and partly related to the practical and emotional difficulties of late termination. Whether to terminate or continue the pregnancy depends crucially on the prognosis. For many parents, the pragmatic approach to a non-recurrent condition with a poor prognosis is to choose termination and try again in a future pregnancy. For those who elect to continue, the main determinants of perinatal outcome in chromosomally and otherwise structurally normal fetuses with PUV are pulmonary hypoplasia and renal dysplasia [18].

Pulmonary hypoplasia

Oligohydramnios is traditionally thought to cause pulmonary hypoplasia by external pressure on the chest; however, new evidence indicates that amniotic pressure is low in oligohydramnios [52,58], suggesting that pulmonary hypoplasia may instead be related to chronic loss of lung liquid by an altered tracheal-amniotic pressure gradient [59]. The prenatal prediction of pulmonary hypoplasia is fraught with difficulty at present [60,61], with most studies involving prolonged premature rupture of membranes (PPROM) rather than renal cases where the pathology is very different. Proposed predictors of pulmonary hypoplasia include fetal breathing movements [62], lung length [63] and chest circumference ratio [61]. Chest/abdominal circumference ratios are reproducible, and a ratio <0.8 can be used to predict pulmonary hypoplasia in PPROM. However, the ratio falls with time, thus limiting its usefulness at initial diagnosis. The potential for preventing or treating pulmonary hypoplasia is limited at present. Amnioinfusion followed by shunting may do this by promoting the accumulation of amniotic fluid (see below). In theory, amnioinfusion may be used to refill the amniotic cavity, but early experience with this is not encouraging [26].

Renal dysplasia

There are two theories about the aetiology of renal dysplasia: that it is *caused* by the obstruction, presumably related to back pressure, or

that it is *associated* with the obstruction due to a common embryological defect in the lower Wolffian duct and ureteric bud.

Theoretical basis for relieving obstruction in utero

Osathanondh and Potter hypothesized that renal dysplasia is caused by early urinary obstruction, raised intraluminal pressure and failure in further nephron induction [64]. Surgical correction of PUV is relatively simple after birth, but mortality is largely related to pulmonary hypoplasia and renal dysplasia. Thus the relief of the obstruction *in utero*, and restoration of normal physiology, has four aims:

1. The prevention of *renal damage* and dysplasia by relief of the obstruction and pressure.
2. The prevention of further *pulmonary hypoplasia* by restoration of amniotic fluid.
3. The reduction of additional *morbidity due to distension* of the abdominal wall and urinary tract causing prune belly, megacystis and megaureter.
4. The avoidance of *pressure deformities*, e.g. talipes, caused by the restriction of movements with oligohydramnios.

A potential pitfall of shunting is that amelioration of the obstruction may result in some otherwise fatal cases being converted into non-fatal cases with residual disease, renal failure requiring dialysis or transplantation and chronic disability.

Lessons from animal studies

The view that obstruction leads to dysplasia, and that its relief can prevent damage, has been supported by ovine fetal studies. Beck surgically induced complete ureteric obstruction in fetal lambs at a variety of gestations and showed that under 70 days this results in cystic dysplasia of the kidney [65]. When obstruction was created after 80 days of gestation, simple hydronephrotic kidneys were produced. Furthermore, relief of an obstruction created at 62–65 days in fetal lambs, at a second operation 20, 40 or 60 days later, resulted in a lesser degree of renal dysplasia. All kidneys showed some postobstructive changes, but these were related to the duration of obstruction. The prevention of renal dysplasia by decompression was inversely proportional to the duration of obstruction. Harrison's group in San Francisco have also shown that complete urinary obstruction in fetal lambs causes renal dysplasia and lung hypoplasia [66] that can be prevented by early decompression [67].

The limitations of animal work are that it is based on sudden, relatively late-onset, surgically induced, complete ureteric obstruction in a normal system. *In vivo*, the obstruction often starts very early in gestation, may have a gradual onset and there may be abnormal renal development and nephrogenesis. The obstruction may not be complete (indeed, it cannot be if amniotic fluid is still present), and could even be intermittent. The situation is complicated by delayed regression and closure of the urachus, which normally occurs by 12 weeks [68], acting as a 'safety-valve' in some cases.

Does obstruction cause dysplasia?

The view that obstruction leads to dysplasia, which can in turn be prevented by overcoming the obstruction mechanically, is challenged by other evidence. Although renal dysplasia co-exists with PUV and other congenital urinary anomalies [39,69–71], it may not be a secondary phenomenon.

Henneberry and Stephens [72] examined the kidneys and urinary tracts in 12 children who died of severe but incomplete obstruction due to PUV and showed that the degree of renal dysplasia was correlated to the position of the ureteric orifice. This has also been shown for duplex kidneys [70]. The suggestion is that renal dysplasia is not caused by the obstruction, but that it accompanies PUV; the two pathologies therefore being concurrent primary developmental malformations due to an abnormal position of the ureteric bud from the Wolffian duct. If the ureteric orifice links with an inappropriate part of the metanephric ridge, the association between PUV and dysplasia can be explained by a common developmental failure rather than a causative association. The natural history of progression of dysplasia is unlikely to be influenced either by any obstruction or its relief. However, there may be additional damage secondary to distension and

pressure, via effects on blood flow, ischaemia or direct damage to the tubules.

The view that dysplasia is not caused by obstruction is also supported by the finding that intravesical pressure may be low in fetuses with low obstructive uropathies [52], although bladder compliance may be artificially concealing raised intrarenal pressure. It might be argued that the intravesical pressure falls in lower urinary tract obstruction when urine production falls once renal dysplasia has occurred, but low pressure (<5 mmHg) has been found both in fetuses with (5/10) and without dysplasia (2/5) [54].

It has been shown that the deviation in urinary electrolytes becomes more pronounced with increasing gestation in those fetuses with obstructive uropathy who have renal dysplasia [45]. This would support the notion that renal damage is a direct effect of obstruction, although it is still possible that the electrolytes appear more deranged as the primarily dysplastic kidney fails to mature normally with increasing gestation.

Selection for *in utero* treatment

Whatever the initial pathology, the working hypothesis is that severe lower urinary tract obstruction diagnosed *in utero* may be amenable to therapy during *in utero* life. If intravesical pressure rises, further damage may be superimposed on dysplasia. Treatment may be limited, depending on the severity of the dysplasia and whether it would have progressed to renal failure. Relief of obstruction may theoretically help renal function by:

1. *Preventing direct damage* (if it is caused by obstruction).
2. *Preventing further damage* superimposed on pre-existing dysplasia (as it is a progressive condition).
3. *Allowing normal maturation* (which might be prevented by distension and malfunction of the ducts).

Dysplasia is not an 'all-or-nothing' condition, and is probably irreversible. Shunting is probably not a treatment for dysplasia, but, rather, prevents secondary damage due to obstruction or distension. Evidence against point 3 above would be that obstructed kidneys

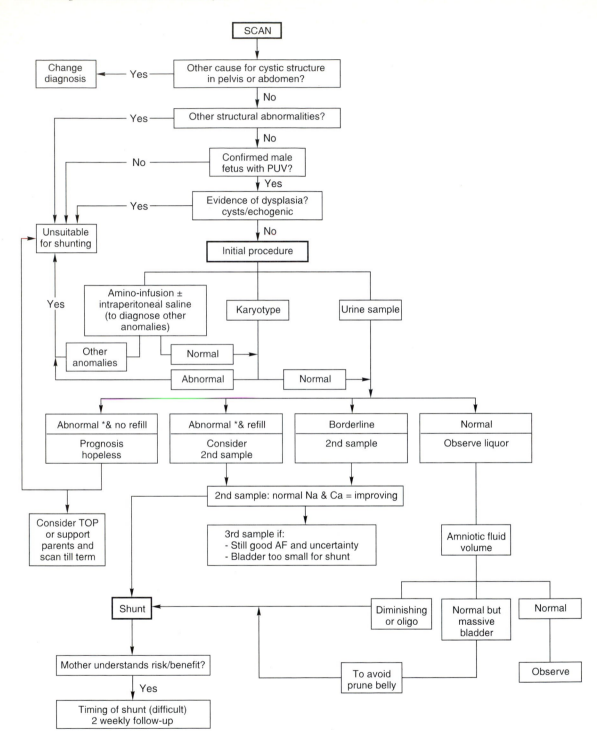

Figure 7.8 Flow diagram to show the selection and assessment for vesicoamniotic shunting.

stop producing urine rather than produce immature urine.

A flow chart that demonstrates our approach to the assessment and selection of cases for shunting is shown in Figure 7.8. This aims to make exclusions to avoid shunting in those fetuses:

1. that have *other abnormalities*;
2. for whom it is *unnecessary*, and
3. for whom it is *too late*.

Fetuses who have an accurate diagnosis of PUV may be considered for shunting. Male genitalia and dilated posterior urethra ('retort' shaped – see Figure 7.4) should be seen to make a diagnosis of PUV. Karyotyping and urine sampling are performed at the first visit and a few days later, the scan is repeated and a decision is made, depending on the earlier results. The karyotype should be normal and renal function should have been assessed as normal (or at least reasonable) or improving significantly. Serial samples may be taken at weekly or 2-weekly intervals before a decision is made to shunt.

Characteristics of fetuses in whom shunting is unnecessary (Group 2 above) are those who will not develop severe renal dysplasia or pulmonary hypoplasia. Fetuses with normal amniotic fluid must have a partial or intermittent obstruction and kidneys that are producing adequate amounts of urine. It is usually not indicated to shunt the upper urinary tract or when the amniotic fluid volume is normal, unless the mechanical compressive effects place the fetus at risk of developing hydrops or polyhydramnios, for example by deviation of the aorta or inferior vena cava. Upper tract dilatation is often not obstructive (PUJ) and the prognosis is moderate to good. However, there is a case for shunting when there is bilateral hydronephrosis and one kidney has poor function and the situation is worsening. Renal shunts may thus rarely be used in hydronephrosis, but only if it is massive, the other kidney appears worse and there is polyhydramnios. In these cases, hydronephrosis may be secondary to a renal defect or PUJ obstruction causing tubular damage, resulting in polyuria secondary to the high sodium content, that causes distension resulting from the high urine flow. That is, there may be a vicious circle, with a form of PUJ distension leading to poly-

uria and further distension which can lead to nephrogenic diabetes insipidus in postnatal life.

Characteristics of fetuses in whom shunting is too late (Group 3 above) are those who already have irreversible renal damage or pulmonary hypoplasia. Fetuses who already have severe renal dysplasia will still die in the neonatal period from renal failure despite shunting, and will not be able to produce enough amniotic fluid to protect themselves from pulmonary hypoplasia. Fetuses with urethral obstruction due to atresia are unlikely to be suitable for shunting as they present early, with severe oligohydramnios, shrunken kidneys and variable dilatation and, in one series, all died postnatally [22].

Few appear to have tried renal biopsy at the time of intervention to see if renal dysplastic changes are already present [73]. This would be relatively easy if open fetal surgery were being performed, but it would be too late to diagnose dysplasia. Renal biopsy has normally been reserved for the diagnosis of congenital Finnish nephrosis, picked up via high maternal serum alpha fetoprotein (AFP), which cannot otherwise be diagnosed by ultrasound or urinary electrolytes, though this may be obviated in the future as the genes for congenital Finnish nephrosis and infantile polycystic kidney disease have recently been mapped, opening the possibility of DNA diagnosis. It is doubtful that *in utero* renal biopsy will aid the prenatal diagnosis of dysplasia and it is very invasive.

Spontaneous resolution of low urethral obstruction, possibly by rupture of the urethral valves [74], also weighs in the decision not to shunt too enthusiastically. Urine aspiration alone may lead to resolution of obstruction [55], possibly by a fall in intravesical pressure, allowing PUVs to open, or by relief of pressure that led originally to a functional obstruction. Serial sampling has an advantage over shunting for this kind of case, provided that there is adequate amniotic fluid for pulmonary development, as well as being appropriate if monitoring for a fall in amniotic fluid volume.

One particular problem is the fetus with obstruction referred early at 16–18 weeks. This would be too early for shunting, as catheter placement is technically difficult under 22 weeks due to the small size, and it is difficult to assess renal function biochemically [47].

The key to selection is thus the assessment of renal function. However, there is no sudden distinction between normal and irreversibly damaged kidneys. The ideal method for selection would be based on predicted *future* rather than *present* renal function, or at least, would use a marker of early and worsening damage.

Techniques for permanently relieving *in utero* obstruction

Urinary diversion can be performed either percutaneously with a shunt or by open operation. Most intrauterine fetal shunting procedures have used ultrasound-guided insertion of vesicoamniotic catheters with preliminary amniotic fluid instillation to overcome the technical problems created by oligohydramnios.

Catheters/shunts

A single pigtail catheter (Harrison Fetal Bladder Stent), made of polyethylene (Cook Urological, Spencer, Indiana, USA), has side holes in both ends, a curled bladder end and an amniotic cavity flare, introduced down the outside of the needle [66–75].

An alternative is the double pigtail catheter [76] that we have used since 1982, which has holes in both ends and can be introduced down the inside of a cannula (Figure 7.9). The two pigtails are perpendicular to each other to encourage the catheter to lie flat against the anterior abdominal wall, and thus to minimize the risk of displacement by the fetus. This has subsequently been found to be more successful [76] and has been widely adopted.

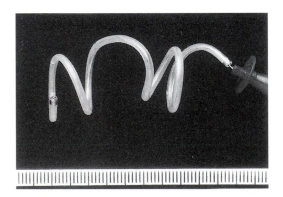

Figure 7.9 Double-pigtail catheter used for shunting.

Technique of inserting vesicoamniotic shunt

Ultrasound is used to choose the site and direction of entry, preferably so that the shunt can be passed into the fetal bladder through the anterior abdominal wall, avoiding the umbilicus. The mother may be sedated and given prophylactic antibiotics. The abdomen is cleaned and draped to ensure sterile conditions. The skin, rectus and peritoneum are anaesthetized with 0.5% lignocaine, and a 20G needle is used to introduce 200 ml of warmed sterile normal saline into the amniotic cavity to improve visualization and ease of shunting, taking care to ensure that it is not extra-amniotic. This needle is then withdrawn and the trochar and 17G cannula (Figure 7.10) are introduced through the mother's abdomen and uterine wall and directed into the fetal bladder. The trochar is removed and pressure can be measured before the shunt is loaded into the cannula. Care must be taken not to allow urine to escape under pressure and the bladder to decompress, as ultrasound localization of the shunt requires a full bladder. Another urine sample should be taken at this point for comparison with previous results. The first pigtail curls up inside the bladder when a short obturator is used to push it out from the end. The shunt is then held steadily in place with a longer obturator, whilst the cannula is withdrawn to ensure the second pigtail curls up on the outside of the fetal abdomen. A good volume of fluid is required in the amniotic cavity to ensure that the outer coil is intra- rather than extra-amniotic.

The bladder empties and the shunt can then only be seen as parallel echogenic lines. Follow-up is performed on a weekly basis to check the shunt placement, the amniotic fluid volume and residual urinary tract dilatation.

Complications of shunting

The insertion of a vesicoamniotic catheter can be technically difficult and complications include insertion failure, fetal trauma and shunt failure. There are a number of pessimistic reports about shunts, including failure to insert catheters at the first attempt of 91% [24], unsuccessful shunt placement in up to 18%; [77] and complications in as many as 44% of cases [77], but the literature is probably

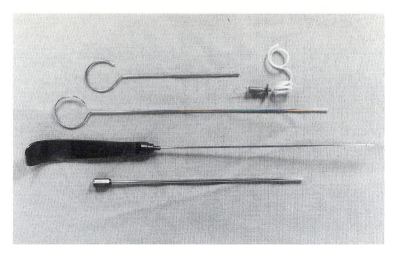

Figure 7.10 Trochar, cannula and obdurators used for insertion of double-pigtail catheter.

distorted by inappropriate selection of cases and single case reports from centres with little experience. In addition, the results may be biased by the use of the wrong shunts and failure to perform preliminary amnioinfusion in the early days. The complications should be much lower, and have been in our experience, although there is a high residual fetal loss rate, probably >5%.

Other rare complications include abdominal wall defect [78], premature labour, urinary ascites, chorioamnionitis, rupture of membranes, haemorrhage, perforation of the fetal jejunum and periureteral scarring [77]. The shunt can fail because it becomes dislodged or blocked. It can migrate out of the fetus or into the peritoneal cavity, secondary to fetal movements and growth, leading to urinary ascites. Occasionally, a second vesicoamniotic shunt has to be reinserted. Rarely, a peritoneal-amniotic shunt has to be inserted if the first shunt dislodges into the fetal abdomen, although there is a risk that the pigtail will wrap around mesentery and bowel.

Open fetal surgery

Under general anaesthesia, the uterus is approached via a transverse incision in the maternal abdomen and opened with a stapling device and a high transverse incision. The fetal trunk is exteriorized and the ureters exposed and marsupialized to the skin via bilateral flank incisions [79]. The fetus is returned to the

amniotic cavity which is filled with Ringer's lactate solution before closure. The operation is covered with prophylactic antibiotics and beta-mimetics. The mother undergoes a caesarean section for delivery [80].

Open surgery necessitates two major operations for the mother and a high risk of premature labour and there is still a chance of uterine rupture and fetal death. It requires a paediatric surgeon with experience of animal surgery and, at present, is not a practical proposition outside one centre in San Francisco. The risk/benefit ratio is difficult to weigh up, and it is uncertain whether there is enough reliable prognostic information to justify such an invasive procedure.

Minimal access surgery

With the development of endoscopic techniques and laser surgery, alternative percutaneous approaches are being tried. Obstruction may be relieved by fetal surgery via the fetal abdomen, or by insertion of stents or laser ablation of urethral valves from within the fetal bladder. These sorts of approaches may enable fetal surgery to be performed at earlier gestations, when smaller catheters than are now available can be developed.

A successful *in utero* cystostomy [81] has been described which was performed at 17 weeks under general anaesthesia using an argon laser via a fetoscope to make two holes in the fetal abdomen. The fetal bladder decompressed immediately and normal amniotic fluid was present until 33 weeks, when the cystostomy closed spontaneously. The following week a healthy infant with prune belly was delivered. There was no significant pulmonary hypoplasia, nor renal dysplasia, although mild pelvic dilatation and bilateral vesicoureteric reflux were demonstrated.

Outcome

Determining the efficacy of vesicoamniotic shunt placement requires knowledge of the natural history of obstructive uropathy diagnosed *in utero* and use of standard criteria for the assessment of renal and pulmonary function.

Harrison et al. [80] reported the first *in utero* decompression at 21 weeks' gestation using bilateral ureterostomies at open fetal surgery. Amniotic fluid never reaccumulated and the infant died of pulmonary hypoplasia. The first successful decompression with a vesicoamniotic catheter was reported the same year [81] in a twin fetus at 32 weeks with ascites, grossly distended bladder, distended ureters and dilated renal pelvises. Amniotic fluid had been normal but was decreasing. The baby underwent bilateral ureterostomies and survived with mild renal dysplasia and prune belly syndrome. Further case reports reported both good [82] and poor outcomes [83].

Elder et al. [77], in a review of the first 57 published reports of intervention for obstructive uropathy, noted a high incidence of complications and that only 21% of fetuses with associated oligohydramnios survived. They were concerned that prenatal treatment was rarely justified and that mothers and fetuses were being exposed to unnecessary risks. The review may have been unduly pessimistic as the final diagnoses were very heterogeneous and only included 15 cases of PUV. The interventions were very mixed, including aspiration and radiological studies. In addition, the early publications were of small numbers of cases from centres with little experience of the techniques. Nevertheless, the conclusion that a prospective randomized trial was needed to compare survival with and without shunt placement has been echoed since [25], although it has not been fulfilled.

In 1986, 73 cases of shunting procedures were reported to the International Fetal Surgery Registry [25] (which has now discontinued). Eleven fetuses were terminated, six with abnormal karyotype and five with renal dysplasia on ultrasound. There were three intrauterine deaths (two traumatic and one in a fetus with central nervous system abnormality). Of 29 neonatal deaths, 27 had pulmonary hypoplasia and two were related to prematurity. Thus the direct loss rate due to shunting can be estimated as 3/73 or 5%. The overall perinatal survival was only 41%, but 11 of these fetuses were terminated after the catheter had been inserted as a primary diagnostic procedure. On the other hand, the success might have been exaggerated as some fetuses with normal amniotic fluid volume were included. The whole series is biased, as 70% of the cases were reported from centres with experience of only one procedure.

Crombleholme et al. [84] described a series of 40 cases of bilateral hydronephrosis which were retrospectively divided into good and poor prognosis groups on the basis of hypotonic urine (sodium $<100\,mEq/l$, chloride $<90\,mEq/l$, osmolarity $<210\,Osm/l$). Some fetuses had decompression procedures and insertion of shunts, although not in a randomized fashion. Survival after intervention was greater in both the good (89% vs 70%) and poor prognosis (30% vs 0%) groups. Although the statistics are dubious and there may have been selection bias, this study does provide some indirect evidence of the usefulness of shunting.

Evans et al. [55], using serial sampling for selection, performed shunting in three out of 11 fetuses with low urethral obstruction and no evidence of renal pathology. All three survived, though two had mild prune belly, one with unilateral hydronephrosis and normal renal function, the other with reflux. The third had multiple anomalies (a non-functioning kidney, talipes and deafness), an iatrogenic abdominal wall defect, thought to be caused by the shunt, and good function from the dilated kidney that required a nephrostomy. Two 'poor prognosis' cases had abnormal urine biochemistry and, despite reaccumulation of urine, the values did not improve. Six cases had normal urine biochemistry and were not shunted. All did well, including one case where the megacystis did not recur.

Why do the results to date seem poor?

Shunting has appeared less useful than it actually is due to:

1. The use of *inappropriate reference ranges* for urinary electrolytes, such that cases were wrongly assigned both for shunting and conservative management. The original cutoffs advised by Glick et al. [46] do not take account of the normal changes in urine electrolytes with gestation [47]. Others have found them inaccurate [48].
2. The *comparison of cases with inappropriate controls*, that is affected fetuses who did well rather than normals.
3. A *long period between urine sampling and outcome*, during which the underlying disease might have been greatly altered.

The initial disappointing results of shunting were based on small numbers of case reports and were probably poorly selected. Thus shunting has acquired a poor reputation at the same time that the indications have been gradually refined. Stricter selection criteria have decreased the use of shunting. Harrison's group found that in a population referred for consideration of treatment, only 5 out of 200 fetuses (2.5%) with bilateral hydronephrosis fulfilled the criteria [85] for open fetal surgery (similar to the strict criteria presently used for shunting).

Future developments

Important developments, to aid present management, would be a better marker of renal function and more accurate assessment of long-term prognosis. As the early enthusiasm has faded, a multicentre prospective randomized controlled trial of shunts versus conservative management after careful assessment is now needed and would be timely. The advent of transvaginal scanning and first-trimester diagnosis [4,86,87] (Figure 7.11) may alter the spectrum of fetal renal disease seen, as well as offering earlier opportunities for intervention. However the natural history may be quite different. In one prospective study of nearly 250 000 first-trimester pregnancies spontaneous resolution of fetal megacystis was seen in 7 out of 12 chromosomally normal cases and 4 progressed to severe obstructive uropa-

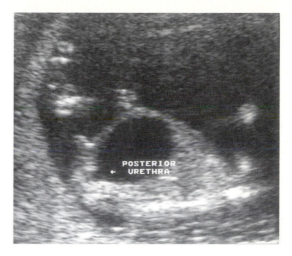

(a)

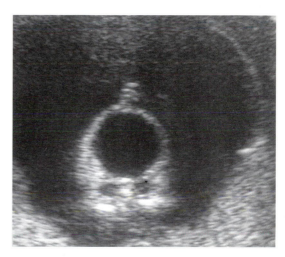

(b)

Figure 7.11 Transvaginal scan of thirteen-week fetus in longitudinal and cross-section showing: (a) megacystis and dilated posterior urethra and (b) megacystis and bilateral hydroureters. Note the normal amount of amniotic fluid.

thy [88]. It may be that earlier and newer methods of drainage (e.g. laser cystostomy) will improve the success rates of shunting. Intrauterine renal transplant could only be considered in cases of renal failure where there was potential for lung development. There may be improvements in postnatal renal treatment, such as the use of growth factors to promote renal growth, or methods of ameliorating or preventing pulmonary hypoplasia that will spur more aggressive treatment of *in utero* lesions in the future.

References

1. Kaback MM. The utility of prenatal diagnosis. In: Rodeck CH, Nicholaides KH (eds) *Prenatal Diagnosis. Proceedings of the 11th Study Group of the RCOG.* London: Wiley, 1984; pp 1–12.
2. Romero R, Cullen M, Grannum P et al. Antenatal diagnosis of renal anomalies with ultrasound: III Bilateral renal agenesis. *Am J Obstet Gynecol* 1985; **151**: 38–53.
3. Greig JD, Raine PAM, Young DG et al. Value of antenatal diagnosis of abnormalities of the urinary tract. *Br Med J* 1989; **298**: 1417–1419.
4. Bronshtein M, Yoffe N, Brandes JM, Blumfeld Z. First and early second-trimester diagnosis of fetal urinary tract anomalies using transvaginal sonography. *Prenat Diag* 1990; **10**: 653–666.
5. Nakamura Y, Hosokawa Y, Yano H et al. Primary causes of perinatal death. An autopsy study of 1000 cases in Japanese infants. *Hum Pathol* 1982; **13**: 54–61.
6. Flake AW, Harrison MR, Sauer L, Adzick NS, de Lorimier AA. Ureteropelvic junction obstruction in the fetus. *J Pediatr Surg* 1986; **21**: 1058–1063.
7. Arger PH, Coleman BG, Mintz MC et al. Routine fetal genitourinary tract screening. *Radiology* 1985; **156**: 485–489.
8. Smith D, Egginton JA, Brookfield DSK. Detection of abnormality of fetal urinary tract as a predictor of renal tract disease. *Br Med J* 1987; **294**: 27–28.
9. King LR. Posterior urethra. In: Kelalis PP, King LR, Belman AD (eds) *Clinical Paediatric Urology.* Philadelphia: WB Saunders, 1985; pp 527–558.
10. Reuss A, Wladimiroff JW, Niermeijer MF. Antenatal diagnosis of renal tract anomalies by ultrasound. *Pediatr Nephrol* 1987; **1**: 546.
11. Garlinger P, Ott J. Prune-belly syndrome – possible genetic implications. *Birth Defects* 1974; **10**: 173–180.
12. Nunn IN, Stephens FD. The triad syndrome: a composite anomaly of the abdominal wall, urinary system and testes. *J Urol* 1961; **86**: 782–794.
13. Hutson JM, Beasley SW. Aetiology of the prune belly syndrome. *Aust Paediatr J* 1987 **23**: 309–310.
14. Beasley SW, Bettenay F, Hutson JM. The anterior urethra provides clues to the aetiology of prune belly syndrome. *Pediatr Surg Int* 1988; **3**: 169–172.
15. Fisk NM, Dhillon HK, Ellis CE, Nicolini U, Tannirandorn Y, Rodeck CH. Antenatal diagnosis of megalourethra in a fetus with the prune belly syndrome. *J Clin Ultrasound* 1990; **18**: 124–126.
16. Tsingoglou RR, Dickson JAS. Lower urinary obstruction in infancy. A review of lesions and symptoms in 165 cases. *Arch Dis Child* 1972; **47**: 215–217.
17. Nakayama DK, Harrison MR, de Lorimer AA. Prognosis of posterior urethral valves presenting at birth. *J Pediatr Surg* 1986; **21**: 43–45.
18. Harrison MR, Golbus MS, Filly RA et al. Management of the fetus with congenital hydronephrosis. *J Paediatr Surg* 1982; **17**: 728–740.
19. Parker RM. Neonatal urinary ascites. A potentially favourable sign in bladder outlet obstruction. *Urology* 1974; **111**: 589–593.
20. Kay R, Brereton RJ, Johnston JH. Urinary ascites in the newborn. *Br J Urol* 1980; **52**: 451–454.
21. Adzick NS, Harrison MR, Flake AW, de Lorimer AA. Urinary extravasation in the fetus with obstructive uropathy. *J Pediatr Surg* 1985; **20**: 608–615.
22. Reuss A, Wladimiroff JW, Stewart PA, Scholtmeijer RJ. Non-invasive management of fetal obstructive uropathy. *Lancet* 1988; **ii**: 949–951.
23. Reuss A, Wladimiroff JW, Scholtmeijer RJ, Stewart PA, Sauer PJJ, Niermeijer MR. Prenatal evaluation and outcome of renal obstructive uropathies. *Prenat Diag* 1988; **8**: 93–102.
24. Manning FA, Harrison MR, Rodeck CH and members of the International Fetal Medicine and Surgery Society. Catheter shunts for fetal hydronephrosis and hydrocephalus. *N Engl J Med* 1986; **315**: 336–340.
25. Nicolini U, Santolaya J, Hubinont C, Fisk N, Maxwell D, Rodeck C. Visualization of fetal intra-abdominal organs in second-trimester severe oligohydramnios by intraperitoneal infusion. *Prenat Diag* 1989; **9**: 191–194.
26. Fisk NM, Ronderos-Dumit D, Soliani A, Nicolini U, Vaughan J, Rodeck CH. Diagnostic and therapeutic transabdominal amnioinfusion in oligohydramnios. *Obstet Gynecol* 1991; **78**: 270–278.
27. Cheng HH, Nicholaides KH. Renal and urinary tract abnormalities. In: Brock DJH, Rodeck CH, Ferguson-Smith MA (eds) *Prenatal Diagnosis and Screening.* Edinburgh: Churchill Livingstone, 1992; pp 257–270.
28. Reuss A, Wladimiroff TW, v d Wijngaard JA, Pijpers L, Stewart PA. Fetal renal anomalies; a diagnostic dilemma in the presence of intrauterine growth retardation and oligohydramnios. *Ultrasound Med Biol* 1987; **13**: 619–624.
29. Gembruch V, Hansmann M. Artificial instillation of amniotic fluid as a new technique for the diagnostic evaluation of cases of oligohydramnios. *Prenat Diag* 1988; **8**: 33–45.
30. Quetel TA, Mejides AA, Salman FA, Torres-Rodriguez MM. Amnioinfusion: an aid in the ultrasonographic evaluation of severe oligohydramnios in pregnancy. *Am J Obstet Gynecol* 1992; **167**: 333–336.
31. Phelan JP, Smith CV, Broussard P, Small M. Amniotic fluid volume assessment with the four-quadrant technique at 36–42 weeks' gestation. *J Reprod Med* 1987; **32**: 540–542.
32. Bruner JP, Reed GW, Sarno AP, Harrington RA, Goodman MA. Intra and interobserver variability of the amniotic fluid index. *Am J Obstet Gynecol* 1993; **168**: 1309–1313.
33. Lind T. The biochemistry of amniotic fluid. In: Sandler M (ed) *Amniotic Fluid and its Clinical Significance.* New York: Marcel Dekker, 1979; pp 1–25.
34. Nicolaides KH, Cheng HH, Snijders RS, Moniz DF. Fetal urine biochemistry in the assessment of obstruc-

tive uropathy. *Am J Obstet Gynecol* 1992; **166**: 932–937.

35. Mahoney BA, Filly RA, Callen PW, Hricak H, Golbus MA, Harrison MR. Fetal renal dysplasia: sonographic evaluation. *Radiology* 1984; **152**: 143–146.

36. Clarke NW, Gough DCS, Cohen SJ. Neonatal urological ultrasound: diagnostic inaccuracies and pitfalls. *Arch Dis Child* 1989; **64**: 578–580.

37. Glazer GM, Filly RA, Callen PW. The varied sonographic appearance of the urinary tract in the fetus and newborn with urethral obstruction. *Radiology* 1982; **144**: 563–568.

38. Bernstein J. Renal hypoplasia and dysplasia. In: Edelmann DM (ed) *Pediatric Kidney Disease* vol II. Boston: Little, Brown, 1978; pp 547–554.

39. Rattner WH, Meyer R, Bernstein J. Congenital abnormalities of the urinary system. IV. Valvular obstruction of the posterior urethra. *J Pediatr* 1963; **63**: 84–94.

40. Campbell S, Wladimiroff JW, Dewhurst DJ. The antenatal measurement of fetal urine production. *J Obstet Gynaecol Br Cmwlth* 1973; **80**: 680–686.

41. Wladimiroff JW. Effect of furosamide on fetal urine production. *Br J Obstet Gynaecol* 1975; **82**: 221–224.

42. Golbus MS, Filly RA, Callen PW, Glick PL, Harrison MR, Anderson RL. Fetal urinary tract obstruction: management and selection for treatment. *Semin Perinatol* 1985; **9**: 91–97.

43. Tassis BMG, Trespidi L, Tirelli AS et al. Serum β_2-microglobulin in fetuses with urinary tract anomalies. *Am J Obstet Gynecol* 1997; **176**: 54–57.

44. Notte SH. Assessment of fetal renal function by determination of serum microprotein levels. In: *Symposium: Fetus as a Patient* (abstracts) 1988; p. 171.

45. Nicolini U, Fisk NM Rodeck CH, Beacham J. Fetal urine biochemistry: an index of renal maturation and dysfunction. *Br J Obstet Gynaecol* 1992; **99**: 46–50.

46. Glick PL, Harrison MR, Golbus MS et al. Management of the fetus with congenital hydronephrosis. II: Prognostic criteria and selection for treatment. *J Pediatr Surg* 1985; **20**: 376–387.

47. Rodeck CH, Nicolini U. Physiology of the mid-trimester fetus. In: Whitelaw A, Cooke RWI (eds) *The Very Immature Infant Less than 28 Weeks' Gestation*. Edinburgh: Churchill Livingstone *Br Med Bull* 1988; **44**: 826–849.

48. Wilkins IA, Chitkara U, Lynch L, Goldberg JD, Mehalek KE, Berkowitz RL. The nonpredictive value of fetal urinary electrolytes: preliminary report of outcomes and correlations with pathological diagnoses. *Am J Obstet Gynecol* 1987; **157**: 694–698.

49. Elder JS, O'Grady JP, Ashmead G, Duckett JW, Philipson E. Evaluation of fetal renal function: unreliability of fetal urinary electrolytes. *J Urol* 1990; **144**: 574–578.

50. Lipitz S, Ryan G, Samuell C et al. Fetal urine analysis for the assessment of renal function in obstructive uropathy. *Am J Obstet Gynecol* 1992; **167**: 174–179.

51. Nicolini U, Rodeck CH, Fisk N. Shunt treatment for fetal obstructive uropathy. *Lancet* 1987; **ii**: 1338–1339.

52. Nicolini U, Fisk NM, Talbert DG et al. Intrauterine manometry: technique and application to fetal pathology. *Prenat Diag* 1989; **9**: 243–254.

53. Nicolini U, Rodeck CH. Fetal urinary diversion. In: Chervenak F, Isaacson G, Campbell S (eds) *Textbook of Ultrasound in Obstetrics and Gynecology*. New York: Little Brown, 1992; pp 1277–1282.

54. Nicolini U, Tannirandorn Y, Vaughan J, Fisk NM, Nicolaidis P, Rodeck CH. Further predictors of renal dysplasia in fetal obstructive uropathy: bladder pressure and biochemistry of 'fresh' urine. *Prenat Diag* 1991; **11**: 159–166.

55. Evans MI, Sacks AJ, Johnson MP, Robichaux AD, May M, Moghissi KS. Sequential invasive assessment of fetal renal function and the intrauterine treatment of fetal obstructive uropathies. *Obstet Gynecol* 1991; **77**: 545–550.

56. Foxall PJD, Bewley S, Robson SC, Rodeck CH, Neild GH, Nicholson JK. High resolution NMR spectroscopic measurements of fetal urine: a novel method to monitor renal abnormalities in utero. *J Am Soc Nephrol* 1992; **3**: 468.

57. Eugene M, Muller F, Dommergues M, Le Moyec L, Dumez Y. Evaluation of postnatal renal function in fetuses with bilateral obstructive uropathy by proton nuclear magnetic resonance spectroscopy. *Am J Obstet Gynecol* 1994; **170**: 595–602.

58. Nicolini U, Fisk NM, Rodeck CH, Talbert DG, Wigglesworth JS. Low amniotic pressure in oligohydramnios – is this the cause of pulmonary hypoplasia. *Am J Obstet Gynecol* 1989; **161**: 1098–1101.

59. Fisk NM. Oligohydramnios-related pulmonary hypoplasia. *Cont Rev Obstet Gynaecol* 1992; **4**: 191–201.

60. Blott M, Greenough A, Nicolaides KH, Campbell S. The ultrasonographic assessment of the fetal thorax and fetal breathing movements in the prediction of pulmonary hypoplasia. *Early Hum Dev* 1990; **21**: 143–151.

61. D'Alton M, Mercer B, Riddick E, Dudley D. Serial thoracic versus abdominal circumference ratios for the prediction of pulmonary hypoplasia in premature rupture of the membranes remote from term. *Am J Obstet Gynecol* 1992; **166**: 658–663.

62. Blott M, Greenough A, Nicolaides KH. Fetal breathing movements in pregnancies complicated by premature rupture of membranes in the second trimester. *Early Hum Dev* 1990; **21**: 41–48.

63. Roberts AB, Mitchell JM. Direct ultrasonographic measurement of fetal lung length in normal pregnancies and pregnancies complicated by prolonged rupture of membranes. *Am J Obstet Gynecol* 1990; **163**: 1560–1566.

64. Osathanondh V, Potter EL. Pathogenesis of polycystic kidneys, Type 1 due to hyperplasia of interstitial portions of collecting tubules. *Arch Pathol* 1964; **77**: 510–512.

65. Beck AD. The effect of intra-uterine urinary obstruction upon the development of the fetal kidney. *J Urol* 1971; **105**: 784–789.

66. Glick PL, Harrison MR, Noall RA, Villa RL. Correction of congenital hydronephrosis *in utero*. II: Early mid-trimester ureteral obstruction produces renal dysplasia. *J Pediatr Surg* 1983; **18**: 681–687.

67. Glick PL, Harrison MR, Adzick NS, Noall RA, Villa RL. Correction of congenital hydronephrosis *in utero*. IV: *In utero* decompression prevents renal dysplasia. *J Pediatr Surg* 1983; **19**: 649–657.

68. Moore KL. *Before We Are Born. Basic Embryology and Birth Defects*, 3rd edn. Philadelphia: WB Saunders, 1989; p 186.

69. Risdon RA. Renal dysplasia. I. A clinico-pathological study of 76 cases. *J Clin Pathol* 1971; **24**: 57–65.

70. Mackie GG, Stephens FD. Duplex kidneys: a correlation of renal dysplasia with position of the ureteral orifice. *J Urol* 1975; **114**: 274–280.

71. Cussen LJ. Cystic kidneys in children with congenital urethral obstruction. *J Urol* 1976; **106**: 939–941.

72. Henneberry MO, Stephens FD. Renal hypoplasia and dysplasia in infants with posterior urethral valves. *J Urol* 1980; **123**: 912–915.

73. Greco P, Loverro G, Caruso G, Clemente R, Selvaggi L. The diagnostic potential of fetal renal biopsy. *Prenat Diag* 1993; **13**: 551–556.

74. Hecher K, Henning K, Spernol R, Szalay S. Spontaneous remission of urinary tract obstruction and ascites in a fetus with posterior urethral valves. *Ultrasound Obstet Gynecol* 1991; **1**: 426–430.

75. Golbus MS, Harrison MR, Filly RA, Callen PW, Katz M. *In utero* treatment of urinary tract obstruction. *Am J Obstet Gynecol* 1982; **142**: 383–388.

76. Rodeck CH, Nicolaides KH. Ultrasound guided invasive procedures in obstetrics. *Clin Obstet Gynaecol* 1983; **10**: 515–539.

77. Elder JA, Duckett JR, Snyder HM. Intervention for fetal obstructive uropathy: has it been effective? *Lancet* 1987; **ii**: 1007–1010.

78. Robichaux III AG, Mandell J, Greene MF, Benacerraf BR, Evans MI. Fetal abdominal wall defect: a new complication of vesicoamniotic shunting. *Fetal Diag Ther* 1991; **6**: 11–13.

79. Crombleholme TM, Harrison MR, Anderson RL et al. Congenital hydronephrosis: early experience with open fetal surgery. *J Pediatr Surg* 1988; **23**: 1114–1121.

80. Harrison MR, Golbus MS, Filly RA et al. Fetal surgery for congenital hydronephrosis. *N Engl J Med* 1982; **306**: 591–593.

81. MacMahon RA, Renou PM, Shekelton PA, Paterson PJ. *In-utero* cystectomy. *Lancet* 1992; **340**: 1234.

82. Manning FA, Harman CR, Lange IR, Brown R, Decter A, MacDonald N. Antepartum chronic fetal vesicoamniotic shunts for obstructive uropathy: a report of two cases. *Am J Obstet Gynecol* 1983; **145**: 819–822.

83. Berkowitz RL, Glickman MG, Walker Smith GJ et al. Fetal urinary tract obstruction: what is the role of surgical intervention *in utero*? *Am J Obstet Gynecol* 1982; **144**: 367–375.

84. Crombleholme TM, Harrison MR, Golbus MS et al. Fetal intervention in obstructive uropathy: prognostic indicators and efficacy of intervention. *Am J Obstet Gynecol* 1990; **162**: 1239–1244.

85. Longaker MT, Adzick NS, Harrison MR. Fetal obstructive uropathy. *Br Med J* 1989; **299**: 325–326.

86. Hill LM, Rivello D. Role of transvaginal sonography in the diagnosis of bilateral renal agenesis. *Am J Perinatol* 1991; **8**: 395–397.

87. Cazorla E, Ruiz F, Abad A et al. Prune belly syndrome – early antenatal diagnosis. *Eur J Obstet, Gynecol, Reprod Biol* 1997; **72**: 31–33.

88. Sebire NJ, Vonkaisenberg C, Rubio C et al. Fetal megacystis at 10–14 weeks of gestation. *Ultra-sound Obstet Gynecol* 1996; **8**: 387–390.

8

Incidence: facts and figures

D.F.M. Thomas and A.P. Barker

Non-lethal congenital anomalies occur more frequently in the genitourinary tract than in any other system. Two categories of genito-urinary anomalies can be conveniently defined, i.e. visible anomalies (affecting predominantly the external genitalia of male infants) and 'internal' or 'invisible' abnormalities of the male and female urinary tracts of which there is little, or no, outward evidence. In the past this second group of anomalies generally came to light only when complications or symptoms had supervened; however, following the introduction of routine ultrasound into obstetric practice, they are now being increasingly recognized *in utero*.

External anomalies

Penis

Phimosis

An estimated 21 000 circumcisions are performed annually in England and Wales [1], the most commonly cited indication being 'congenital' phimosis with or without infection (balanoposthitis). Approximately 7% of boys can expect to lose their foreskins for 'medical' as opposed to religious reasons before the age of 15. Despite the scale on which congenital phimosis is being diagnosed, it is highly doubtful whether it should be regarded as a genuine congenital anomaly.

Hypospadias

The incidence of hypospadias in the general male population has been estimated at 3–4 per 1000 live births, i.e. 0.25–0.3% [2,3]. Genetic factors have been implicated and one study [4] identified hypsopadias in 14% of siblings and other close relatives of index cases with hypospadias.

Certain other congenital abnormalities of the penis, e.g. chordee without hypospadias, fall within the hypospadias spectrum, but their relative rarity precludes any reliable estimates of incidence. The same is true of other rare penile anomalies such as urethral duplication, penile duplication, micropenis, etc.

Undescended testis

The most reliable picture of the current incidence of cryptorchidism in the UK is provided by the study of 7500 consecutive births in Oxford undertaken by the John Radcliffe Hospital Cryptorchidism Study Group [5]. Birth weight and gestational maturity were found to have an important bearing on incidence, the cryptorchidism rate at birth in babies weighing less than 2000 g, 2000–2499 g and 2500 g or more being 45.4, 13.4 and 3.8%, respectively. At 3 months of age the incidence of cryptorchidism in the same birthweight groups was 7.7, 2.5 and 1.4%. Spontaneous descent of the testis occurs to a small degree in the first year of life but not thereafter. For practical purposes the most reliable current estimate of the incidence of cryptorchidism is probably around 1–2%.

External manifestations of urinary tract malformation

The characteristic Potter's facies, with low-set ears and other manifestations of moulding deformity, resulting from oligohydramnios, are perhaps the best-known manifestations of serious underlying urinary tract pathology. Congenital abnormalities such as oesophageal atresia which are known to be associated with a high incidence of coexistent anomalies in other systems (e.g. VATER syndrome) call for investigation of the urinary tract as a matter of routine. Similarly, the presence of syndromes such as Down syndrome and Turner's syndrome are regarded as an indication for routine postnatal ultrasound examination of the urinary tract in most specialist centres.

Prune belly syndrome

This sporadic anomaly of varying severity is characterized by hypoplasia of the abdominal wall musculature, massive urinary tract dilatation and bilateral cryptorchidism. The features of prune belly syndrome almost certainly result from severe bladder outflow obstruction at an early stage in gestation. Following the advent of prenatal ultrasound, the birth of an infant with prune belly syndrome is becoming an increasingly rare event, presumably because prenatal detection of massive urinary tract dilatation generally results in termination of pregnancy. For this reason it is difficult to put a figure on the incidence in the liveborn population.

Abdominal masses

The genitourinary tract is the most common source of abdominal masses in the neonatal period. Reviewing 117 neonatal abdominal masses, Griscom [6] noted that 63 originated within the urinary tract (and that hydronephrosis and multicystic dysplastic kidney accounted for 45 abdominal masses). A further 15 arose within the female genital tract, i.e. hydrocolpos, ovarian cyst. In many countries

it is now relatively uncommon for an infant to be born with an unsuspected mass since the majority, particularly when fluid filled, are detected prenatally.

Bladder exstrophy

Our experience of a relatively static population in the Yorkshire region (population 3.5 million; 50 000 live births per annum) suggests an incidence of around 1 in 40 000 live births. Males outnumber females by a ratio of 5 : 1. Primary epispadias, a manifestation of the exstrophy complex confined to the urethra, striated sphincter and external genitalia, occurs with an incidence of approximately 1 in 25 000 live births in males, whereas the female variant is extremely rare, e.g. approximately 1 in 250 000.

Anomalies of the female external genitalia

Congenital anomalies of the female external genitalia are uncommon but include, for example, phallic enlargement associated with intrauterine virilization (congenital adrenal hyperplasia, etc.), hymenal tags, imperforate hymen, cloacal anomalies and prolapsed ectopic ureterocele. Labial adhesions, arguably the most common problem affecting the external female genitalia, are acquired rather than congenital in aetiology.

Urinary tract anomalies

The true incidence of invisible anomalies affecting the kidneys, ureters, bladder and urethra is difficult to gauge.

Historically three methods have been employed to estimate their incidence:

1. *Clinical series* based on patients presenting with symptoms, urinary infection, pain, etc.
2. *Radiological surveys*.
3. *Autopsy data*.

To these we must now add a fourth, i.e.

4. *Prenatal ultrasound screening*.

Since each method is subject to differing sources of error, it is not surprising that they yield varying estimates of incidence.

Clinical series

Published series of clinically presenting cases represent an unreliable basis upon which to establish the true incidence of anatomical abnormalities of the urinary tract. Until recently, these series consisted almost exclusively of cases which had come to light because of infection or other symptomatic complications. Series of this nature often shed little light on the true incidence of the underlying anomaly in the asymptomatic population. In pelviureteric (PUJ) obstruction, for example, it is becoming apparent that only a proportion (perhaps between a third and a half) of all cases previously presented clinically in childhood. A further limitation of clinical series relates to the fact that most are published from specialist centres attracting referrals from a wide and poorly defined catchment population.

Radiological surveys

Radiological surveys cast the net wider by including asymptomatic anomalies identified incidentally during the investigation of unrelated symptoms. Typically anomalies such as asymptomatic ureteric duplication or unilateral renal agenesis are discovered during the investigation of unrelated haematuria or prostatic symptoms in adult life. Nevertheless, most radiological surveys do entail a degree of selection bias since they are based on symptomatic patients rather than the general low-risk population.

Autopsy data

Unfortunately not even autopsy can be regarded as a reliable final arbiter of the true incidence of congenital abnormalities of the urinary tract. Autopsies are not performed according to uniform criteria but rather when doubt exists about the cause or circumstances of death. Asymptomatic abnormalities are likely to be missed by this approach. Analysing data collected more consistently from 245 000 autopsies in US service personnel, Ashley and Mostofi [7] reported an incidence of renal anomalies of 1 in 650, a figure broadly corresponding to that previously published by Bell [8], i.e. 1 in 519. Although Ashley and Mostofi's data were inevitably skewed by the disproportionate number of males of service age, they did include significant numbers of infants born to service families. Thus of 364 renal anomalies discovered at autopsy, 104 (28.6%) were either in stillbirths or liveborn infants who had died during the neonatal period. Bilateral renal agenesis was cited as the most frequent pathological diagnosis in this subgroup, accounting for 47 (45%) of all lethal renal abnormalities.

Calculations of incidence based on paediatric autopsies will inevitably exclude those renal anomalies which are destined to result in death in adult life. Furthermore, since congenital anomalies are the single most frequent cause of death in childhood and are frequently multiple, a relatively high incidence of renal anomalies will be uncovered even if they are unrelated to the cause of death. For these reasons data derived from paediatric autopsies cannot be reliably extrapolated to the general paediatric population.

At the other end of the age spectrum, data derived from adult autopsies inevitably fail to include renal anomalies which have already resulted in death in childhood. Similarly, autopsy in adult life may uncover little evidence of anomalies such as PUJ obstruction or vesicoureteric reflux (VUR) in individuals in whom these conditions have undergone spontaneous resolution in childhood or early adult life.

Terminated pregnancies

Recently the findings of earlier autopsy studies have been complemented by data derived from pregnancies terminated for severe fetal anomalies. In the Yorkshire Region (approximately 50 000 live births per annum) a 3.5-year prospective study [9] identified 2261 ultrasound-detected anomalies, of which 369 (16%) resulted in termination. Post-mortem examination of the aborted fetus was undertaken in 357 cases (97%). CNS anomalies predominated, accounting for 47.9% of terminations for fetal anomaly. The genitourinary tract, however, ranked second, i.e. 35 terminations (9.9%). The distribution of anomalies by system, together with a breakdown of post-mortem diagnoses in the urinary tract, is detailed in Table 8.1.

Table 8.1 Final diagnosis following post-mortem and cytogenetics in 357 fetuses following termination of pregnancy for fetal anomaly

Final diagnosis	No.	%
CNS	171	47.9
Urinary tract	35	9.9
Bilateral renal agenesis	10	
Bilateral multicystic displastic		
kidney	9	
Unilateral multicystic dysplastic		
kidney/contralateral agenesis	3	
Infantile polycystic	1	
Outflow obstruction	10	
Dysplasia	1	
Complex	1	
Complex	30	8.5
Chromosomal	25	7
Cardiac	23	6.4
Musculoskeletal	14	3.9
Gastrointestinal	7	2
Pulmonary	6	1.7
Tumour	1	0.3
Twin related	2	0.8
Miscellaneous		
(unknown aetiology)	41	11.5

From reference [9].

Incidence – comparison of alternative methods

Accepting the limitations outlined above, a measure of the incidence of some of the more common anomalies of the urinary tract can be derived from the published estimates of incidence summarized in Table 8.2 [10–27]. Where estimates of incidence derived from prenatal ultrasound have been published, these are also included in Table 8.2.

Prenatal ultrasound

As a method of determining the true incidence of urinary tract anomalies, prenatal ultrasound has the advantage that it now constitutes a *de facto* screening programme of the general, low-risk fetal population in many western countries.

Prenatal ultrasound suffers from two major drawbacks, however, both as a clinical screening test and as a means of establishing the true incidence of urinary tract anomalies:

1. The detection rate is closely linked to the gestational age at which ultrasound screening is routinely performed.
2. Mild dilatation, the most frequently reported 'abnormality', is a finding of uncertain clinical significance. The point at which dilatation denotes genuine underlying pathology has yet to be established.

Routine scanning in the later stages of pregnancy yields a higher incidence of fetal

Table 8.2 Incidence of urinary tract malformations

	Clinical series	Radiological surveys	Autopsy	Prenatal ultrasound
Bilateral renal agenesis	1 : 4800 [10] births		1 : 3571 [11]	1 : 3228 [12]– 1 : 6292 [13]
Unilateral renal agenesis	1 : 1200 [14] births	1 : 1500 [15] IVUs	1 : 1610 [16]	1 : 2400 [17]– 1 : 3146 [12]
Multicystic dysplasia				1 : 4300 [18]
Pelviureteric junction obstruction	1 : 7300 [19] paediatric admissions			
Ureteric/renal duplication		1 : 37–1 : 50 [20]	1 : 125 [16]	1 : 3146 [12]– 1 : 11 986 [17]
Vesicoureteric junction obstruction (obstructed megaureter)	3.5 [21]–7.5 [22] cases/year			1 : 3600 [23]
Vesicoureteric reflux	0.66 [24]–1 : 55 [25] 'normal' children*			1 : 3146 [23]
Posterior urethral valves	1 : 4000 [26]– 1 : 7500 [27] births			1 : 5400 [24]– 1 : 11 986 [17]

* MCUs performed as screening investigations in normal babies and children.

uropathy than routine scanning at an earlier gestational age. Similarly, centres which report mild degrees of dilatation as an abnormal finding will encounter a higher apparent incidence of fetal uropathy. The importance of gestational age was highlighted by Helin and Persson [17] in a single centre study of 11 986 pregnancies scanned at 17 weeks and 33 weeks. In total, 33 urological abnormalities were identified, but of these only three were apparent at 17 weeks, the remaining 30 (91%) only being evident on the second scan at 33 weeks. In another single centre study from Scandinavia reported by Rosendahl et al. [28], 4586 fetuses were routinely scanned at 18 and 34 weeks. In this study the upper limit of normality was defined as an anteroposterior renal pelvis diameter of 1 cm. Clinical follow-up was maintained for 2–4 years. The incidence of urinary tract malformations detected by ultrasound screening was 0.48%, rising to an overall total of 0.57% when those presenting clinically in the first 2–4 years of life were included in the figures. Rosendahl claimed a sensitivity of 84.6%, a specificity of 99.9% and a positive predictive value of 81.5% for antenatal screening. Livera et al. [12] screened 6292 pregnancies at 28 weeks' gestation, defining 'abnormality' as a renal pelvis diameter of 1 cm or more. On this basis abnormalities of the urinary tract were reported in 92 fetuses, although significant pathology was confirmed in only 42 postnatally. In the remaining 47 infants (52%) postnatal ultrasound revealed either a normal urinary tract or a simple extrarenal pelvis. During follow-up extending to up to 18 months, a further seven children presented clinically with renal abnormalities that had been missed on prenatal ultrasound. Thus,

Table 8.3 Published incidence of prenatally detected uropathies: six European cities

Incidence	Centre	Authors
1 : 1200	Lund	Kullendorf et al. 1984 [29]
1 : 935	Derby	Watson et al. 1988 [30]
1 : 600	Leeds	Arthur et al. 1989 [31]
1 : 330	Malmo	Helin and Persson, 1986 [17]
1 : 208	Hameenlinna	Rosendahl, 1990 [28]
1 : 154	Stoke	Livera et al. 1989 [12]

Livera et al. derived an incidence of abnormalities detected by prenatal screening of 0.65%, with an overall incidence at 18 months follow-up of 0.76%. In Leeds, a policy of routine second-trimester ultrasound combined with further ultrasound where indicated in later pregnancy identified 78 fetuses with an important urinary tract anomaly from a total of 46 775 pregnancies, i.e. 1 in 600 pregnancies [31]. Figures for the incidence of prenatally detected uropathy reported from studies undertaken in six European cities are listed in Table 8.3.

Limitations of second-trimester ultrasound screening

It is becoming increasingly evident that second-trimester ultrasound fails to detect a substantial proportion of cases of non-lethal uropathy. In most instances this failure stems not from technical error or inexperience, but rather from the fact that the underlying anomaly has given rise to detectable dilatation at that stage in gestation. In a study designed to explore the correlation between gestational age at detection and functional outcome of PUJ obstruction [32] (see below), it was noted that of 35 cases of prenatally detected unilateral hydronephrosis, 24 were associated with dilatation at a mean of 19 weeks' gestation. Eleven of the 35 hydronephrotic kidneys (31%), however, had appeared entirely normal at 19 weeks and it was only on scanning in later pregnancy that dilatation became apparent.

Even posterior urethral valves, a severe form of obstructive uropathy associated with a fixed anatomical obstruction present from the seventh to ninth week of gestation, may not be associated with detectable dilatation in the second trimester. Dineen et al. [33] analysed the antenatal histories of 42 patients with posterior urethral valves whose mothers had all been scanned at least once with ultrasound during pregnancy. Despite this, fetal uropathy was detected in only 19 cases. In the 36 pregnancies scanned before 24 weeks' gestation, fetal uropathy was detected in only three. In our own series [26] of 31 prenatally detected cases of posterior urethral valves, dilatation had been evident in the second trimester in 17 cases, but in 14 the ultrasound appearances of the fetal urinary tract had been normal before

24 weeks' gestation. If their mothers had not been scanned in later pregnancy, these cases would have been missed – as indeed others were when ultrasound had been limited to the second trimester.

On the available evidence it seems improbable that a formal screening policy based around a second, i.e. third-trimester scan, would be cost-effective in terms of reducing the economic burden of urinary infection, renal scarring and chronic renal failure. In reality, however, obstetricians are increasingly resorting to the use of third-trimester ultrasound for obstetric indications and as this practice becomes more widespread, so the detection of non-lethal fetal uropathies will continue to increase.

Is gestational age at onset of dilatation a predictor of functional outcome?

Logic would suggest that the earlier dilatation becomes apparent in pregnancy (and, by inference, the greater the duration of exposure of the fetal kidney to obstruction or reflux), the worse the prognosis for function in the affected kidney. An early study from Bristol [34], involving 28 pregnancies, demonstrated a clear difference in outcome between those cases detected in the second trimester and those in whom the second-trimester scan had been normal. The sensitivity of real-time ultrasound has improved in subsequent years and more subtle degrees of dilatation can be detected than was possible with the equipment of the early 1980s. We have studied the possible correlation between second-trimester ultrasound appearances and postnatal functional outcome for two conditions, PUJ obstruction and posterior urethral valves. For PUJ obstruction, a broad correlation was observed between the mean value for differential function in the affected kidney and the severity of dilatation documented on second-trimester ultrasound scan. However, this correlation only acquired statistical significance in the small group of kidneys that were already severely dilated (i.e. renal pelvis diameter $>15\,mm$) in the second trimester. Despite a broad correlation for mean values of differential function, the figures for differential function in individual kidneys in each category was subject to considerable scatter (Table 8.4). The heterogeneity of PUJ

Table 8.4 Correlation between severity of dilatation on second-trimester ultrasound and renal function in prenatally detected hydronephrosis (PUJ obstruction): 35 kidneys

Ultrasound appearances (median 19 weeks)	Renal pelvis AP diameter (mm)	Number of kidneys	Mean differential function DTPA or MAG 3
Normal	< 5	11	48.2%
'Mild' dilatation	6–10	15	42.7%
'Moderate' dilatation	11–15	4	37.3%
'Severe' dilatation	> 15	5	26.5%*

* $P < 0.01$.
From reference [32].

obstruction appears to limit the predictive value of second-trimester ultrasound for the purposes of prenatal counselling.

Unlike obstruction at the PUJ, the anatomical basis for obstruction associated with posterior urethral valves is believed to date from a more consistent point in gestation, i.e. the seventh week when the regressing wolffian ducts interact with the developing urogenital sinus. Despite the uniformity of embryology and anatomy, however, the severity of the resulting obstruction can vary considerably. At one end of the spectrum are the lethal obstructive uropathies associated with renal dysplasia and pulmonary hypoplasia, whilst at the other are the boys whose posterior urethral valves only come to light during the investigation of voiding dysfunction in later childhood. The correlation between gestational age at which dilatation became apparent and the functional outcome in 31 boys with prenatally detected posterior urethral valves is illustrated in Table 8.5.

Deaths (from pulmonary hypoplasia or early renal failure) was confined to those boys in whom there had been evidence of dilatation in the second trimester. The likelihood of subsequent development of chronic renal failure was also significantly higher in this group. In contrast, all the boys with prenatally detected posterior urethral valves whose second-trimester scans were normal survived, with the majority (93%) having normal values for plasma creatinine at follow-up.

Table 8.5 Correlation between gestational age at appearance of dilatation and outcome in 31 boys with prenatally detected posterior urethral valves

	Gestational age at detection of dilatation			
	< 24 weeks		> 24 weeks (normal appearances on second-trimester scan)	
	No.	%	No.	%
Patients (no.)	17		14	
Deaths	4	24	0	0
Chronic renal failure	5	29	1	7
Alive/normal creatinine	5	47	13	93

From reference [26].

How useful is prenatal diagnosis?

Although the majority of prenatally detected uropathies are being detected in normal, asymptomatic infants, there are occasions when prenatal ultrasound simply pre-empts the diagnosis of a condition that would have been immediately apparent at delivery, e.g. prune belly syndrome, large renal mass, etc. In these instances it is difficult to argue that prenatal detection has been of tangible benefit – except in the possible context of parental counselling.

In an early study of 145 [35] liveborn neonates with prenatally detected uropathies, it was found that 24 (17%) had relevant physical signs or associated syndromes that rendered the prenatal diagnosis largely irrelevant. In a separate study [31] clinical signs or coexistent pathology were found in 26% of cases of prenatally detected bilateral uropathy but in only 3% of children with isolated unilateral uropathy. Analysing 258 cases of clinically unsuspected prenatally detected uropathies (D.F.M. Thomas, unpublished data), we judged prenatal detection to have been of 'definite' clinical value in only 44 infants (17%), i.e. obstruction or high grade reflux occurring bilaterally or in a solitary kidney. In 96 cases (37%) prenatal diagnosis was judged to have been of 'probable' clinical value, i.e. by identifying significant pathology occurring unilaterally in the presence of a normal contra-

lateral kidney. As such, there was no potential threat to overall renal function. In a final group of 118 cases (46%), prenatal diagnosis was deemed of 'doubtful' benefit, i.e. detection of mild dilatation or pelvicaliectasis of uncertain clinical significance.

Pattern of prenatally detected uropathies

The final urological diagnoses of 426 liveborn infants with significant prenatally detected uropathy referred to a regional paediatric urological unit are listed in Table 8.6. Infants with mild pelvicalyceal dilatation or rare anomalies such as crossed fused renal ectopia have been excluded from this analysis. In addition, it is important to note that the figures relate to children referred to a paediatric urologist and the relative proportion of potentially 'surgical' conditions may be unrepresentative of the broader picture. Children with unilateral renal agenesis, for example, would not necessarily be referred for a surgical opinion and the relative incidence of prenatally detected renal agenesis may be considerably higher than these figures suggest. PUJ obstruction, nevertheless, emerges as the single most important condition, accounting for 35% of prenatally detected uropathies referred to our unit.

Causes of end-stage renal failure in childhood

By the time children or young adults progress onto end-stage renal failure and transplantation programmes, it may be extremely difficult

Table 8.6 Final urological diagnosis in 426 liveborn infants with significant prenatally detected uropathy

Urological diagnosis	No.	%
Pelviureteric obstruction	150	35.2
Vesicoureteric reflux	83	19.5
Multicystic dysplastic kidney	64	15
Vesicoureteric junction obstruction	42	9.8
Posterior urethral valves	37	8.6
Duplex systems	36	8.4
Renal agenesis	14	3.3

D.F.M. Thomas, unpublished data, 1994.

to establish the pathological basis for their renal failure. This is particularly true of reflux nephropathy where it may be impossible to distinguish the consequences of congenital renal dysplasia from postinfective scarring. One of the most instructive insights into the aetiology of end-stage renal failure in childhood comes from the North American Paediatric Renal Transplant Co-operative Study [36]. Spanning a 6-year period from 1987 to 1993, the Report details information derived from 3223 children and adolescents of 17 years and less, receiving a total of 2819 renal transplants in 82 participating centres in the USA and Canada. In children under 5 years of age, congenital uropathies accounted for approximately 50% of cases of end-stage renal failure, whilst in the older age group acquired glomerulonephritis was the single most important aetiology. Sixty per cent of the transplant patients were male. The male predominance was seen most clearly in the youngest age groups, with males accounting for 69% of transplant recipients under the age of 1 year and 66% of those between the ages of 2 and 5 years. These data reflect the high incidence of renal aplasia/hypoplasia/dysplasia (62%) and obstructive uropathy (88%) in the male paediatric transplant population and the increased importance of these diagnoses in the younger age groups.

Over the entire paediatric age group, the five most common primary diagnoses in children undergoing renal transplantation were aplasia, hypoplasia, dysplasia (17.2%), obstructive uropathy (17.1%), focal segmental glomerulosclerosis (FSGS) (11.1%), reflux nephropathy (5.6%) and systemic immunological disease 4.6%.

The importance of dysplasia and obstructive uropathy as a cause of end-stage renal failure in young male children has also been documented in European centres. Between 1969 and 1988, the European Dialysis and Transplant Association Registry [37] recorded 296 children (67% males, 33% females) commencing renal replacement therapy before their second birthday. In European children under the age of 2 years, the main causes of end-stage renal failure were hypoplasia and dysplasia (24%), haemolytic uraemic syndrome (17%), focal sclerosis and pyelonephritis superimposed upon urinary tract obstruction (14%) and glomerulonephritis (14%).

Fetal surgery is unlikely to make any positive contribution to a reduction in the burden of chronic renal failure in childhood. Indeed it may add to it by contributing to the survival of infants with severe renal dysplasia who might otherwise have died of pulmonary hypoplasia in the neonatal period. Conversely, the increasing use of termination when severe obstructive uropathy is detected in the second trimester may reduce the relative importance of obstructive uropathy as a cause of renal failure in early childhood – particularly in males. For boys at the less severe end of the posterior urethral valves spectrum, prenatal detection may prove beneficial, by identifying the need for chemoprophylaxis and early surgical relief of infravesical obstruction. Until recently, posterior urethral valves most commonly presented with urinary infection, often associated with severe systemic infection and profound metabolic disturbance. It is now uncommon for the condition to present in this fashion. By preventing severe pyelonephritis and pyenephrosis, prenatal ultrasound may reduce the ultimate burden of chronic renal impairment associated with this condition.

Similarly, one study [38] has identified a lower incidence of renal damage in children with prenatally detected VUR when compared with the incidence of reflux nephropathy in children with clinically presenting VUR. Even when prenatal detection fails to prevent the subsequent development of urinary infection associated with an underlying urological anomaly, the findings of our study indicate that prenatal detection has the effect of reducing its severity [39]. Although some of the early enthusiasm for the prenatal ultrasound detection of urinary tract anomalies was misplaced, evidence is accumulating to refute those critics who have dismissed it as an entirely worthless, or positively harmful, byproduct of routine obstetric practice. Quite apart from its impact on clinical paediatric practice, prenatal ultrasound will make a continuing contribution to our understanding of the genetic basis and epidemiology of genitourinary anomalies.

References

1. Rickwood AMK, Walker J. Is phimosis over-diagnosed in boys and are too many circumcisions performed in consequence? *Ann R Coll Surg Eng* 1989; **71**: 275–277.

2. Sweet RA, Schrott HG, Kurland R et al. Study of the incidence of hypospadias in Rochester, Minnesota 1940–70, and a case control comparison of possible etiologic factors. *Mayo Clin Proc* 1974; **49**: 52–59.

3. Chung CS, Myriantholpoulos NC. Racial and prenatal factors in major congenital malformations. *Am J Hum Genet* 1968; **20**: 44–60.

4. Bauer SB, Retik AB, Colodny AH. Genetic aspects of hypospadias. *Urol Clin North Am* 1981; **8**: 559–564.

5. John Radcliffe Hospital Cryptorchidism Study Group. Cryptorchidism: a prospective study of 7500 consecutive male births, 1984–8. *Arch Dis Child* 1992; **67**: 892–899.

6. Griscom BT. The roentgenology of neonatal abdominal masses. *Am J Roentgenol* 93: 447–463.

7. Ashley DJB, Mostofi FK. Renal agenesis and dysgenesis. *J Urol* 1960 83: 211–230.

8. Bell ET. Renal Diseases, 2nd edn. Philadelphia: Lea & Febiger, 1950.

9. Brand IR, Kaminopetros P, Cave M, Irving CH, Lilford RJ. Specificity of antenatal ultrasound in the Yorkshire Region: a prospective study of 2261 ultrasound detected anomalies. *Br J Obstet Gynaecol* 1994; **101**: 392–397.

10. Potter EL. Bilateral absence of ureters and kidneys: a report of 50 cases. *Obstet Gynecol* 1965; **25**: 3–12.

11. Davidson WM, Ross GIM. Bilateral absence of the kidneys and related congenital anomalies. *J Pathol Bacteriol* 1954; **68**: 459–474.

12. Livera Ln, Brookfield DSK, Egginton JA, Hawnaur JM. Antenatal ultrasonography to detect foetal renal abnormalities: a prospective screening program. *Br Med J* 1989; **298**: 1421–1423.

13. Gunn TR, Mora JD, Pease P. Outcome after antenatal diagnosis of upper urinary tract dilatation by ultrasonography. *Arch Dis Child* 1988; **63**: 1240–1243.

14. Sheih CP, Hung CS, Wei CF, Lin CY. Cystic dilatations within the pelvis in patients with ipsilateral renal agenesis or dysplasia. *J Urol* 1990; **144**: 324–327.

15. Longo VJ, Thompson GJ. Congenital solitary kidney. *J Urol* 1952; **68**: 63–68.

16. Campbell MF, Harrison JH (eds). *Anomalies of the Kidney in Urology*, 3rd edn. Philadelphia: WB Saunders, 1970; pp 1417–1422.

17. Helin I, Persson PH. Prenatal diagnosis of urinary tract abnormalities by ultrasound. *Pediatrics* 1986; **78**: 879–883.

18. Gordon AC, Thomas DFM, Arthur RJ, Irving HC. Multicystic dysplastic kidney: Is nephrectomy still appropriate? *J Urol* 1988; **140**: 1231–1234.

19. Williams DI, Karlaftis CM. Hydronephrosis due to pelviureteric obstruction in the newborn. *Br J Urol* 1966; **38**: 138–144.

20. Dees JE. Clinical importance of congenital anomalies of the upper urinary tract. *J Urol* 1941; **46**: 659–666.

21. Pfister RC, Hendren WH. Primary megaureter in children and adults. *Urology* 1978; **12**: 160–165.

22. Rabinovitch R, Barken M et al. Surgical treatment of the massively dilated primary megaureter in children. *Br J Urol* 1979; **51**: 19–23.

23. Thon W, Schlickenrider JA, Thon A, Aitweir JE. Management and early reconstruction of urinary tract abnormalities detected *in utero*. *Br J Urol* 1987; **59**: 214–217.

24. Peters PC, Johnston DE, Jackson JH. The incidence of vesicoureteric reflux in the premature child. *J Urol* 1960; **84**: 69–70.

25. McGovern JH, Marshall VF, Paquin A Jr. Vesicoureteral regurgitation in children. *J Urol* 1960; **83**: 122–149.

26. Hutton KAR, Thomas DFM, Arthur RJ, Irving HC, Smith SEW. Prenatally detected posterior urethral valves: is gestational age at detection a predictor of outcome? *J Urol* 1994; **152**: 698–701.

27. Atwell JD. Posterior urethral valves in the British Isles: a multi-centre BAPS review. *J Pediatr Surg* 1983; **18**: 70–74.

28. Rosendahl H. Ultrasound screening for fetal urinary tract malformations: a prospective study in general population. *Eur J Obstet Gynecol Reprod Biol* 1990; **36**: 27–33.

29. Kullendorf CM, Larson LT, Jorgenson C. The advantages of antenatal diagnosis of intestinal and urinary tract malformation. *Br J Obstet Gynaecol* 1984; **91**: 144–147.

30. Watson AR, Readett D, Nelson CS et al. Dilemmas associated with antenatally detected urinary tract abnormalities. *Arch Dis Child* 1988; **63**: 719–722.

31. Arthur RJ, Irving HC, Thomas DFM, Watters JK. Bilateral fetal uropathy: what is the outlook? *Br Med J* 1989; **298**: 1419–1420.

32. Barker AP, Cave MM, Thomas DFM et al. Fetal PUJ obstruction: predictors of outcome. *Br J Urol* 1995; **76**: 649–652.

33. Dineen MD, Dhillon HK, Ward HC et al. Antenatal diagnosis of posterior urethral valves. *Br J Urol* 1992; **72**: 364–369.

34. Pocock RD, Witcombe JB, Andrews HS et al. The outcome of antenatally diagnosed urological abnormalities. *Br J Urol* 1985; **57**: 788–792.

35. Thomas DFM, Gordon AC. The management of prenatally diagnosed uropathies. *Arch Dis Child* 1989; **64**: 58–63.

36. Avner ED, Chavers B, Sullivan EK, Tejani A. Renal transplantation and chronic dialysis in children and adolescents: the 1993 annual report of the North American Pediatric Renal Transplant Co-operative Study. *Pediatr Nephrol* 1995; **9**: 61–73.

37. Ehrich JHH, Rizzoni G, Brunner FP, et al. Renal replacement therapy for end-stage renal failure before 2 years of age. *Nephrol Dial Transplant* 1993; **7**: 1171–1177.

38. Sheridan M, Jewkes F, Cough DCS. Reflux nephropathy in the first year of life. *Pediatr Surg Int* 1991; **6**: 214–216.

39. Lakhoo K, Thomas DFM, D'Cruz AJ, Fuenfer M. Failure of prenatal ultrasound to prevent urinary tract infection associated with underlying urological abnormalities. *Br J Urol* 1996; **77**: 905.

9

Renal function in the infant and management of renal failure

J.T. Brocklebank

Maturation of renal function

During early fetal life the excretory role of the kidney is minimal. Thus the anephric fetus with bilateral renal dysplasia enjoys biochemical haemostasis. Birth immediately imposes a functional role on the kidney. The kidneys of term infants, although immature when compared with the kidneys of adults, are well adapted for the demands of normal postnatal life. Their functional capacity, however, can easily be overwhelmed by the stresses of illness or therapeutic excesses. In contrast, the renal function of the very low birth weight infant is much more immature and the maintenance of normal fluid and electrolyte balance, even in normal circumstances, may be difficult. The medical management of the newborn infant requires some knowledge of the effects of maturation on the physiological functions of the kidney.

Expressing renal function

It is readily apparent that many functions of the kidneys of newly born infants are less than those of adults. Before it can be assumed that the reduced function is due to immaturity, it is necessary to make some allowance for the differences in body size between infants and adults. This standard correction should also allow meaningful comparisons to be made between serial estimations of renal function during growth, so that the natural history of a disease can be described and comparisons made between different disease groups. In paediatric medicine it is conventional to correct renal function to a standard body size of $1.73 \, m^2$, which represents the average body surface area of a standard man. There are, however, theoretical and physiological limitations inherent in the use of this correction. First, the surface area calculation is a derived figure which introduces the possibilities of errors and inaccuracies. Second, the physiological significances of surface area in infancy is unclear as both metabolic rate and renal function increase more rapidly than surface area. It has been suggested that body weight is the best standard for glomerular filtration rate in the newborn [1], but this is unreliable because the newborn has a tendency to lose weight in the first 10 days of life which will result in an apparently rapid increase in GFR/ml/kg. It is more meaningful for absolute values of glomerular filtration rate (GFR) to be used, as this avoids the problems associated with changes in body size due to the effects of disease and growth. Percentile charts for absolute values of GFR measured by insulin clearance have been derived for children aged between 2 weeks and 12 years and can be used as a means of following the progression of renal disease in the same way growth charts are used [2]. Their clinical value has yet to be established, but it may be expected that children whose body weight is on the 90th centile will have a GFR on the same centile. Inulin clearance averages $10 \, ml/min$ at 14 days of age and increases rapidly during the first year to an average of 30 ml/min. There is a slow linear increase thereafter to 12 years when the average normal adult's GFR of 100 ml/min is attained. Absolute values for GFR for boys and girls of different ages who are at the 10th or 50th centile in weight for age are shown in Figure 9.1. The pattern of maturation of GFR when corrected for body surface area is entirely different. It averages 30 ml/min/1.73 m^2 at birth and increases rapidly during the first 2 years of life, reaching the adult value of 127 ml/min/1.73 m^2 at age 5 years (Figure 9.2).

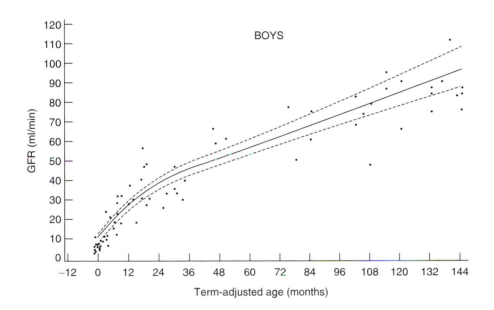

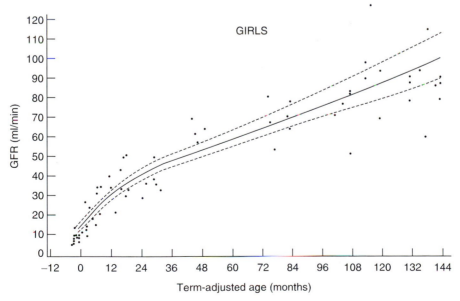

Figure 9.1 Absolute values for glomerular filtration rate (ml/min) related to age for boys and girls. (From reference [2].)

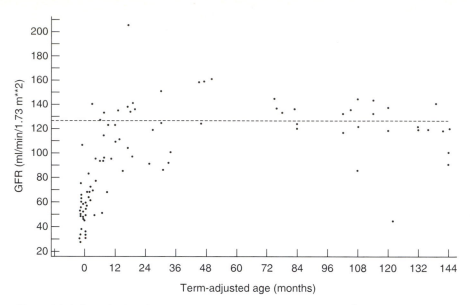

Figure 9.2 Adjusted values for glomerular filtration rate (ml/min/1.73 m²) related to age.
Average value for adults is shown (- - - - - - -). (From reference [2].)

GFR, renal blood flow and renal tubular handling of sodium and other solutes are significantly affected by changes in the extracellular fluid (ECF) volume or, more specifically, circulating blood volume. These and other body fluid spaces change in a non-linear fashion during growth. When expressed as a percentage of body weight, total body water (TBW) is greatest at birth (80%) and decreases to 60% by 6 months of age and thereafter remains constant until puberty where sex differences are observed [3], probably because of the greater deposition of fat in females which lowers the percentage of body weight represented by water. The newborn infant is therefore in a state of relative overhydration compared with an adult. For this reason, and because the kidney's primary function is the biochemical haemostasis of body fluids, it has been suggested that glomerular filtration rate should be corrected for TBW or ECF volume. When this is done, a completely different pattern of GFR maturation is observed [4]. There are, as yet, no simple, accurate and reproducible methods of measuring body fluid spaces in routine clinical practice and, until there are, it is suggested that glomerular filtration rate is expressed in absolute values. GFR is usually measured to assess the progress of disease and this can be done by calculation of the absolute values rather than by introducing another

factor such as surface area, which adds to the inaccuracies of the estimation.

Factors influencing the maturation of glomerular filtration rate

In the human infant nephrogenesis is complete by 34 weeks of intrauterine life when there is a full complement of 1 million nephrons, and by 10 weeks' gestation fetal urine production begins. At term GFR, measured by inulin clearance, varies 10-fold between 0.5 and 5.71 ml/min. It increases rapidly and doubles by the third week of life [1]. In the preterm infant GFR averages 0.6 ml/min at 26 weeks, and increases in a pre-ordained way to 1.4 ml/min at 33 weeks postconceptual age [5].

Studies in experimental animals have shown that the immaturity of glomerular filtration rate in the newly born is under the influence of many different factors. First, the intraglomerular capillary hydrostatic pressure is reduced due to the lower systemic blood pressure of the newborn and increased glomerular afferent arteriolar resistance. The net effect of these factors is to reduce the hydrostatic force for filtration and, as a consequence, the glomerular capillary surface area for filtration is also reduced. Second, the intrarenal blood flow is shunted away from the cortical nephrons in favour of the deeper medullary nephrons. Finally, clearance studies of dextrans of various molecular size have shown that the glomerular capillary permeability is reduced in the developing kidney when compared with the adult.

Measurement of glomerular filtration rate in infancy

Glomerular filtration rate is defined as the volume of plasma completely cleared of a solute by the kidney in unit time. Inulin is used as the reference solute because it is cleared completely by glomerular filtration and neither secreted nor reabsorbed by the renal tubules. There are many technical problems surrounding the use of inulin in the newborn [6] and it is not generally used in clinical practice. Using the technique of inulin infusion, GFR in the newborn of between 27 and 40 weeks' gestation varied from 0.5 to 5.71 ml/min. There was less variability when expressed per unit of body weight (0.59–1.56 ml/min/kg). Radiopharmaceuticals have been substituted, including ^{99m}Tc-DTPA (diethylenetriamine penta-acetic acid), ^{125}I-iothalamate and ^{51}Cr EDTA (ethane D-amine tetra-acetic acid) each has its limitations, including concerns about the administration of radioisotopes and the tendency to underestimate GFR because of reabsorption by the renal tubules. They are not routinely employed in infancy, when an accurate measurement of GFR is not generally clinically important.

Plasma creatinine in infancy

Creatinine originates in muscles, its rate of production is a function of muscle mass and it is excreted only by the kidney. In steady-state conditions when its rate of production and elimination are equal, then the plasma concentration of creatinine will be constant. In adult patients this is largely true and the plasma creatinine concentration has been shown to have an exponential or reciprocal relationship with GFR. In contrast, in children plasma creatinine concentration increases as muscle mass increases because of growth. GFR

Table 9.1 Normal plasma creatinine concentrations of children according to age

Age	Plasma creatinine concentration ($\mu mol/l$)	
	Mean	*Range*
Term at birth	75	188–17
5 days	35	12–62
0.3–2.9 y	33	15–73
3–7.9 y	47	35–63
8–12 y	53	33–86

From references [7] and [8].

increases because of maturation, and thus this simple relationship between plasma creatinine concentration and GFR does not exist. It is therefore necessary to have access to normal plasma creatinine concentrations of children of different chronological and gestation ages (Table 9.1).

At birth the plasma creatinine concentration in term infants approximates to that of the mother and averages 75 μmol/l. The concentration falls rapidly during the first week and by the second week of life averages 35 μmol/l. There is then a slow increase in plasma creatinine concentration as body muscle mass increases, reaching normal adult values at the age of 12 years. In the preterm infant plasma creatinine concentrations tend to be higher (Figure 9.3). Schwartz et al. [10] have derived a formula which can be used to calculate the GFR corrected to 1.73 m² body surface and for term infants after the first month of life:

$$\text{GFR (ml/min per 1.73 m}^2) = \frac{48.6 \times \text{length (cm)}}{\text{Plasma creatinine} (\mu mol/l)}$$

The disadvantage of this method is that the result depends upon the accuracy of the length measurement and it is necessary to refer to normal data corrected for body surface area.

The interpretation of the plasma creatinine concentration during the neonatal period is further complicated by problems with its chemical analysis. Conjugated bilirubin causes falsely low creatinine concentration and, in contrast, ketones and some drugs, such as cephalosporins, will result in falsely high concentrations.

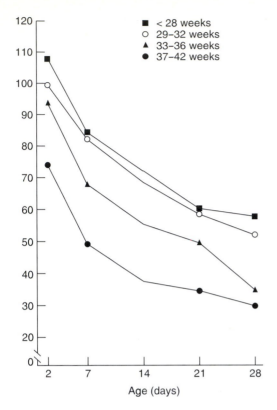

Figure 9.3 Relationship between mean plasma creatinine levels and postnatal age group in different gestational age groups. (From reference [9])

Urine-concentrating ability

The kidney conserves water, achieving increased urine concentration, by two mechanisms. First, by increasing the permeability of the renal collecting tubule to water under the influence of antidiuretic hormone and, second, by maintaining a high osmotic gradient within the renal medullar. Studies in the human infant [11] have shown that the newborn infant can maximally concentrate urine to 700 mosmol/l (compared to an adult of 1200 mosmol/l). This is due to the low renal medullary osmolality around the collecting tubule. The rate of increase in medullary osmolality can be influenced by diet, as infants fed a high protein diet or a diet (cows' milk) supplemented with urea can achieve a higher urine osmolality. Other factors which may explain the inability of kidneys of newborns to concentrate urine include relatively short loops of Henle and increased synthesis of prostaglandin PGE by the neo-

natal kidney. The distal tubular response to antidiuretic hormone is intact. When fluid intake is restricted and vasopressin administered, a normal infant does not achieve a maximum urine osmolality greater than 100 mosmol/l until 2 years of age [12]. This puts the infant at increased risk of dehydration in situations when there is excessive fluid loss, such as gastroenteritis.

In addition to the inability to maximally concentrate urine, the newborn kidney has a reduced capacity to excrete a fluid load. An adult given a water load will have excreted the majority of it in 2 hours. In contrast, a newborn will excrete only 15% of the water load in this time. There is a progressive increase in the speed with which a water load is excreted with increasing age and term infants over 2 weeks of age respond to a fluid load in a manner similar to adults [13]. There is a delay of 20 minutes in the onset of the diuresis when the fluid load is administered orally rather than intravenously. A term infant would be expected to be able to excrete urine volumes 10–15% of the GFR. As GFR is the major limiting factor affecting the newborn kidneys' ability to excrete a water load, it is safer and more physiological to express the expected urine flow rate as a fraction of GFR rather than to use the arbitrarily chosen urine flow rate of 1 ml/kg/h. Thus a term infant weighing 3.5 kg would be expected to have a GFR $3.5 \times 0.86 = 3$ ml/min and a maximum urine flow rate of $(3 \times 10 \times 60)/100 = 18$ ml/ph. Appropriate adjustments have to be made in patients with renal insufficiency.

Renal sodium excretion

Several factors participate in the regulation of sodium excretion. These include sodium intake, glomerular filtration rate, aldosterone and atrial naturetic factor. In the term neonate, the fractional excretion of sodium is increased at birth but by the third day of life a newborn infant is able maximally to conserve sodium in a similar way to the adult, i.e. 1% of filtered load. In contrast, the ability to excrete a sodium load is blunted, probably because of the high circulating plasma aldosterone level and the relatively low GFR.

In contrast, the very low birth weight baby (VLBW) behaves as a salt loser and is only able to conserve up to 5% of the filtered load of sodium, and urine losses up to 20 mmol/kg/day have been described [5]. This high urine sodium loss is probably due to proximal renal tubular immaturity of Na-K ATPase activity, and partial resistance of the distal tubule of the VLBW infant to aldosterone. Hyponatraemia is a common problem in the very low birth weight neonate and sodium supplements are usually necessary. It has been found that a maintenance daily sodium intake of at least 3 mmol/kg is needed to maintain balance.

Acid–base balance

The newborn infant becomes acidotic very readily in stressful situations. The net acid excretion (NAE), i.e. the sum of hydrogen ion excreted as ammonium and titratable acidity minus bicarbonate, is reduced at birth but matures within the first 3 weeks of life. NAE is lower in the preterm than the term infant. The normal plasma bicarbonate in a term infant is low, averaging 20 mmol/l. By 12 months of age the plasma bicarbonate concentration is 22 mmol/l and reaches the normal adult range 24–26 mmol/l in the second year of life. In contrast, the preterm infant plasma bicarbonate averages 17 mmol/l. These differences are due to age-related effects on the renal bicarbonate threshold [14], i.e. the plasma concentration above which the plasma bicarbonate is spilled into the urine. It is important to recognize these differences, because attempts to increase the plasma bicarbonate above the renal threshold by infusing bicarbonate will be unsuccessful, yet every mmol of bicarbonate is accompanied by 1 mmol of sodium and there is a risk of sodium overload.

Excretion of organic anions

Organic anions are excreted both by glomerular filtration and secreted by the proximal tubule. They are an important group of solutes and include many metabolites such as keto-acids and drugs, including many antibiotics such as the penicillins and cephalosporins, and diuretics such as frusemide. The renal handling of these organic acids can be examined using a representative organic anion, para amino hippurate (PAH). Studies in experimental animals have shown that PAH extraction by the renal tubule averages 60% of the normal adult value at term and approaches adult values by 6 months of age. Its rate of maturation can be influenced by diet. A low protein intake will delay and substrate stimulation by penicillin accelerates its rate of maturation [15]. It is important to bear this in mind when administering drugs in the neonate [16], as blood levels of antibiotics excreted by this mechanism have been shown to fall during treatment as the excretory pathways are stimulated.

Urinary composition

The fetal kidney has no excretion responsibilities but urine is formed from the ninth to twelfth week of gestation, increasing progressively throughout gestation. Fetal urine is the major constituent of amotic fluid. The urine flow rate in the neonate is determined mainly by the GFR and has been discussed above. Urine is normally passed within the first 48 hours of birth. A normal urine flow is reported to vary between 0.5 and 5.0 ml/kg/h. Oliguria is generally defined arbitrarily as a urine flow rate less than 0.5 ml/kg/h. The urine osmolality varies between 60 and 700 mosmol/l.

Proteinuria is rare in the newborn and is abnormal when the albustix result exceeds 100 μg/dl [17]. False positives using the dipstik method may be found when specimens are contaminated with disinfectants based upon the quarternary ammonium compounds or chlorhexidine. The urinary excretion of the low molecular weight protein β_2 microglobulin and urinary enzyme *N*-acetyl glucosaminidase are increased in the neonatal period, suggesting proximal renal tubular immaturity.

Haematuria is an unusual finding but 10% of neonates may have up to 1+ on dipstik testing. Urine pH shows a large range (5.0–7.0), and all infants can achieve a urine pH below 5.4 by the second week of life.

Hormonal regulation

Plasma concentration of renin, aldosterone and angiotensin are high in the newborn and decrease during the first months of life [18].

Prostaglandin synthesis is increased but production decreases following birth. The importance of the renin–angiotensin system in the development of renal function is illustrated when anuria occurs in a neonate whose mother was treated with an angiotensin-converting enzymes inhibitor [19].

Renal failure in infancy

Definition

Renal failure is said to have occurred when the GFR falls to a level at which normal plasma homeostasis is not maintained. This generally does not become a major clinical problem until the GFR has fallen to around 10% of normal. It is said to be acute when this occurs over a period of days or weeks and chronic when it happens over months or years. but it is more important to consider whether it is reversible or irreversible. Renal failure in the newborn is unique, as it occurs after a period of intrauterine life and in a setting of immature renal function where major anatomical abnormalities such as bilateral renal agenesis may present as acute renal failure, yet are irreversible.

Diagnosis

The diagnosis of renal failure is generally based upon the urine flow rate and the plasma creatinine concentrations. A urine flow rate less than 0.5 ml per kilogram body weight per hour is arbitrarily defined as oliguria. However, it is important to recognize that renal failure can occur with a high urine flow rate. Oliguria may occur not only when GFR is reduced, but also as a consequence of inadequate fluid intake. Undetected voiding during delivery may give the impression of oliguria.

Oliguria may occur due to inadequate fluid intake. Typically the maintenance water requirement at term is 80 ml/kg/day. This increases daily to a rate of 150 ml/kg/day by 5–7 days of age. This fluid requirement may increase by 30% when infants are nursed under radiant heaters when insensible fluid losses are increased. Phototherapy significantly increases fluid loss. Recognition of these factors should avoid oliguria occurring. When present, a cautious fluid challenge (10 ml/kg) will help to determine whether oliguria is due to dehydration or renal failure. The clinical assessment of fluid status in the neonate is often very difficult, especially if daily accurate weight measurements are not possible. In this situation the calculation of the fractional excretion of sodium or renal failure index may help to distinguish between renal failure and dehydration.

1. The fractional excretion of sodium (FE_{Na}):

$$= (U/P_{Na})/(U/P_{creat})$$

2. Renal failure index (RFI):

$$= (U_{Na})/(U/P_{creat})$$

Where U and P are respectively the urine and plasma concentrations of sodium (Na) and creatinine (creat).

The normal value for both is the same and a Fe_{Na} or RFI greater than 3 in the newborn is said to represent parenchymatous renal disease, but the tests have poor specificity. Many babies, particularly very low birth weight babies with oliguria may not, due to renal failure, yet have high urinary sodium excretion particularly during the early neonatal period.

Examination of the urine for the presence of increased amounts of blood and protein usually gives more useful information. Microscopy of a fresh urine sample for the presence of red cells and broad granular casts is very suggestive of parenchymatous renal disease.

A high plasma creatinine concentration is often the first indication of renal failure. Interpretation can be difficult in the first 2 weeks of life when the plasma concentration reflects maternal levels and plasma creatinine concentrations greater than $100\,\mu mol/l$ may be normal (Figure 9.3). In this situation it is more helpful to obtain serial blood tests when a plasma creatinine concentration increasing by more than $20\,\mu mol/l$ a day is suggestive of renal failure. Blood urea concentration is not a good measure of GFR, as many other factors influence the level. These include dietary protein and energy intake, increased catabolism, reduced urine flow rate and dehydration. A blood urea concentration which is inappropriately high in relation to the plasma creatinine suggests attention should be paid either to the dietary energy intake or increasing the rate of fluid administration.

Incidence

It is difficult to estimate the true incidence of renal failure in the neonatal period and during infancy. It has been calculated that 6% of babies admitted to a neonatal intensive care unit had renal failure [20]. In another study, it was calculated that 0.2 newborns per 1000 live births required dialysis treatment because of renal failure [21]. There are, of course, many more infants who have renal failure who do not require dialysis. Renal failure in the first year of life outside the neonatal period is much less common.

Aetiology

Some of the factors which may cause renal failure in the first year of life are outlined in Table 9.2. It is convenient to classify the aetiologies into prerenal, renal and postrenal. This is because the management of the three groups is different. In the prerenal group, management is designed to restore renal perfusion, the treatment of renal causes requires specific measures such as withdrawal of the offending nephrotoxic agent, and surgery may be required for

Table 9.2 Causes of renal failure in the first year of life

Prerenal
Reduced renal perfusion:
  Hypotension
  Sepsis
  Cardiac failure/congenital heart disease
  Hypoxia/asphyxia
  Placental separation
  Renal venous thrombosis
  Treatment with ACE inhibitors (mother or baby)

Renal
Congenital malformations:
  Bilateral renal dysplasia
  Infantile polycystic kidney diseases
Acute tubular necrosis
Acute cortical necrosis
Nephrotoxic drugs
Glomerular nephritis
  Viral infections
  Congenital nephrotic syndrome
Metabolic disease
  Oxalosis
Acute pyelonephritis
Haemolytic uraemic syndrome

Postrenal
Bladder outlet obstruction
Neurogenic bladder

obstructive uropathies. Often there may be more than one factor present in the same patient, for instance, prerenal failure due to dehydration may progress to acute tubular necrosis. Similarly, acute pyelonephritis often complicates an obstructive uropathy.

The most frequent single cause of renal failure in the neonatal period is cardiac surgery for congenital heart disease, followed by sepsis complicating prematurity. Outside the neonatal period the haemolytic uraemic syndrome is the commonest cause of renal failure.

Investigations and management

The investigation of renal failure is conveniently categorized into three areas: to establish the presence of renal failure, to determine its cause and to detect complications.

Established renal failure is present when there is oliguria which is unresponsive to a fluid challenge of 10 ml/kg of isotonic saline and the plasma creatinine concentration is greater than 150 μmol/l and the level is rising.

The cause of renal failure is usually apparent from a carefully taken history and physical examination. Dehydration which is sufficient to cause renal failure usually implies at least 15% loss of body weight and may be detected clinically. Blood pressure measurement is essential in the evaluation of all sick infants and may be low in patients who are shocked or dehydrated.

A history of exposure to nephrotoxic drugs should be sought and it is always wise to examine the drug chart carefully. Nephrotoxic drugs should be stopped, those which are excreted by the kidney should be administered in reduced dosages and, where possible, blood concentrations measured.

The urine should be examined for blood, protein and bacteria. Gross haematuria may suggest renal venous thrombosis, lesser amounts are found in cortical and tubular necrosis. Proteinuria up to 2+ albustix is found in renal failure, but heavy proteinuria suggests glomerulonephritis and then a renal biopsy is necessary.

Haemolytic uraemic syndrome is common in the toddler age group but is rare in the first year of life. It is suggested by a history of blood-stained diarrhoea, pallor, bruising or purpura. Infants may present with generalized seizures. The diagnosis can be confirmed when the blood film shows typical fragmentation of the red blood cells and thrombocytopenia.

Postrenal failure is now unusual during the first year of life because antenatal ultrasound examination of the fetus will usually detect these abnormalities and they can be dealt with early, before renal failure develops. It is, however, wise to perform a renal ultrasound on all children with renal failure to exclude obstruction and identify other renal anomalies such as renal dysplasia or polycystic kidney disease. Bladder outflow obstruction may not always be detected by renal ultrasound when there is established renal failure and a reduced urine flow rate. A micturating cystourethrogram (MCU) may be necessary to detect urethral valves.

The major complications of renal failure are sepsis, haemorrhage, hypertension, anaemia and biochemical disturbances, all of which may be fatal unless they are detected and dealt with. A successful outcome to the management of children with renal failure requires attention to the details of all these.

Sepsis should be considered at every stage in the management. Blood and urine cultures should be obtained at the initial assessment and repeated during the course of the illness whenever necessary. Central venous catheters and long parenteral blood lines should be removed at the earliest opportunity.

Abnormalities of blood clotting are frequently found in renal failure and may be treated with fresh frozen plasma or specific clotting factors whenever necessary. Similarly, platelet transfusions may also be required. However they should be infused cautiously because of the risk of volume overload. It is often preferable to limit their use to those patients who are bleeding. If blood transfusions are required to maintain haemoglobin levels it is better to give frequent small volumes, 10–20 ml/kg body weight, rather than to try to correct totally the anaemia with one larger transfusion. If clotting factors or transfusions are required then early renal replacement treatment is required to make room for the extra fluid infused.

Hypertension should be treated promptly. Hydralazine (1–4 mg/kg/24h) has the advantage of maintaining renal perfusion and is the initial drug of choice. Nifedipine (0.25 mg/kg) may be given sublingually and labetolol by infusion (1–4 μg/kg/min). Sodium nitropresside

infusion is difficult to use and requires special precautions during administration. Hypertension in acute renal failure is often due to fluid overload and is best treated by early dialysis treatment and strict attention to fluid balance.

It is essential to maintain adequate renal and cerebral perfusion by restoring circulatory blood volume and perfusion pressure. This is facilitated by central venous pressure monitoring. The use of ionotropic drugs is necessary when hypotension persists, despite adequate replacement of the circulating blood volume. This is a common problem in acute renal failure associated with sepsis. Maintenance of fluid balance is achieved by replacing fluid losses (insensible and other losses). Insensible fluid loss in the newborn is 50 ml/kg body weight per day and 400 ml/m^2/day in older children, but is reduced by one-third when pulmonary losses are absent during artificial ventilation. Insensible fluid loss increases by 10% for every 1°C of fever and radiant heaters will increase it by up to 30%.

Hyperkalaemia is aggravated by poor nutrition, catabolism and acidosis. Conservative measures should be taken to maintain plasma potassium within the normal range by adequate nutrition with energy supplements and a low potassium diet. Glucose infusion, ion-exchange resins and nebulized salbutamol may be used to control potassium concentration whilst preparations are being made for dialysis. Acidosis can be corrected with sodium bicarbonate, but it is important to remember that 1 mmol of sodium is given with each mmol of bicarbonate and this increases the risk of fluid overload, hypertension and cerebral haemorrhage. Severe acidosis is best treated by early dialysis. Hypocalcaemia is a frequent finding in acute renal failure. Rapid correction of the acidosis will result in a fall in the ionized calcium concentration with a risk of seizures. The maintenance of adequate nutrition is important. If enteral feeding is not possible, then intravenous nutrition should be given. It is often necessary to start dialysis treatment early, in order to make room for the extra fluids required to achieve adequate nutrition.

Dialysis treatment is indicated when there is fluid overload resulting in cardiac failure, difficulties with pulmonary ventilation and oedema, or there is a risk of inducing fluid overload because of high volumes of intravenous fluid support. Acidosis (pH less than 7.2) and hyperkalaemia (K greater than 6 mmol/l) resistant to conservative treatment should be managed by dialysis.

Peritoneal dialysis remains the method of choice in infancy. The soft peritoneal catheters which are introduced percutaneously over a guidewire have proved to be safe and effective. In neonates the catheter is inserted lateral to the rectus abdominus muscle to avoid damaging the umbilical vessels. It is inserted just below the umbilicus in older children and guided into the pelvis. Dialysate volumes of between 25 and 50 ml/kg body weight are used. Low volumes are preferred so that venous return to the heart is not compromised causing hypotension during the abdominal filling phase. This can be a problem causing hypotension in children after cardiac surgery. Perforation of an abdominal organ or blood vessel (usually the inferior vena cava), peritonitis and dehydration are the major complications. Peritonitis is usually due to *Staphyllococcus albus* infection; *E. coli* and pseudomonas infections may also occur. Until microbiological help is available, treatment with vancomycin and a cephalosporin antibiotic is usually sufficient. Dehydration and hyperglycaemia will occur very easily when high glucose containing dialysis fluids are used. Careful attention to fluid balance is essential. Regular weighing will give an indication of the rate of fluid removal.

Haemodialysis, variations of continuous haemodiafiltration and slow dialysis techniques may all be used in infancy with success. Vascular access can be obtained using double lumen subclavian venous catheters (size 7 French). The umbilical vessels can be catheterized in the newborn (size 5 French). Occasionally femoral veins may be used, but they have an increased risk of sepsis. These techniques require the support of specialized paediatric renal dialysis and intensive care teams and should not be attempted otherwise.

Prognosis

The outcome of acute renal failure in infancy is largely determined by the underlying cause. Overall the mortality is around 60% in the neonatal period. When it is secondary to cardiac disease the prognosis is particularly bad

[22]. Over 90% of children with haemolytic uraemic syndrome survive. Recovery is associated with the onset of a diuresis which commences between 2 and 4 weeks after the original insult. This can be a difficult period as dialysis may still be necessary to maintain biochemical stability and fluid and electrolyte losses in the urine may be excessive requiring appropriate replacement.

Renal damage, which may progress to chronic renal insufficiency, may occur in 27% of the survivors [22]. It is wise to keep all survivors under long-term review.

Chronic renal failure

Renal failure is said to be chronic when it occurs over a period of weeks or months. All of the conditions listed in Table 9.2 may progress to chronic renal failure and for that reason it is more practical to refer to irreversible renal failure.

Clinical features and management

Irreversible renal insufficiency is generally relatively asymptomatic and it is not until GFR approaches 15% of normal that clinical symptoms develop and end-stage renal failure is said to be present. There are many features of chronic renal failure.

The anaemia of chronic renal failure has many causes. Iron deficiency is frequent because of poor nutrition and anorexia. In renal failure iron deficiency is present when the plasma ferritin is less than $100 \mu g/l$ [23]. When anaemia persists despite attention to these factors, then erythropoietin is a very effective treatment. It is administered by subcutaneous injection three times a week in a dose of 40 units/kg. Hypertension and hypercoaguability are important complications.

The kidneys' ability to produce 1,25-dihydroxycholecalciferol is impaired in renal failure. This results in renal rickets. Furthermore, as renal function deteriorates, phosphate retention stimulates secondary hyperparathyroidism. True rickets with bone deformity does not develop until the infant is weight bearing but radiological and biochemical features are apparent much earlier.

Muscle weakness is often a feature of advanced renal bone disease causing delay in walking and in achieving other motor milestones. Treatment with adequate doses of 1,25-di-hydroxycholecalciferol, dietary phosphate restriction with phosphate-binding drugs such as calcium carbonate, aiming to maintain normal plasma Ca and P concentrations, is usually effective in healing renal bone disease. The degree of hyperparathyroidism can be confirmed by measurement of the plasma concentration of the hormone. The normal range in children is 11–35 μg/l [24].

Hypertension is a major problem in chronic renal failure and is treated with drugs, dietary salt and often fluid restriction. A no added salt diet, avoiding foods containing excessive salt such as potato crisps and tinned foods, is tolerable. Treatment with hydralazine 1–4 g/kg/day or a beta blocker is usually adequate. The use of angiotensin-converting enzyme inhibitors is effective when the hypertension is severe, but there is a risk of precipitating a rapid reduction in the GFR, and the plasma creatinine should be measured frequently at the onset of treatment.

Growth velocity is often poor in children with renal failure. It is particularly important in infants, as height lost in the first 2 years of life cannot be regained. The major factor which determines growth rate is adequate dietary energy intake, and the target is to achieve the recommended dietary intake for age. Children with renal failure eat poorly and additional nutritional supplements containing high energy glucose polymers or fat are necessary. Despite these supplements, energy intake may still be inadequate and then nasogastric or gastrostomy feeding at night is necessary to maintain a steady growth rate.

Other factors may contribute to poor growth, including anaemia, hyponatraemia, acidosis and severe renal bone disease. The onset of puberty is often delayed in both boys and girls with renal failure and this also contributes to their shortness of stature. Growth hormone treatment has been shown to increase the height velocity in children with renal failure, but it is expensive and should only be used when all the other factors known to interfere with growth have been corrected.

Dietary management of infants with renal failure is difficult [25]. It is usually necessary to restrict fluid and dietary protein sodium, potassium and phosphorus intakes, and provide energy supplements. This makes dietary management a very skilled procedure and a paediatric renal dietician is essential.

When conservative management of chronic renal failure can no longer maintain an adequate quality of life, dialysis treatment is necessary. Both peritoneal and haemodialysis treatment is possible in infants and small children. Although there have been no studies comparing the two, it is generally accepted that peritoneal dialysis treatment offers the best quality of life [26]. It may be delivered by continuous ambulatory peritoneal dialysis (CAPD) or continuous cycling peritoneal dialysis (CCPD). In CAPD the required volume (30–50 ml/kg) of dialysis fluid is run into the peritoneal cavity and left for a period of 4 hours and then drained out and replaced. This process continues throughout the day, but stops at night-time. It works well in small children and can maintain satisfactory fluids and electrolyte status.

In CCPD an automatic cycling peritoneal dialysis machine is used to infuse and drain the dialysis fluid during the night-time whilst the patient is asleep. This technique has the advantage of leaving the daytime free for other activities but it is a much more expensive treatment than CAPD. Both of these peritoneal dialysis techniques can be done at home by the parents, with support from the hospital centre.

The major complication of peritoneal dialysis is peritonitis, usually due to *Staphylococcus albus*, requiring appropriate antibiotic treatment. Fluid retention and oedema can be treated by strict fluid restriction and the use of a hyperosmolar dialysis fluid to achieve greater ultrafiltration.

Haemodialysis treatment requires vascular access to a major vessel. Usually a double-lumen catheter is placed surgically into the right subclavian vein. A blood flow rate of between 3–5 ml/kg/min is necessary to achieve adequate dialysis in these small children. Dialyser selection is determined by the size of the patient and the prescribed urea clearance [27]. Treatment lasts for a period of 3–4 hours, three times a week. It is a very specialized technique in young children and should only be carried out in specialized dialysis centres, with the staff who possess the necessary skills to treat them.

Renal transplantation

Renal dialysis and transplantation are complementary modes of treatment. A successful renal transplant is the best treatment option as it provides a better quality of life, increased growth velocity and is a significantly less expensive treatment.

Patient selection

Every child entered onto the renal replacement programme should be a candidate for kidney transplantation. There is a greater risk of failure in children under 5 years where 50% of kidneys are functioning at 2 years. The results using living related donors are better than cadaver kidneys [28]. The results are particularly poor when kidneys from donor children under 5 years are transplanted into young recipients. The reasons for poor results in children under 5 years of age are many. First, technical difficulties related to the size of the vessels increase the risk of vascular thrombosis and postoperative acute tubular necrosis. Second, small children may be more immunologically active than older children and adults, making rejection more likely. Third, children metabolize cyclosporin more rapidly than adults, consequently higher doses are necessary to achieve therapeutic blood levels which increase the risk of inducing nephrotoxicity. Finally, children are more likely to have a primary renal disease which will adversely affect graft function. This occurs in about a third of children with renal failure due to focal segmental glomerular sclerosis, mesangiocapillary glomerulonephritis and IgA nephropathy. It is generally recommended that a period of time of at least a year should elapse before transplantation in patients with these diseases to reduce the risk of recurrence. When renal failure is due to congenital urological abnormalities such as urethral valves, functional abnormalities of the bladder may compromise graft function. Urinary infections also occur more frequently in this group of patients. If the infection cannot be controlled by prophylactic antibiotics, then native nephroureterectomy may be necessary.

Donor selection

The use of living related donors is controversial and is criticized mainly on ethical grounds. Nevertheless, the results of living donor are superior to cadaver kidneys. The procedure can be planned around important events such as school examinations. Primary renal function is more likely to occur because of short kidney ischaemia times. The risks to the donor are minimal providing adequate selection and counselling has occurred, although it does mean time away from work and the family.

Cadaver kidneys are preferred. It is important to select the donors carefully to avoid transplanting kidneys which are diseased or which may transplant infections or malignancy along with the kidney. The transmission of cytomegalovirus requires special precautions in young children.

It is generally accepted that ABO blood group compatibility is important and optimum HLA matching improves graft survival.

Postoperative care

The improvement in the results of transplantation in small children has occurred mainly due to better postoperative care. They are best managed in an intensive care ward where appropriate monitoring facilities are available Rigorous fluid management is the key to success and this should be controlled by central venous pressure monitoring, maintaining it between 6 and 10 mmHg. Intermittent infusions of albumin or blood may be necessary to achieve this.

It is now generally accepted that the best results are achieved by triple immunosuppression therapy using prednisolone, azathioprine and cyclosporine in combination.

Opportunistic infections are a major risk because of the intensive immunosuppression. The risks can be avoided by early removal of intravenous lines. Many units routinely prescribe cotrimoxazole as prophylaxis against *Pneumocystis carinii*.

Cytomegalovirus (CMV) infection occurs in about 50% of patients receiving solid organ transplants, but only a minority develop serious CMV-related disease where treatment with CMV hyperimmune globulin and ganciclovir may be necessary.

Prognosis

The results of living related donor kidney transplantation in children under 2 years of age are improving, the 1-year graft survival rate averages 80%. However, the results for cadaver donor kidneys is less good 50% [27].

Growth velocity improves providing the dose of prednisolone can be kept below the growth-suppressant age of 0.1 mg/kg/day.

The quality of life is much improved after a successful kidney transplant, but it is always necessary to be alert to the possibility of an acute rejection episode, particularly in the first year following transplantation. Usually this can be reversed by prompt treatment with intravenous methylprednisolone. Chronic vascular rejection, a slow deterioration in renal function which is resistant to treatment, accounts for the majority of transplanted kidneys which fail in the later years. The nature and treatment of this chronic rejection is unknown but the development of newer immunosuppressant drugs may improve the long-term prognosis.

References

1. Coulthard MG, Hey EN. Weight is the best standard for glomerular filtration rate in the newborn. *Arch Dis Child* 1984; **59**: 373–375.
2. Heilbran DC, Holliday MA, Al-Dahwi Amira, Kogan BA. Expressing glomerular filtration rate in children. *Pediatr Nephrol* 1991; **5**: 5–11.
3. Fris Hansen. Body water compartments in children: changes during growth and related changes in body composition. *Pediatrics* 1961; **2**: 169–181.
4. McCance RA, Widderson EM. The correct physiological basis on which to compare infant and adult renal failure. *Lancet* 1952; **ii**: 860–862.
5. Wilkins BH. Renal function in sick very low birth weight infants. 1. Glomerular filtration rate. *Arch Dis Child* 1992; **67**: 1140–1145.
6. Coulthard MG, Hey EN. Comparison of methods of measuring renal function in preterm babies using inulin. *J Pediatr* 1983; **102**: 923–930.
7. Feldman H, Guignard JP. Plasma creatinine in the first month. *Arch Dis Child* 1982; **57**: 123–126.
8. Parkin A, Smith HC, Brocklebank JT. Which routine test for kidney function. *Arch Dis Child* 1989; **64**: 1261–1263.
9. Rudd PT, Hughes EA, Placzek MM. Reference ranges for plasma creatinine during the first month of life. *Arch Dis Child* 1983; **58**: 212–215.
10. Schwartz GJ, Feld LG, Langford DJ. A simple estimate of glomerular filtration rate in full-term infants during the first year of life. *J Pediatr* 1984; **104**: 849–854.
11. Edelmann CH, Barnett HL, Troupkou V. Renal concentrating mechanisms in newborn infants, effect of dietary protein and water content, role of urea and responsiveness to antidiuretic hormone. *J Clin Invest* 1960; **39**: 1062–1069.
12. Potacek E, Voiel J, Nengebauerova M, Sebkova J, Vechetova E. The osmotic concentrating ability in healthy infants and children. *Arch Dis Child* 1965; **40**: 291–295.
13. Ames RG. Urinary water excretion and neurohypophyseal function in full-term and premature infants shortly after birth. *Pediatrics* 1953; **12**: 272–282.
14. Edelmann CM Jr, Rodriguiz-Soriano J, Baidius H, Gruskin AB, Acosta M. Renal bicarbonate reabsorption and hydrogen ion excretion in infants. *J Clin Invest* 1967; **46**: 1309–1317.
15. Cole BR, Brocklebank JT, Capps RG, Murray BN, Robson AM. Maturation of *p*-aminohippuric acid transport in the developing rabbit kidney: interrelationships of the individual components. *Pediatr Res* 1978; **12**: 992–997.
16. Swartz GJ, Higgs T, Spitzer A. Subtherapeutic dicloxacillin levels in a neonate: possible mechanisms. *J Pediatr* 1976; **89**: 310–312.
17. Rhodes PG, Hammel CL, Berman LB. Urinary constituents of the newborn infant. *J Pediatr* 1962; **60**: 18–23.
18. Kotchen TA, Strideland AL, Rice TW et al. A study of the renin–angiotensin system in newborn infants. *J Pediatr* 1972; **80**: 938–946.
19. Guignard JP, Burgew F, Calane A. Persistent anuria in a neonate: a side-effect of captopril. *Int J Pediatr Nephrol* 1981; **2**: 133–134.
20. Norman HC, Asadi FK. A prospective study of acute renal failure in the newborn. *Pediatrics* 1979; **63**: 475–479.
21. Brocklebank JT. Renal failure in the newly born. *Arch Dis Child* 1988; **63**: 991–994.
22. Shaw NJ, Brocklebank JT, Dickinson DF, Wilson N, Walker DR. Longterm outcome for children with acute renal failure following cardiac surgery. *Int J Cardiol* 1991; **31**: 161–166.
23. MacDougall IC, Hutton RD, Cavill I, Coles GA, Williams JD. Treating renal anaemia with recombinant erythropoietin: practical guidelines and a clinical algorithm. *Br Med J* 1990; **300**: 655–659.
24. Shaw NJ, Wheeldon J, Brocklebank JT. Tubular maximum for calcium reabsorption: a normal range in children. *Clin Endocrinol* 1992; **36**: 193–195.
25. Brocklebank JT, Wolfe S. Dietary treatment of renal insufficiency. *Arch Dis Child* 1993; **69**: 704–708.
26. Brownbridge G, Fielding DM. Psychosocial adjustment to end-stage renal failure: comparing haemodialysis continuous ambulatory peritoneal dialysis

and transplantation. *Pediatr Nephrol* 1991; **5**: 612–616.

27. Evans JHC, Smye SW, Brocklebank JT. Mathematical modelling of haemodialysis in children. *Pediatr Nephrol* 1992; **6**: 349–353.

28. McEnery PT, Stabrein DM, Arbus G, Tejani A. Renal transplantation in children: a report of the North American Pediatric Renal Transplant Co-operation Study. *N Engl J Med* 1992; **326**: 1727–1732.

10

Urinary tract infection in the first year of life

M.J. Ellison, F. Jewkes and K. Verrier Jones

Introduction

During the first year of life bacterial infection of the urinary tract is both common and serious. Over the past 30 years there has been an increased awareness of the possibility of urinary infection in infancy and the widespread use of effective antibiotics has undoubtedly reduced the morbidity and mortality of infant urinary tract infection [1–3]. Early reviews of urinary tract infection fail to distinguish clearly between acute and chronic pyelonephritis, making it difficult to disentangle the results of severe acute or chronic infection from the resultant renal damage. There was clear evidence of severe morbidity and a high mortality rate [4]. Reflux nephropathy is the commonest preventable cause of end-stage renal failure in children and adults. In spite of advances in knowledge of the long-term risks and presenting symptoms, many doctors in primary care responsible for infant welfare are still either unaware of the possibility of this diagnosis or do not have access to urine culture in the emergency situation unless the child is referred to hospital. In some areas, urine is still not examined for infection in every sick infant, even in hospital [5]. This has led to a delay in initiating treatment and an increased risk of permanent renal damage. Generally, however, urinary tract infection (UTI) is now diagnosed earlier than it was in previous decades, leading to a change in the severity of the clinical picture and probably a reduction in the residual renal damage produced. Increasing health awareness and rising expectations of the general public have influenced the level of communication with parents, so that some will now expect urinary tract infection to be excluded each time their infant is ill. Doctors have access to a range of effective antibiotics and a better knowledge of the antibiotic sensitivity of the commonest organisms.

The role of ureteric reimplantation in prevention of urinary tract infection and renal damage has been questioned and fewer children now undergo this procedure even when severe reflux is present. The use of prophylactic antibiotics has been widely accepted as an effective means of substantially reducing the risk of infection in children with increased susceptibility to UTI. Although there may be no universal agreement on the most appropriate radiological investigation, there is broad consensus that vesicoureteric reflux (VUR) is an important risk factor for the development of both infection and renal scarring, and the need for thorough investigation of every infant after the first infection is generally accepted.

The widespread use of ultrasound during pregnancy with resultant antenatal diagnosis of fetal uropathy has created further opportunities for the prevention of infection in those most at risk, using prophylactic antibiotics, and for early detection and treatment of intercurrent infection when it occurs. It is also clear that VUR runs in families and that those most often affected are newborn infants. Such families are often highly motivated to use prophylaxis and to ensure that intercurrent infections are treated promptly, since they have usually had previous experience with a sick infant or have reflux nephropathy themselves.

Epidemiology

During the first month of life, UTI is significantly more common in boys than in girls, in contrast to the pattern after 6 months of age and throughout childhood when infection is more common in girls [6]. However, in both sexes the commonest time for the first infection to occur is the first month of life [7] (Figure 10.1). It has been suggested that infection is more common in preterm infants and in infants born to mothers with prolonged rupture of membranes, following assisted delivery and birth asphyxia [8]. After appropriate treatment relapsing or persisting infection is uncommon and when it does occur is an indication of a significant underlying abnormality, whereas reinfection with a different organism, is relatively common. In practice if serotyping

has not been carried out it may be impossible to differentiate between a relapse and a reinfection.

Girls are prone to develop reinfections throughout childhood, while in boys reinfections are less common but are often clustered soon after the initial infection when they do occur. From his studies Winberg calculated that the risk of developing a UTI before the age of 11 years was 1.1% for boys and over 3% for girls, with the period of greatest risk for the first infection being the first year of life for both sexes [6].

When bacteriuria is detected as a result of screening programmes or in healthy people, it is termed asymptomatic or covert. On close questioning mild symptoms are sometimes present. Covert bacteriuria has been detected in 4% of term infants and 9.8% of preterm infants [9]. The female preponderance noted in school age children is absent in the neonatal period. The prevalence of asymptomatic bacteria in early childhood is shown in Table 10.1. In a prospective study of covert bacteriuria in infancy, Wettergren showed that the infection resolved spontaneously in many cases, while in others it persisted without giving rise to renal damage or symptoms [10]. However, two infants became acutely unwell and were treated.

Pathogenesis

The development of UTI occurs when pathogenic organisms colonize the infant and then invade the urinary tract, triggering the inflammatory response, resulting in symptoms and, in some cases, renal damage. Successful pathogens must also have the ability to survive and multiply in the urinary tract. The commonest pathogen is *E. coli* which has been shown to have a variety of virulence factors.

Colonization and route of entry

At birth the infant is normally sterile, the exceptions being those cases of infection of the amniotic fluid following premature rupture of the membranes or following other maternal infections including acute pyelonephritis. Soon after birth, normal commensal organisms colonize the skin and mucous membranes, particularly the gastrointestinal tract, which is rapidly colonized with *E. coli*. Septicaemia is thought

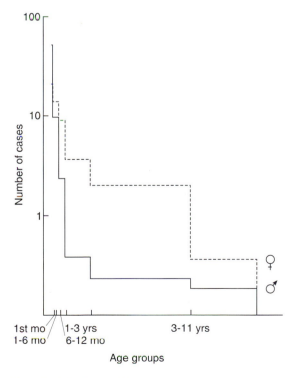

Figure 10.1 Incidence of first urinary tract infections in relation to age in infants and children (Winberg et al. 1974).

Table 10.1 Prevalence of asymptomatic bacteriuria in infancy and early childhood

Age	Sex	Collection method	%	Number screened	Author
Preterm	M, F	SPA	9.8	102	Pendarvis [11]
Preterm	M, F	Bag and SPA	2.9	206	Edelmann [12]
Term	M, F	Bag and SPA	0.7	836	Edelmann [12]
Term	M, F	Bag and SPA	1.0	1460	Abbott [13]
Term	F	Glass bottle	0	286	Lincoln [14]
	M	Glass bottle	2.7	298	
0–12 months	F	Bag and SPA	1.1⎫	3581	Wettergren [10]
	M	Bag and SPA	1.2⎭		

SPA = suprapubic aspiration.

to occur when these gut organisms breach the intact mucosa and enter the blood stream. This occurs mainly in the first month of life when IgA levels are at their lowest. Later the prepucial sac and periurethral region are colonized with *Proteus* and *E. coli* in uncircumcised but not in circumcised male infants. In female infants the periurethral region is normally colonized with multiple species of *E. coli*, *Enterobacteriacae*, *staphylococci* and *enterococci* from a few days of life. Winberg observed that in girls prone to recurrent infection the periurethral area became colonized with *E. coli* prior to the development of infection and that ampicillin altered the normal flora in favour of *E. coli*. The usual route of entry to the urinary tract in the first month of life is believed to be via the blood stream, whereas ascending infection is believed to occur thereafter. It is interesting to note that urinary tract infection is less common in circumcised than in uncircumcised male infants. Wiswell [15] suggested that colonization of the prepucial sac and the ascending route are important as a source of infection and route of entry in infant boys.

Survival in the urinary tract

Once within the urinary tract, bacteria are able to grow and multiply in the urine and, in some cases, in the renal parenchyma. Energy for growth is derived from urinary glucose and it is interesting to note that glycosuria is prominent in the first few days of life (M. James Ellison, unpublished data, 1993), and in premature sick infants it is particularly heavy [16]. Bacteria can multiply more rapidly between pH 5 and 7 than at the extremes and when the osmolality is 200–500 mosmol/kg [17]. These

conditions are often present for long periods in infant urine which does not vary much throughout the day because of the frequent intake of milk and lack of variation in the diet.

Frequent micturition in infants will eliminate a proportion of the bacteria often preventing the colony count reaching the 100 000/cfu/ml usually regarded as indicative of infection. However, it has been shown that many infants do not completely empty the bladder and that complete bladder emptying does not occur regularly until after 2 years of age [18]. Thus bacteria ascending the urethra may easily multiply in the infant urinary tract and are less likely to be eliminated by micturition than in older children, although the colony count may sometimes be relatively low [19]. Some bacteria have adhesive properties mediated by fimbria which facilitate colonization and survival within the bladder.

Ascent to the kidneys

Following colonization of the bladder, the bacteria may proceed to colonize the ureters and eventually the kidneys. This is more likely to occur if vesicoureteric reflux (VUR) is present or if there is outflow obstruction. VUR is more often present in infants than older children and tends to improve or disappear with time as the child grows. The presence of intrarenal reflux in some infants is associated with upper tract infection and subsequent scar formation at the site of the lesion [20]. The resulting acute pyelonephritis may be followed by septicaemia. *E. coli* bearing p fimbria have been shown to be particularly prone to cause acute pyelonephritis, even in the absence of anatomical host factors such as VUR [21]. The production of endotoxin has been shown to reduce ureteric peristalsis or cause dilatation and may contribute to upper tract involvement in some cases [22].

The inflammatory response

The inflammatory response is initiated by contact between the bacteria and the host, resulting in the release of chemotactic mediators which encourage the influx of polymorphs. *E. coli* bearing p fimbria have been shown to invade the tissues and to trigger an inflammatory response in the normal urinary tract. Mannose-sensitive fimbria have been shown to activate the inflammatory burst of polymorphs and have been implicated in scar formation [23].

Host defence and immunity

Since urine is an effective culture medium and the urinary tract communicates with the perineum via the urethra, it is clear that there must be effective mechanisms preventing colonization or infection of the urinary tract, otherwise the urine would be colonized from a few days after birth in the majority of infants (Figure 10.2). The act of micturition undoubt-

edly plays a part in washing out bladder bacteria but since micturition is incomplete in many infants and children under 2 years old, this cannot be the only factor.

Secretory IgA in the urine may have an important role in preventing infection and it has been shown that girls with *E. coli* colonization of the perineum had low levels of secretory IgA in vaginal secretions. Similarly low levels of urinary SIgA have been found in children with recurrent UTI [24]. Breast feeding which is associated with higher urinary IgA levels than bottle feeding, is associated with a lower risk of bacterial infection [25,26]. At birth urinary IgA and SIgA are undetectable, although the free secretory component is present [27]. This may account in part for the increased risk of urinary tract infection in the newborn and premature infant.

A serum antibody response to *E. coli* occurs following upper tract infections in infants and children but is absent in the first 2 months of life. Elevated antibodies to lipid A were closely related to subsequent scar formation in older children but not in children under 2 years [28]. Little is known about the role of cellular immunity in infant urinary tract infection.

The secretion of water-soluble carbohydrate blood group substances in the urine appears to have a protective effect against infection. This characteristic is inherited as an autosomal dominant but is independent of the inheritance of the ABO blood group and closely linked to Lewis antigen status [29]. The presence of p1 antigens on individuals expressing the p1 blood group, predisposes to colonization with p fimbriated organisms in individuals of blood group B, who also seem to be particularly prone to urinary tract infection.

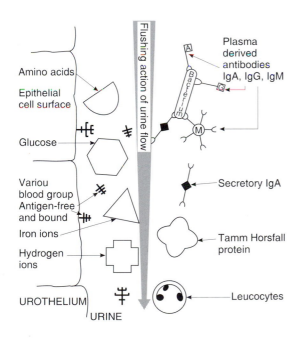

Figure 10.2 Host defence mechanisms in the urinary tract.

The invading organism

The commonest invading organism at all ages is *E. coli*; however, in the neonatal period a number of other organisms have been grown including *Staphylococcus aureus*, *Staphylococcus epidermidis*, streptococci, *Klebsiella* and *Proteus* spp. *Proteus* spp. are important pathogens because of their ability to split urea to ammonia, lowering the urinary pH and predisposing to stone formation. These infections are more common in male infants, possibly because the reservoir for *Proteus* is under the

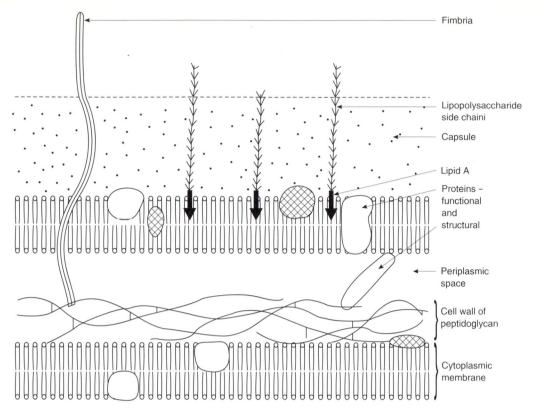

Fimbria

Lipopolysaccharide
side chaini

Capsule

Lipid A

Proteins –
functional
and
structural

Periplasmic
space

Cell wall of
peptidoglycan

Cytoplasmic
membrane

Figure 10.3 Structure of the cell wall and outer structures of *E. Coli.*

foreskin. *E. coli* have been studied extensively for the virulence factors which enable them to colonize, invade, survive, and cause inflammation and damage within the urinary tract (Figure 10.3).

Bacterial virulence factors

Some bacteria, notably *E. coli*, have the ability to adhere to the urothelium, while some can also invade the tissues and trigger the inflammatory and immune responses.

Mannose-resistant or p fimbriae are hair-like projections which enable the organism to adhere to p blood group receptors expressed on the urothelium. P fimbriate *E. coli* have been associated with systemic symptoms and invasion of the upper tracts causing acute pyelonephritis, but have not been linked closely with permanent renal damage or scar formation [30]. On the other hand, mannose-sensitive fimbriae adhere to mannose residues on the urothelial cells or on Tamm Horsfall protein. Organisms bearing these characteristics have

often been found in cases of asymptomatic bacteriuria and in the presence of underlying urological abnormalities including VUR. These fimbriae appear to be capable of causing inflammation and permanant renal damage. Lipid A, an endotoxin released during bacterial lysis, has been held responsible for ureteric dilatation and reduced ureteric motility [22], and when released within the blood stream causes endotoxic shock. It is also responsible for activating the complement cascade. Bacteria bearing the K or Capsular antigen have increased ability to invade the kidney and cause acute pyelonephritis, can inhibit phagocytosis, and are more resistant to the cidal effect of serum. Haemolysin and aerobactin are bacterial proteins which trap iron, essential for bacterial growth. Bacteria producing these proteins have increased cytotoxicity to host inflammatory cells and renal tissue. Aerobactin producing *E. coli* variants are also commonly associated with septicaemia.

The expression of virulence factors may vary with the environment so that features demonstrated *in vitro* may not always represent the situation *in vivo*. In addition, *E. coli* can undergo phase variation, a spontaneous re-arrangement of genetic material, which allows certain virulence characteristics to be expressed or suppressed in different situations, increasing the ability of the organism to survive, multiply and spread in a changing environment. Furthermore, genetic material can be ex-changed from one bacterium to another, thus rapidly transferring characteristics such as anti-biotic resistance [31].

Effect of age and sex on host–parasite relationship

The most obvious difference between the sexes in the infant urinary tract is the greater length of the male urethra and presence of the fore-skin. The observations by Wiswell that infec-tion is much less common in circumcised than uncircumcised male infants suggests that the prepucial sac acts as an important reservoir for infection [15]. However, there is an increase in morbidity from serious blood-borne infection in male infants compared to female infants in the first month of life, which cannot be accounted for by these anatomical differences. This presumably represents some undefined delay in maturation of the immune system or an alteration in other host factors.

The most severe illness associated with UTI tends to occur in the youngest infants and they are also most vulnerable to renal damage. The reason for increased susceptibility of infants to scarring is not known, although rapid renal growth, severity of infection and immaturity of the collagen and basement membranes and the presence in infants of intrarenal reflux [32] have been postulated as contributing factors.

Symptoms

Symptoms of UTI are diverse and rarely loca-lized to the urinary tract before 2 years of age (Figure 10.4). In the neonate, severe illness

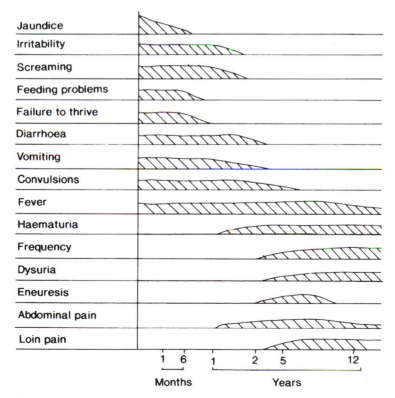

Figure 10.4 Age distributions of common childhood symptoms of urinary tract infection.

with septicaemia may occur, giving rise to symptoms such as irritability, vomiting, convulsions, apnoea, hypoglycaemia, unstable temperature and collapse. In these very ill babies severe electrolyte disturbance, disseminated intravascular coagulation and acute renal failure may be present and signs of other organ involvement may occur such as meningitis or, less commonly, osteomyelitis. Jaundice may be the only symptom of *E. coli* UTI and may indicate infection with an organism with specific ability to cause haemolysis.

Failure to thrive may be the presenting symptom of infection in infancy and may often be associated with a significant degree of transient renal functional impairment or electrolyte dysfunction which resolves after antibiotic treatment. More commonly, infants have other features of poor health such as vomiting, anorexia, abdominal pain or recurrent low grade fever [33]. These symptoms are often attributed to viral infections unless the urine is cultured.

After 6 months of age a significant number of febrile convulsions are caused by UTI [34]. Hyponatraemia, acidosis and elevated urea and creatinine suggest upper tract involvement or severe underlying abnormality.

Diagnosis of infection

Precise bacteriological diagnosis is mandatory because symptoms and physical signs are inconclusive, and even misleading. Urine should be collected as a matter of urgency from every sick infant for microscopy, culture, colony count and antibiotic sensitivity of the infecting organism. Unless this is done, it is not possible to start treatment promptly and to ensure that the most appropriate antibiotic is used. Failure to collect urine before the start of antimicrobial therapy will obscure the diagnosis resulting in a false-negative result, and important investigations for underlying renal pathology will be overlooked. Alternatively, a false-positive result from a contaminated sample will lead to unnecessary invasive tests being carried out. It is usual to accept a colony count of $>10^5$ cfu/ml as indicative of UTI, but occasionally the count may be lower, particularly if there is acute pyelonephritis which often leads to a concentrating defect and frequent bladder emptying.

Suprapubic aspiration of urine should always be carried out in any sick infant prior to the start of antibiotic therapy. The use of ultrasound to check that urine is present is helpful. If no urine is obtained and the baby is sufficiently sick to merit immediate treatment with antibiotics, a catheter sample should be collected. In a less sick child, bag urine samples are often used but their value is limited by the high contamination rate. Their greatest value is in excluding UTI when negative. Ideally two samples should be collected. Clean catch specimens may have less contamination but bacteria under the foreskin in males are still a common source of contamination.

Dipslides are useful in primary care since the dipslide can be inoculated with urine in the home prior to being sent to the laboratory but does not permit microscopy. Bottles containing boric acid are also useful but must be filled with the correct amount of urine otherwise the concentration of boric acid either fails to prevent bacterial multiplication of contaminants or inhibits growth of the infecting organism on the culture plate [35]. The use of impregnated sticks to test for blood and protein is of no value in establishing the presence of infection. The use of the nitrite test is also unhelpful, since there is a high incidence of false-negative results in infants with acute infection, although a positive result is highly significant.

Level of infection

Some indication of the level of infection can be obtained from clinical observation. Renal involvement is more likely to be present if the child is systemically ill, has a fever or has tender enlarged kidneys. Upper tract involvement is usually associated with a raised white cell count in the blood, raise erythrocyte sedimentation rate and raised C-reactive protein and sometimes electrolyte disturbance, acidosis or elevation of urea and creatinine. The urine is more likely to show evidence of tubular proteinuria, enzymuria and a concentration defect when there has been renal involvement. Transient filling defects on DMSA scan are highly suggestive of upper tract infection; however, no test has been shown to be totally reliable in making a level diagnosis in infants [36].

Management of the acute illness

In addition to urine culture the sick infant may require a blood culture, white blood count, urea electrolytes, creatinine, blood gases and lumbar puncture, depending on the severity of the illness and the mode of presentation. Intravenous fluids and parenteral antibiotic, usually gentamycin and ampicillin should be used initially [37,38]. If renal function is impaired, the gentamycin dose should be adjusted and levels monitored. If the baby is not significantly better after 48 hours, there is an urgent need to review the sensitivity of the organism and to look for underlying pathology in the urinary tract by an ultrasound examination. In many cases the infant will be much improved and in the older infant a change to the most appropriate oral antibiotic can be made. In the first 2 months of life it is usual to continue intravenous treatment for 5 days. Trimethoprim is the oral antibiotic most often used in the management of UTI and may be used in an infant who is not seriously ill; however, increasing resistance may limit its value in the future. After completion of the therapeutic course, usually 5–10 days of oral therapy, prophylactic trimethoprim or nitrofurantoin 1–2 mg/kg at night should be started and continued until all relevant investigations of the urinary tract have been completed.

Supportive treatment is often needed in the more seriously ill babies. In particular failure of conservation of electrolytes and water can require careful adjustment of fluid and electrolyte balance using intravenous or oral supplements. Urine culture should be taken at the end of treatment to ensure that the infection has been eradicated [39].

Investigation of underlying abnormalities

It is recommended that all children and infants should have investigation of the urinary tract and kidneys following the first proven infection to assess renal damage and to look for underlying pathology such as VUR, obstruction or dilatation, which may predispose to further infection or damage [32]. Although the need for full investigation of the older child is controversial, most paediatricians agree that infants should undergo micturating cystourethrography, as well as a DMSA scan and ultrasound examination.

The initial examination is usually made using ultrasound, which is a simple non-invasive procedure which can establish the presence, size and position of the kidneys and dilatation of the urinary tract. However ultrasound is unreliable as a means of establishing the presence or absence of VUR or of renal damage in infants and small children [40]. Enlarged kidneys are often found soon after acute pyelonephritis (Figure 10.5). Small kidneys may be due to renal scarring or congenital renal dysplasia.

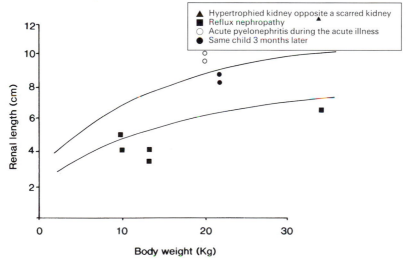

Figure 10.5 Normal range for renal length on ultrasound vs weight and observations on kidney size in children with reflux nephropathy and acute pyelonephritis.

It is recommended that all infants with UTI should have a conventional micturating cystourethrogram to establish the presence or absence of VUR, to look at the size and shape of the bladder and in males with dilatation of the urinary tract, to exclude urethral valves at the same time [41]. Direct radionuclide cystography can be used as an alternative in girls but indirect cystography using DTPA, ^{99}Tc^m or MAG3 is unreliable in this age group. Prophylactic antibiotics should be given to prevent the introduction of infection during catheterization.

DMSA ^{99}Tc^m scanning is used to demonstrate renal involvement and scar formation, which is characterized by filling defects which are often not visible on ultrasound examination [42]. Transient filling defects lasting a few weeks are seen to correspond with areas of acute pyelonephritis, while renal scars give rise to permanent abnormalities (Figure 10.6). The total dose of radiation from a DMSA scan is lower than for intravenous urography, although the radiation to the gonads is higher.

Intravenous urography remains the best investigation to demonstrate precise anatomical detail and to define the level of obstruction and is used when significant pelvicalyceal or ureteric dilatation is seen on ultrasound. However poor function in preterm infants and during the first few weeks of life limit the value of this test in early infancy.

Long-term management

Obstructive lesions will usually require surgical correction and should be referred urgently to the paediatric urologist. Occasionally an acutely ill infant with obstruction will have to be managed conservatively with nephrostomies or suprapubic catheter, intravenous fluids and antibiotics until fit for definitive surgery. Such cases should always be managed in collaboration with a paediatric surgeon.

When investigations have been completed and providing no abnormalities have been detected, it is reasonable to discontinue prophylactic antibiotics in children over 6 months of age. However, in infants under 6 months, it is wise to continue prophylaxis for at least 6 months because of the high risk of recurrence even if no underlying abnormalities have been seen. The role of circumcision in preventing recurrent infection has not been evaluated fully, but may have a place in infant boys with complicated urological abnormalities.

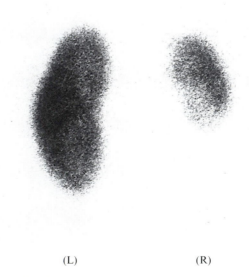

(L)   (R)

Figure 10.6 DMSA Scan showing hypertrophied left kidney (L) and small scarred right kidney (R) following recurrent urinary tract infections in infancy.

VUR is present in one-third of infants with UTI and scarring will occur in some, mainly in those cases where infection has developed very early, and when there has been a delay in starting treatment [43]. For these reasons prophylaxis must be continued until reflux and obstruction have been excluded. When reflux is present, prophylaxis should be continued long term unless an antireflux procedure is carried out or reflux resolves spontaneously. There is no clear-cut point at which it is safe to discontinue prophylaxis when reflux is present and it is often convenient to continue until the child is at least 5 years of age [44]. After this age it is relatively easy to collect urine samples and to diagnose and treat infections promptly. The practice of repeated cystography to confirm the resolution of VUR has never been evaluated in prospective studies and is unpopular with the patients. However, this is still commonly done. The role of reimplantation is also in doubt [45,46], but is certainly helpful in some children who are unable to comply with medical treatment. Antireflux procedures are discussed in depth elsewhere in this book.

Prophylactic antibiotic therapy

The use of a small dose of trimethoprim or nitrofurantoin 1–2 mg/kg/day has been shown to reduce the risk of further infections in infants and children prone to infection. To obtain the maximum benefit from this treatment it should be started immediately after completion of the therapeutic course of antibiotic given to treat the first infection. It should not normally be stopped during treatment with other drugs or antibiotics. Common causes of poor results from prophylaxis are failure to give the drug regularly, failure to obtain repeat prescriptions and stopping prophylaxis during courses of antibiotics such as Amoxil given for intercurrent infections. Breakthrough infection with a sensitive organism suggests failure to give the prophylactic agent, whereas breakthrough with a resistant organism is usually due to incomplete bladder emptying or underlying dilatation or obstruction of the urinary tract which may need surgical treatment.

Much of the success of treatment in recent years has been due to better communication between doctors, nurses and parents with heightened awareness of the need for urine culture, early treatment of infection, and better understanding of how to use prophylactic therapy.

Prognosis

Recurrent infection

A small proportion of boys and a larger proportion of girls will develop further UTI during childhood. Those with VUR or dilatation of the urinary tract are at greatest risk and some may develop further renal damage.

Renal damage

Reflux nephropathy develops in 7–25% of infants and children with UTI [47]. The risk of further scar formation is greatest in those with reflux and when there is a delay in starting treatment after an infection. Scarred kidneys are smaller and function less well than normal kidneys. If bilateral scarring has occurred the total GFR will often be reduced [48]. In 5–20% of cases hypertension will develop, particularly in those with bilateral scarring and reduced renal function. The development of proteinuria is an ominous sign and is an indication of progressive renal damage and hyperfiltration of the remaining glomeruli. Children with reduced renal function and persistent proteinuria usually become hypertensive and almost invariably progress to end-stage renal failure. Reflux nephropathy was the commonest preventable cause of end-stage renal failure in childhood and in adults [49], but there is some evidence that the prevalence of this condition is declining in Sweden following better management of infant UTI [50].

Women with scarred kidneys are at increased risk of hypertension when taking oral contraceptives and during pregnancy [51]. All women with a past history of UTI have an increased risk of further infection precipitated by sexual activity.

VUR is probably inherited by autosomal dominance. There is a 50% risk that infant siblings and offspring will be affected and therefore that they too will have an increased risk of UTI [52,53]. Appropriate counselling on the risk, management and detection of infection and reflux will reduce the morbidity in subsequent babies. The risk of infection in the first

2 years of life can be reduced by giving prophylactic antibiotics to those high-risk infants
from the first day of life.

References

1. Verrier Jones K. Lower and upper urinary tract infection in the child. In: Cameron S, Davidson A et al.
   (eds) *Oxford Textbook of Clinical Nephrology*, vol. 3.
   Oxford: Oxford University Press, 1992; pp 1699–1719.
2. Winberg J. Clinical aspects of urinary tract infection.
   In: Barratt TM, Holliday MA, Vernier RL (eds)
   Paediatric Nephrology, 2nd edn. Baltimore: Williams
   & Wilkins, 1987; pp 626–646.
3. Verrier Jones K, Asscher AW. Urinary tract infection
   in paediatric kidney disease. In: Edelmann CM,
   Bernstein J, Meadow R et al. (eds). 2nd edn. Boston:
   Little Brown, 1992; pp 1943–1991.
4. Steele RE, Leadbetter GW, Crawford JD. Prognosis
   of childhood urinary tract infection. *N Engl J Med*
   1936; **269**: 883–889.
5. van der Voort J, Edwards A, Roberts R, Verrier
   Jones K. The struggle to diagnose UTI in children
   under two in primary care. *Family Practice* 1997; **14**:
   44–48.
6. Winberg J, Bergstrom T, Jacobsson B. Morbidity, age
   and sex distribution, recurrences and renal scarring in
   symptomatic urinary tract infection in childhood.
   Kidney Int 1975; **8**:101–106.
7. Bergstrom T, Larson H, Lincoln K, Winberg J.
   Studies of urinary tract infections in infancy and
   childhood. XII. Eighty consecutive patients with neonatal infections. *J Paediatr* 1972; **80**: 858–866.
8. Littlewood JM. 66 infants with urinary tract infection
   in the first month of life. *Arch Dis Child* 1972; **47**:
   218–226.
9. Edelmann CM, Ogwo JE, Fine BP, Martinez AB.
   The prevalance of bacteriuria in full term and premature new born infants. *J Pediatr* 1973; **82**: 125.
10. Wettergren B, Jodal U. Spontaneous clearance of
    asymptomatic bacteriuria in infants. *Acta Paediatr
    Scand* 1990; **79**:300–304.
11. Pendarvis BCJ, Wenzl JE, Chitwood L. Bacteriuria in
    premature infants detected by aspiration cultures.
    Interscience Conference on microbial agents and
    chemotherapy, Washington D.C. *Paediatric News*
    1970; **4**: 33.
12. Edelmann CM, Ogwo JE, Fine BP, Martinez AB.
    The prevalence of bacteriuria in full term and prema-
    ture new born infants. *J Pediatr* 1973; **82**: 125.
13. Abbott GD. Neonatal bacteriuria: a prospective study
    of 1,460 infants. *Br Med J* 1972; **1**: 267–269.
14. Lincoln K, Winberg J. Studies of urinary tract infec-
    tion in infancy and childhood. II. Quantitative esti-
    mation of bacteriuria in unselected neonates with
    special reference to the occurrence of asymptomatic
    infections. *Acta Paediatr Scand* 1964; **53**: 307–316.

15. Wiswell TE, Smith FR, Bass JW. Decreased incidence
    of urinary tract infection in circumcised male infants.
    Pediatrics 1985; **75**:901–903.
16. Wilkins BH. Renal function in sick, very low birth
    weight infants: 4. Glucose excretion. *Arch Dis Child*
    1992; **67**: 1162–1165.
17. Asscher AW. *The Challenge of Urinary Tract Infec-
    tion*. London: Academic, 1980.
18. James Ellison M, Verrier Jones K. Bladder emptying
    in infancy and childhood: a possible host factor for
    urinary tract infection. *Pediatric Rev Commun* 1994;
    7: 285–286. (Abstract)
19. Bollgren I, Engstrom CF, Hammarlind M, Kallenius
    G, Ringertz H, Svenson SB. Low urinary counts of
    p-fimbriated *Escherichia coli* in presumed acute
    pyelonephritis. *Arch Dis Child* 59; 102–106.
20. Rolleston GL, Maling JMJ, Hodson J. Intrarenal
    reflux and the scarred kidney. *Arch Dis Child* 1974;
    49: 531–539.
21. Lomberg H, Hansson LA, Jacobsson B, et al. Corre-
    lation of P blood group, vesicoureteral reflux and
    bacterial attachment in patients with recurrent
    pyelonephritis. *N Engl J Med* 1983; **308**: 1189–1192.
22. Roberts JA. Etiology and pathophysiology of
    pyelonephritis. *Am J Kidney Dis* 1991; **XVII**: 1.
23. Matsumoto T, Mitzunoe Y, Ogata N, Tanaka M,
    Takahasi K, Kumazawa J. Antioxidant effect on renal
    scarring following infection of Mannose-sensitive-
    piliated bacteria. *Nephron* 1992; **60**: 210–215.
24. Fliedner M, Mehls O, Rauterberg EW, Ritz E. Urin-
    ary sIgA in children with urinary tract infection.
    Pediatrics 1986; **109**: 416.
25. Prentice A. Breast feeding increases concentrations of
    IgA in infants' urine. *Arch Dis Child* 1987; **62**: 792–
    795.
26. Tacket CP, Losonsky G, Link H. Protection by milk
    immunoglobulin concentrate against oral challenge
    with enterotoxigenic escherichia coli. *N Engl J Med*
    1988; **318**: 1240.
27. Ellison MJ, Topley N, Verrier Jones K. Urinary
    secretory IgA and mucosal immunity during the first
    6 months of life. *Nephrol Dial Transplant* 1994; **9**:
    856–857. (Abstract)
28. Mar PJ, Marget W, Schneider K et al. Relevance of
    vesicoureteric reflux in development of lipid A anti-
    bodies in recurrent urinary tract infections in children
    – a preliminary study. *Eur J Pediatr* 1987; **146**: 51–55.
29. Sheinfeld J, Cordon-Cardo C, Fair WR, Wartinger
    DD, Rabinowitz R. Association of Type 1 blood
    group antigens with urinary tract infections in chil-
    dren with genitourinary structural abnormalities.
    J Urol 1990; **144**: 469–473.
30. Harber MJ, Asscher AW. Virulence of urinary
    pathogens. *Kidney Int* 1985; **28**: 717–721.
31. Kroll JS. Bacterial virulence: an environmental
    response. *Arch Dis Child* 1991; **66**: 361–363.
32. Ransley PG, Risdon RA. Renal papillary morphology
    in infants and young children. *Urol Res* 1975; **3**: 111.

33. Smellie JM, Hodson CJ, Edwards D. Clinical and radiological features of urinary infection in childhood. *Br Med J* 1964; **2**: 1222–1226.

34. Lee P, Verrier Jones K. Urinary tract infection in febrile convulsions. *Arch Dis Child* 1991; **66**: 1287–1290.

35. Jewkes FEM, McMaster DJ, Napier WA, Houston IB, Postlethwaite RJ. Home collection of urine specimens – boric acid bottles or dipslides? *Arch Dis Child* 1990; **65**: 286–289.

36. Jodal U, Lindberg U, Lincoln K. Level diagnosis of symptomatic urinary tract infections in childhood. *Acta Paediatr Scand* 1975; **64**: 201–208.

37. Jodal U, Winberg J. Management of children with unobstructed urinary tract infection. *Pediatr Nephrol* 1987; **1**: 647–656.

38. Verrier Jones K. Antimicrobial treatment for urinary tract infections. *Arch Dis Child* 1990; **65**: 327–330.

39. Haycock GB. Investigation of urinary tract infection. *Arch Dis Child* 1986; **61**: 1155–1158.

40. Li Volti S, Di Bella D, Garozzo R, Di Fede GF, Mollica F. Imaging of urinary tract malformations: intravenous urography and/or kidney ultrasonography? *Child Nephrol Urol* 1991; **11**: 96–99.

41. Report of a Working Group of the Research Unit, Royal College of Physicians. Guidelines for the management of acute urinary tract infection in childhood. *J R Coll Phys Lond* 1991; **25**: 36–42.

42. Goldraich NP. Reflux nephropathy: the place of the DMSA renal scan. In: Bailey R (ed) *Second C J Hodson Symposium on Reflux Nephropathy*, 2nd edn. Christchurch: Design Printing Services, 1991; pp 9–13.

43. Smellie JM, Ransley PG, Normand ICS, Prescod N, Edwards D. Development of new renal scars; a collaborative study. *Br Med J* 1985; **290**: 1957–1960.

44. Arant BS Jr. Vesicoureteric reflux and renal injury. *Am J Kidney Dis* 1991; **17**: 491–511.

45. Birmingham Reflux Study Group. Prospective trial of operative versus non-operative treatment of severe vescioureteric reflux in children: five years' observation. *Br Med J* 1987; **295**: 237–241.

46. Smellie JM, Tamminem-Mobius T, Olbing H et al. Five year study of medical or surgical treatment in children with severe reflux: radiological renal findings. The International Reflux Study in Children. *Pediatr Nephrol* 1992; **6**: 223.

47. White RHR. Vesicoureteric reflux and renal scarring. *Arch Dis Child* 1989; **64**: 407–412.

48. Verrier Jones K, Asscher AW, Verrier Jones ER et al. Glomerular filtration rate in schoolgirls with covert bacteriuria. *Br Med J* 1982; **285**: 1307–1310.

49. Brunner FP, Brynger H, Chantler C et al. Combined report on regular dialysis and transplantation in Europe IX 1978. In: Robinson RHB, Hawkins JB, Naik RB (eds) *Proceedings of The European Dialysis Transplant Association*, vol. 16. Bath: The Pitman Press, 1979; pp 4–73.

50. Helin I, Winberg J. Chronic renal failure in Swedish children. *Acta Paediatr Scand* 1980; **69**: 607–611.

51. Sacks S, Verrier Jones K, Roberts R, Leddingham JGG, Asscher AW. Outcome of pregnancy in women with childhood bacteriuria. *Lancet* 1987; **ii**: 991–994.

52. Kenda RB, Kenig T, Budihna N. Detecting vesico-ureteral reflux in asymptomatic siblings of children with reflux by direct radionuclide cystography. *Eur J Pediatr* 1991; **150**: 735–737.

53. Aggarwal VK, Verrier Jones K. Vesicoureteric reflux: screening of first degree relatives. *Arch Dis Child* 1989; **64**: 1538–1541.

11

Pathophysiology and diagnosis of upper tract obstruction in the newborn and infant

Y.L. Homsy and R. Lambert

The subject of this chapter is currently undergoing rapid changes and causing a lively debate between proponents and opponents of early surgical intervention, as opposed to observation alone for apparent ureteropelvic (UPJ) and ureterovesical junction (UVJ) obstruction. The main difficulty lies in recognizing obstruction that is truly harmful to the kidney in the newborn and infant. Current diagnostic techniques fall short of providing an accurate evaluation of the multiple functions of the newborn and infant kidney and the degree to which they may be impaired. Available diagnostic modalities are too frequently overstretched in their interpretation, leading to confusion in the significance of one test or the other. Management decisions are more often based on the individual practitioner's bias, judgement and experience, and can sometimes become speculative. The diagnostic tools that can be used in upper tract obstruction will be reviewed, and put in perspective with the current state of understanding of the subject as it relates to the newborn and infant.

Obstructive anomalies of the ureteropelvic junction

Aetiology

The most common congenital anomaly of the ureteropelvic junction is known as ureteropelvic junction (UPJ) obstruction. This is really a misnomer as complete obstruction seldom occurs. The anomaly is due to restrictive outflow of urine from the renal pelvis. The condition is manifested by hydronephrosis which is often detected antenatally by maternal ultrasonography. Aetiological factors may be intrinsic or extrinsic. Intrinsic factors consists of interruption of the smooth muscle layer and its replacement by collagen (Murnaghan, Foote, Gosling, Tanagho) [1–4]. Hanna et al. have shown that transmission of peristalsis may be hindered by the disruption of intercellular bridges or nexi located in the immediate vicinity of the UPJ [5]. Extrinsic factors include bands, kinks, crossing aberrant vessels or high insertion of the ureter on the pelvis. Detection usually occurs only later in life, as the obstructive effect of extrinsic factors tends to become more accentuated with a self-perpetuating distension of the renal pelvis. A review of contributory aetiological factors in 47 cases of hydronephrosis seen before the age of 2 years at Hôpital Sainte-Justine in Montreal, Canada revealed that extrinsic elements that contributed to hydronephrosis were present in one-third (16/47) of cases. They were not found to be more often associated with reduced individual renal function than when those extrinsic factors were not found. (S. Renda, R. Lambert and Y.L. Homsy, 1992, unpublished data).

Definition of obstruction

With the advent of pressure-perfusion studies and diuretic renography in the 1970s, it has become recognized that urinary tract dilatation does not necessarily indicate the invariable presence of obstruction. Management of the dilated upper urinary tract in the asymptomatic subject has become increasingly complex. Nowhere are these difficulties more evident than in the newborn and infant. There is general consensus at present that little benefit is to be derived from antenatal intervention in the absence of oligohydramnios. Although it would be expected that obstruction should manifest itself by dilatation, it is not as yet entirely clear how much of the dilatation could persist if the cause for obstruction was to be removed, spontaneously or otherwise. The impact that potentially obstructive anomalies of the UPJ may have on renal function is felt to be rather presumptive at the present time. Neither is it clear whether persistent dilatation might be due to residual obstruction. It therefore becomes necessary to observe the *effects* of obstruction (morphological and functional) over a period of time, that should not be permanently detrimental to the kidney, before ascertaining whether the presence of dilatation and/or obstruction is indeed harmful.

For clinical purposes, obstruction has been defined as *any restriction to urinary outflow that, left untreated, will cause progressive renal deterioration* [6]. The use of such a definition requires very close monitoring of renal function which becomes desirable in order to avoid significant deterioration. Recuperation, by the appropriate timing of corrective surgery, of whatever function that may have been lost in the monitoring process, has been shown to occur [7–9]. This definition is less than ideal but it does have practical clinical applications. It may change when more sophisticated indices of renal damage become available.

Prenatal diagnosis

Maternal ultrasonography has rendered detection of fetal hydronephrosis possible, as the condition was only detectable postnatally before ultrasonography became available in the late 1970s. The reported incidence varies from 1 in 100 to 1 in 500 pregnancies, depending on the timing of ultrasonography and the degree of hydronephrosis [10]. At 28 weeks the incidence is 1.4% but drops to 0.65% after birth [11]. Anomalies of the UPJ are the most frequent causes of neonatal hydronephrosis. They were responsible for 64% of 187

hydronephrotic kidneys detected by antenatal ultrasonography at Hôpital Sainte-Justine. Anomalies of the UVJ were next in frequency (13.4%) [12]. In the past, hydronephrosis would manifest itself by the presence of a renal mass, haematuria or infection. The varying degrees of renal damage that were found were attributed to delayed diagnosis in postnatal life which led to nephrectomy for poor function in 5–24% of cases. A sense of urgency emerged in the management of the anomaly, and surgical correction was recommended in an attempt to relieve symptoms and to prevent further renal damage. Symptomatic improvement was the rule. The majority of patients showed improvement on intravenous pyelography (IVP), but more accurate recovery of function could not be documented. It appeared logical to apply the same approach in asymptomatic newborns as in older subjects, as they were felt to be running a high risk of deterioration of renal function. With the advent of antenatal diagnosis, however, the number of cases of pyelocaliectasis brought to medical attention rose from 22 to 41% [13]. It was realized that many cases exhibited a transitional form of hydronephrosis before stabilizing or resolving spontaneously [12,14].

Characteristics on ultrasound

In 1986 Grignon et al. established a classification of hydronephrosis in the fetus based on over 34 000 maternal ultrasonograms done after the twentieth week of gestation. There were 92 fetal hydronephrotic kidneys. Shortly after birth dilatation persisted in only 45 kidneys. The degree of caliectasis and pyelectasis were related to that of cortical thinning. Hydronephrosis was graded in five groups according to these three parameters [15,16]. Other sonographic classifications have emerged, all with their merits and drawbacks, the most recent being that of Maizels et al. [17] which is based on findings described in postnatal kidneys. This classification was adopted by The Society for Fetal Urology with the aim of striving for uniformity in clinical assessment. Uniform ultrasonographic evaluation may provide useful criteria for non-invasive follow-up of morphological changes such as degree of caliectasis and cortical thickness. Of course, it is essential to distinguish between hydronephrotic and multicystic kidneys at the outset, as outlined by Stuck and co-workers [18]. The initial ultrasonographic study does have some predictive value when considering either improvement or deterioration of hydronephrosis. In one report, no deterioration occurred in mildly hydronephrotic units, whereas 14% of moderately hydronephrotic and 32% of markedly hydronephrotic units showed further deterioration in cases that were followed over a period of 12 months. Predictions could however not be made specifically in individual cases. In Maizels' study, when the value to predict obstruction was set at grade 3 hydronephrosis or greater, sensitivity was 88% and specificity 95% [17].

Postnatal clinical presentation

About one-third of hydronephrotic kidneys will escape antenatal detection and present postnatally, particularly in instances where maternal ultrasonography is not performed routinely. The most usual postnatal presentation is by an upper abdominal mass detected at birth or shortly thereafter. Haematuria or urinary tract infection may be the first symptom. In a small proportion of cases vomiting or hypertension may first bring the condition to medical attention. It is not uncommon for hydronephrosis to be associated with oesophageal atresia, imperforate anus or cardiac anomalies.

Developmental histopathology

Stereomorphometric studies show that smooth muscle architecture at the UPJ in normal human subjects changes from a circular pattern in neonates to an oblique mesh in adults and that longitudinal muscle fibres only emerge at the age of 2 years in the subepithelial layer. These patterns are either ambiguous or lacking in hydronephrotic subjects where segmental muscular hypoplasia, disarrangement of bundles or lack of longitudinal fibres were considered to correlate closely with obstruction by Kaneto et al. [19] On the other hand, dell'Agnola and co-workers have related duration and severity of obstructive hydronephrosis and the histological structure of smooth musculature at the UPJ in prenatally diagnosed cases. They found a close correlation between the duration of hydronephrosis from the time

of first detection *in utero* to the time of surgery and the volume of the hydronephrotic kidney. The larger the volumes, the more severe the muscular damage. However, in the long term, poor results after surgery were only obtained in 5 of the 19 newborns who exhibited severe hypotrophy and fibrosis of the pelvis [20].

The musculature of the normal ureter matures much in the same way as a spring would be seen to slowly uncoil. The process may take up to 2 years to be completed [19]. In the course of this uncoiling process, various incidents may occur that could result in structural smooth muscle anomalies such as segmental hypoplasia, disarrangement of fibres or the lack of development of longitudinal fibres. Kinks may occur along the course of the fetal ureter that may either persist or dissipate as development progresses.

Investigations

Ultrasonography

As mentioned earlier, ultrasonography has become very widespread in the diagnosis and follow-up of hydronephrosis both antenatally and postnatally. Although there are a number of grading systems available that are indicative of the extent of dilatation and parenchymal thinning, no reliable data can be obtained from the ultrasonogram in relation to function. Diuretic Doppler ultrasonography with measurement of resistive indices (RI) has been attempted but has not gained widespread acceptance, as there are some difficulties with the technique when applied to young children [21]. The use of the resistive index ratio (RIR) which relates the RI of the affected kidney to that of the healthy side seems to correlate better with diuresis renography in this population [22]. Pyelectasis alone may probably be treated conservatively, whereas the presence of pyelocalyectasis could require a more aggressive approach expending upon corroborative evidence of renal damage. Although higher degrees of obstruction might be necessary to cause calyceal distension, the ultrasonogram cannot supply the information required to indicate the presence or persistence of obstruction, unless sequential examinations were to be performed under the same circumstances of hydration and diuresis every time. Higher grades of hydronephrosis are less susceptible to show spontaneous improvement [12]. It would seem advantageous to couple ultrasonography with other diagnostic modalities for the follow-up of such cases. For example, contralateral renal growth as measured ultrasonographically has been used as an indication of severity of obstruction in the hydronephrotic kidney. Diuretic Doppler ultrasonography may show some promise as a sensitive indicator of obstruction.

Diuretic renography

This modality was introduced by Rado et al. in 1968, but it was not until clinical reports by O'Reilly et al. in 1978 and Koff et al. in 1979 that the technique gained wide acceptance [23–25]. Four patterns characterized the diuretic response: normal, dilated non-obstructive, obstructive and equivocal. Subsequently, Majd et al. described a quantitative method of measuring the clearance half-time of the injected radioisotope from the renal pelvis and called it $T_{1/2}$ [26]. If the value was less than 10 minutes, this indicated the absence of obstruction. A $T_{1/2}$ over 20 minutes was definitely obstructive, whereas a $T_{1/2}$ situated between 10 and 19 minutes was equivocal. It soon became obvious that several factors could alter the diuretic response, the degree of renal function being first and foremost. Other factors include: state of hydration, compliance of the collecting system, large hydronephrotic volume and last, but not least, the method of measuring $T_{1/2}$. Indeed there are no less than eight methods currently defined to measure $T_{1/2}$ [27]. Some protocols in current use call for injection of furosemide 15 minutes prior $(F - 15)$ to radioisotope injection, 20 minutes after $(F + 20)$ or only when the renal pelvis is considered to be full [28]. The $F - 15$ protocol was introduced by English and co-workers on the premise that furosemide could take up to 15 minutes to reach its peak activity [29]. Further experience with this protocol was shown to reduce the equivocal response rate from 17 to 3% in 50 adult patients [30]. O'Reilly has shown that patients exhibiting a delayed double peak on their renogram (Homsy's sign) indicated the presence of intermittent obstruction at the UPJ and would decompensate under the increased flow rate of an $F - 15$ protocol [28]. We have been able to experience the advantages of this protocol in cases that exhibited a pattern of intermittent obstruction, when these were seen to convert to completely obstructive patterns. However all our patients were well past their infancy so that we cannot, as yet, draw any final conclusions on the usefulness of this protocol in neonates and infants [31].

In an attempt to standardize the method of performing diuretic renography so that equivalent results might be obtained, the 'well-tempered' diuretic renogram was devised by Conway [27]. This method has been endorsed by the Society of Fetal Urology and the Pediatric Nuclear Medicine Council of the Society of Nuclear Medicine.

Three radiopharmaceuticals are currently employed for diuretic renography, radio-hippuran (^{123}I or ^{131}I hippurate), ^{99m}Tc-DTPA ([99m] technetium-diethylene triamine pentacetic acid) and ^{99m}Tc-MAG3 ([99m] mercuroacetyltri-glycine). The choice lies with individual preference in each laboratory, although it is expected that MAG3 is likely to improve data from laboratories using DTPA, owing to its capacity to reduce background uptake of the radio-isotope, as it is eliminated after a single passage through the kidney. At present, in Montreal, we are comfortable using ^{99m}Tc-DTPA as our basic isotope.

Despite its drawbacks and pitfalls diuretic renography provides a reasonably accurate estimate of renal function and drainage. The affected side must always be compared to the normal side to maximize the information that the test can deliver, particularly in very young subjects. Estimates of absolute total function can be derived by other tests but individual kidney function may be compared from one examination to the other by correlating the early scintigraphic images and the acquisition phase of the renogram curve. There have been problems with the determination of percent differential renal function for each kidney; in some obstructed kidneys values may either be normal or higher than the normal side, particularly in neonates. The exact reason for this is unclear. It may be related to the selection of the 'region of interest' for background subtraction. This is usually done in the interval between 60 seconds and initial appearance of radiotracer in the calices, but may be subject to erroneous interpretation, particularly with larger kidneys and smaller babies [27]. It is also possible that 'functional' compensatory hypertrophy on the affected side may manifest itself in this manner.

Accurate evaluation of renal function can be problematical in neonates and infants, as the difference between depressed values of glomerular filtration rate (GFR) due to loss of function cannot be readily differentiated from that due to immaturity. Upon repeat evaluation GFR values will normally increase unless there is loss of function. Individual kidney GFR may be derived from total GFR which can be estimated by several methods. Most are either inaccurate or require multiple blood sampling and are therefore neither practical nor accurate in very young subjects [32,33]. The value of methods that use a single blood sample and the gamma camera has been questioned [34,35]. Lambert et al. have recently elaborated a single blood sample technique that reproduces the accuracy of multiple sampling without the inconvenience. The technique involves the calculation of external plasma clearance by serial counting on the skull with a thyroid probe to determine plasma clearance of ^{99m}Tc-DTPA after a bolus injection of the isotope. In a prospective study 99 patients aged 0.5–17 years (mean = 10.5 years) were validated against a standard 4-plasma sample mono-exponential technique. There was a correlation of $r^2 = 0.988$ which confirms reliability [36]. In 18 patients aged 0–3 years, the correlation was still the same. We are currently evaluating ^{99m}Tc-MAG3 clearance with this technique and the preliminary results appear promising.

Brown et al. [37] showed a mathematical correlation between urinary output, GFR and effective renal plasma flow (ERPF) which indicates that the furosemide response should be weighted against the functional status of the kidney in the analysis of the diuretic renogram interpretation.

There is some controversy about timing of the initial renogram in the infant. The argument that GFR is too low in the neonate to permit a valid interpretation is not necessarily true if adequate function and drainage data are obtainable from the contralateral normal kidney [38,39]. The expected rapid increases in GFR seen in this age group allow for better monitoring of the maturation process that should be witnessed on subsequent renograms.

Pharmacological boosting of the renogram with agents other than lasix: the future?

The kidney has multiple functions: it controls the composition and volume of extracellular fluid, regulates acid–base balance, eliminates nitrogenous waste products, activates vitamin D, secretes erythropoietin, synthesizes prostaglandins, endothelin, bradykinin and dopamine. Many other hormones may influence renal function, such as vasopressin, parathyroid hormone, aldosterone, catecholamines, glucocorticoids and atrial natriuretic peptide. The renin–angiotensin system has an important role in the regulation of blood pressure. It is becoming clearer that prostaglandins and angiotensin II play an important protective role on the fetal kidney and in the modulation of function that occurs in early postnatal life.

GFR values are known to double in the first 2 weeks of life, secondary to growth of glomeruli, increase in blood pressure, diminution of renal resistance and increase in capillary permeability. These changes are associated with a significant diminution of angiotensin II, prostaglandins, atrial natriuretic peptide and endothelin, which could serve as indices in monitoring the maturation process [40]. The normal kidney possesses a reserve that allows it to increase its filtration rate in response to a variety of conditions. In renal disease, this functional reserve is used to maintain filtration rate by increasing the GFR of residual nephrons. When these can no longer compensate, GFR will show a decrease. Renal reserve seems to be modulated partly by prostaglandins. It can be demonstrated in children and adults by protein loading which will increase GFR by about 30%. The response to protein loading has been shown to be attenuated by the administration of indomethacin [41–43]. Kuhl et al. have shown that there is an increased biosynthesis of prostaglandin E2 and thromboxane A2 [44]. This could suggest that hydronephrotic kidneys may be using up their reserve function and a mechanism of 'functional' compensatory hypertrophy might thus become initiated. It is not obvious at this point whether the increased level of prostaglandins found in the urine originates from the affected kidney or the contralateral kidney.

Performing renography before and after protein loading, or after indomethacin administration (boosted renography), may reveal whether the kidney is using up its reserve function and whether the process of compensatory hypertrophy is being initiated. The study of such mechanisms will certainly provide more insight into the better understanding of obstructive uropathy and assessment of renal reserve function [45].

Experimental evidence now seems to point toward the involvement of growth factors such as TGF-β ribonucleic acid and the renin–angiotensin system. These may influence growth arrest, contralateral hypertrophy and interstitial fibrosis [46]. Currently attempts are in progress to verify the role of ACE-inhibitors such as captopril in the diagnosis and management of significant hydronephrosis [47,48].

Pressure-perfusion studies

Pressure-perfusion studies were introduced by Whitaker in 1973 to measure the resistance offered by obstruction [49]. They are performed by percutaneous kidney puncture and measuring pressure within the collecting system at a constant flow rate of 10 ml/min. The test was found to be accurate in about 80% of cases and equivocal in 20%. Correlation with diuretic renography is wide, ranging from 40 to 85% according to the series. Application of the test to the neonate is limited because of its invasive nature and as yet undetermined values of pressure and perfusion rates in newborns and infants. In older children, the test becomes more useful when interpreted in the perspective of adjuvant data from other tests. Pitfalls of the test are related to needle and tubing size, viscosity and temperature of the injected material, hydronephrotic volume and flow rates. Changes in renal function cannot be monitored by the Whitaker test. We recommend its use in persistently dilated collecting systems associated with poor renal function. In young subjects flow rates should start at 1–2 ml/min and be increased progressively until a rise in pressure is observed.

Biological markers

Biological markers are being increasingly used to monitor disease processes provided that the markers are specific. Prostanoids have been shown to be released by hydronephrotic kidneys in both animals and humans. Kuhl et al. have found increased amounts of prostaglandin E2 (PGE2) and thromboxane A2 (TxA2) to be significantly increased in 12 neonates with hydronephrosis. Surgical decompression caused further increases, which gradually normalized during follow-up. No other renal prostanoids or systemic prostanoid metabolites were consistently elevated. It is suggested that endogenous renal formation of PGE2 and TxA2 is selectively stimulated in the hydronephrotic kidneys of neonates and infants [44]. These prostanoids may be involved in modulating renal function in infants. They may thus become useful parameters in the follow-up of hydronephrosis.

Current difficulties in the management of obstruction

In 1985 a number of neonates with hydronephrosis were reported on, who showed spontaneous improvement by diuretic renography, the condition was called 'transitional hydronephrosis' [14]. Dilatation was associated with equivocal or dilated non-obstructive diuretic response patterns. It was surmised that developmental changes leading to improvement or total resolution of hydronephrosis could still go on after birth, much like closure of an atrial septal defect, resolution of a fetal ureteral anomaly or vesicoureteric reflux.

In the newborn, hydronephrosis without a typically obstructive washout pattern on diuresis renography can show improvement or stabilization over a 12-month period in 80% of cases. Deterioration to significant obstruction was shown to occur in 15–20% [8,12]. Immediate surgical correction is obviously not a plausible solution in such cases. More recent reports have indicated that even when there is no washout on the diuretic renogram, conservative management will not necessarily cause any deterioration in renal function and that as drainage slowly improves spontaneously, so will the function of the affected kidney [50–53]. Renal function that had deteriorated in some patients who were being managed nonoperatively was shown to have returned after surgery, provided that patients were monitored closely [8,14]. Madden et al. concluded that the non-operative management of selected cases of antenatally detected UPJ obstruction was safe [54]. Several other studies have recently demonstrated that function could improve significantly in non-operated children who presented with impaired function in the hydronephrotic kidney [39,48,55]. Improvement in function after pyeloplasty performed in infants cannot be attributed to the effects of surgery alone. In Koff and Campbell's study, there were 15 neonatal hydronephrotic kidneys with significantly impaired renal function (actual glomerular filtration rate ranging from 1.75 to 44 ml per minute per $1.73\,m^2$ – mean 14.8). They were all observed and none underwent surgery. About one-half of the kidneys improved, with complete disappearance of hydronephrosis in two. Washout on diuretic renography improved in all, but became truly non-obstructive in four cases ($T_{1/2}$ less than 15 minutes). All kidneys showed rapid improvement of glomerular filtration rate, more so in younger than older infants, with five kidneys increasing their percent of function to more than 50%. There was no evidence of renal deterioration, no evidence of compensatory hypertrophy contralaterally and no surgery was required over the 2.5 year period of the study. Furthermore, these non-operated obstructed kidneys improved their function more rapidly than those who underwent surgery when a comparison was made with other series where surgery was performed [39]. Such studies are creating a lively controversy at present, as it is being questioned whether the function of the involved kidney truly reflects the degree of obstruction, considering that variables such as pyelovenous and pyelolymphatic backflow all combine to maintain pressure within the system at a low level. It will not be easy to resolve this issue and long-term follow-up will be required to validate these conclusions.

Management considerations

Complete obstruction is readily recognized by dilatation and parenchymal loss which, uncorrected, will result in total parenchymal destruction. Chronic partial obstruction will share some of the signs characteristic of complete obstruction but the evolution may be quite different. The main difficulty in ascertaining the presence or absence of significant obstruction at a given point in time stems from our inability to determine whether causative factors responsible for obstruction are still operative or were compensated for by mechanisms such as muscle hypertrophy or changes in compliance of the renal pelvis, or even by mechanisms such as pyelovenous or pyelolymphatic backflow. These changes might not necessarily be expressed by alterations in pressure or flow rate and would therefore escape detection by current methods of evaluation, whereas dilatation would still persist.

Some authors strongly recommend early surgical correction, founding their arguments on experimental and clinical data in infants and young animals which show compensatory hypertrophy to occur very quickly after unilateral neonatal nephrectomy or in congenital absence of one kidney. It was observed that the eventual size of the remaining kidney is inversely proportional to the age at which the other kidney is lost. Compensatory enlargement of the contralateral kidney was noted to occur experimentally when partial obstruction was briefly applied to cause hydronephrosis in newborn rats. The affected kidneys did not show any signs of damage [56]. King and Hatcher concluded that if correction of a unilateral obstruction is deferred until contralateral hypertrophy occurs, there is less potential for recovery of function in the obstructed kidney [57]. This would probably be true if it could be proved that compensatory hypertrophy only occurred postnatally, but there is no clinical support for this consideration so far. However there is evidence that compensatory hypertrophy occurs *in utero*, in human fetuses with multicystic kidneys who underwent serial antenatal ultrasonograms [58]. This could indicate that when obstruction is severe enough to cause damage to one kidney, compensatory hypertrophy would be expected to occur on the contralateral side, starting even before birth. Glomerular filtration rate is known to increase rapidly in the first 12 weeks of life at a rate that is inversely proportional to age. Increases in glomerular filtration rates seen in infants undergoing early surgery may only be the reflection of expected renal maturation.

It is now clear that morphological criteria cannot be relied upon alone to decide upon management. The washout curve of the diuretic renogram provides useful information when it is non-obstructive. Equivocal and obstructive patterns have not been convincingly shown to interfere with renal growth and maturation, except if associated with decreased glomerular filtration rates (GFR). Even kidneys with decreased GFR have shown improvement in the face of obstructive washout curves.

Management options

Until such a time that obstruction can be diagnosed more accurately, three management options are available. The first is to continue performing surgery as in the past on the grounds of apparent obstruction. This is no longer acceptable as a significant number of neonates would probably undergo unnecessary surgery. They might indeed be affected by non-obstructive hydronephrosis. The few who would need surgery would be sure to benefit as the success rate of pyeloplasty is over 95%. The adepts of this option are therefore expected to decrease. The second option is to follow neonates with more than 35% function in the hydronephrotic kidney with serial ultrasonograms and diuretic renograms at 3-, 6- or 12-month intervals, reserving surgery for those kidneys that clearly show a deterioration of renal function. The third option is to follow all neonates with hydronephrosis by observation at frequent intervals by ultrasonography and renal scans until obstruction can be defined or excluded, and perform surgery accordingly. The second option will probably gain in popularity. The establishment of a definite diagnosis of ongoing obstruction at the UPJ remains perplexing at this time. It will not be possible to improve diagnostic accuracy until more specific tests are developed. A period of uncertainty in terms of providing the therapeutic alternative is inevitable. This will require clinicians involved in the management of hydronephrosis to set their biases aside and to be receptive to the changing concepts of obstructive uropathy. Research activity must be heightened in the realms of the laboratory, imaging techniques as well as technology and continuing long-term prospective clinical studies.

References

1. Murnaghan GF. Mechanism of congenital hydronephrosis with reference to factors influencing surgical treatment. *Ann R Coll Surg Engl* 1958; **23**: 25–28.
2. Foote JW, Blennerhassett JB, Wiglesworth FW, MacKinnon KJ. Observations on the ureteropelvic junction. *J Urol* 1970; **104**: 252–259.
3. Gosling JA. The musculature of the upper urinary tract. *Acta Anat* 1970; **75**: 408–412.
4. Tanagho EA. Ureteral embryology, developmental anatomy and myology. In: Boyarski S, Gottschalk CW, Tanagho EA, Zimskind, PD (eds) *Urodynamics: hydrodynamics of the ureter and renal pelvis*. New York: Academic, 1971; pp. 3–27.
5. Hanna MK, Jeffs RD, Sturgess JM et al. Ureteral structure and ultrastructure. Part II. *J Urol* 1976; **116**: 725–729.
6. Koff SA. Problematic ureteropelvic junction obstruction. *J Urol* 1987; **138**: 390–393.
7. Dhillon HK, Duffy PG, Gordon I, Ransley PG. A randomised clinical trial in infants with prenatally diagnosed unilateral hydronephrosis. In: *Section on Urology, Program for Scientific Sessions, 1992 Annual Meeting AAP, San Francisco*, 1992; **89**: 116 (abstract).
8. Cartwright PC, Duckett, JW, Keating MA et al. Managing apparent ureteropelvic junction obstruction in the newborn. *J Urol* 1992; **148**: 1224–1228.
9. Allen TD. The swing of the pendulum (editorial). *J Urol* 1992; **148**: (Part 2), 534–535.
10. Thomas DFM. Fetal uropathy. *Br J Urol* 1990; **66**: 225.
11. Livera LN, Brookfield DSK, Egginton JA, Hawnaur, JM. Antenatal ultrasonography to detect fetal renal abnormalities: a prospective screening programme. *Br Med J* 1989; **298**: 1421–1424.
12. Homsy YL, Saad F, Laberge I et al. Transitional hydronephrosis of the newborn and infant. *J Urol* 1990; **144**: 579–582.
13. Lebowitz RL, Mandell J. *Pediatr Urol Newslett* 1986; October, **1**: 11–12.
14. Homsy YL, Williot P, Danais S. Transitional hydronephrosis: fact or fantasy? *J Urol* 1985; **136**: 339–341.
15. Grignon A, Filion R, Filiatrault D et al. Urinary tract dilatation in utero: classification and clinical applications. *Radiology* 1986; **160**: 645–648.
16. Grignon A, Filiatrault D, Homsy YL et al. Ureteropelvic junction stenosis: antenatal ultrasonographic diagnosis, postnatal investigation and follow-up. *Radiology* 1986; **160**: 649–652.
17. Maizels M, Reisman ME, Flom LS et al. Grading nephroureteral dilatation detected in first year of life: correlation with obstruction. *J Urol* 1992; **148**: (Part 2), 609–614.
18. Stuck KJ, Koff SA, Silver TM. Ultrasonographic features of multicystic dysplastic kidney: expanded diagnostic criteria. *Radiology* 1982; **143**: 217–219.

19. Kaneto H, Orikasa S, Chiba T et al. Three-D muscular arrangement at the ureteropelvic junction and its changes in congenital hydronephrosis: a stereomorphometric study. *J Urol* 1991; **146**: 909–914.

20. dell'Agnola CA, Carmassi LM, Merlo D et al. Duration and severity of congenital hydronephrosis as a cause of smooth muscle deterioration in pyelo-ureteral junction obstruction. *Z Kinderchir* 1990; **45**: 286–290.

21. Palmer JM, Lindfors KK, Ordorica RC et al. Diuretic Doppler sonography in postnatal hydronephrosis. *J Urol* 1991; **146**: 605–607.

22. Keller MS, Korsvik HE, Piccolello ML, Weiss RM. Comparison of diuretic Doppler sonography with diuretic renography in children with hydronephrosis. In: *Section on Urology, Program for Scientific Sessions, 1992 Annual Meeting AAP, San Francisco,* 1992; **53**: 16 (abstract).

23. Rado JP, Bano C, Tako J. Radioisotope renography during furosemide (Lasix) diuresis. *Nucl Med* 1968; **7**: 212–221.

24. O'Reilly PH, Testa HJ, Lawson RS et al. Diuresis renography in equivocal urinary tract obstruction. *Br J Urol* 1978; **50**: 76–80.

25. Koff SA, Thrall JH, Keyes JW Jr. Diuretic radionuclide urography: a non-invasive method for evaluating nephro-ureteral dilatation. *J Urol* 1979; **122**: 451–454.

26. Majd M, Kass EJ, Gainey MA, Belman AB, Burnette DG Jr. Diuretic augmented radionuclide renography in the evaluation of hydronephrosis in children. *J Nucl Med* 1982; **23**: 14 (abstract).

27. Conway JJ. 'Well-tempered' diuresis renography: its historical development, physiological and technical pitfalls and standardized technique protocol. *Semin Nucl Med* 1992; **22**: 74–84.

28. O'Reilly PH. Diuresis renography: recent advances and recommended protocols. *Br J Urol* 1992; **69**: 113–120.

29. English PJ, Testa HJ, Lawson RS et al. Modified method of diuresis renography for the assessment of equivocal pelviureteric obstruction. *Br J Urol* 1987; **59**: 10–14.

30. Upsdell SM, Testa HJ, Lawson RS. The F-15 diuresis renogram in suspected obstruction of the upper urinary tract. *Br J Urol* 1992; **69**: 126–131.

31. Homsy YL, Mehta P, Danais S. Intermittent hydronephrosis: a diagnostic challenge. *J Urol* 1988; **140**: 1222–1226.

32. Shore RM. Glomerular filtration rate in children: where we have been; where we are going (editorial) *J Nucl Med* 1991; **32**: 1297–1300.

33. Summerville DA, Potter CS, Treves ST. The use of radiopharmaceuticals in the measurement of glomerular filtration rate: a review. In: Freeman LM (ed) *Nuclear Medicine Annual 1990.* New York: Raven, 1990; pp 191–222.

34. Han HR, Piepsz A. Estimation of glomerular filtration rate in infants and in children using a single-plasma method. *J Nucl Med* 1991; **32**: 1294–1297.

35. Peters AM, Myers MJ. Single plasma GFR in children. *J Nucl Med* 1992; **33**: 173–174.

36. Lambert R, Turpin S, Taillefer R, Leveille J. An easy technique for GFR determination in children using ^{99m}Tc-DTPA, one plasma sample and external counting with a thyroid probe. *J Nucl Med* 1993; **34**: 5 (abstract).

37. Brown SC, Upsdell SM, O'Reilly PH. The importance of renal function in the interpretation of diuresis renography. *Br J Urol* 1992; **69**: 121–125.

38. Koff SA, McDowell GC, Byard M. Diuretic radionuclide assessment of obstruction in the infant: guidelines for successful interpretation. *J Urol* 1988; **140**: 1167–1168.

39. Koff SA, Campbell K. Nonoperative management of unilateral neonatal hydronephrosis. *J Urol* 1992; **148**: (Part 2), 525–531.

40. Guignard JP. Le rein immature. *Méd/Sci* 1993; **9**: 289–296.

41. Anders A, Zimmerman L, Bergstrom J. Potential role of a liver-derived factor in mediating renal response to protein. *Blood Purif* 1988; **6**: 276–278.

42. Krishna GG, Newell G, Miller E. et al. Protein-induced glomerular hyperfiltration: role of hormonal factors. *Kidney Int* 1988; **33**: 578–583.

43. Ruilope LM, Rodicio J, Garcia Robles R et al. Influence of a low sodium diet on the renal response to amino acid infusions in humans. *Kidney Int* 1987; **31**: 992–999.

44. Kuhl PG, Schonig G, Schweer H et al. Increased renal biosynthesis of prostaglandin E2 and thromboxane B2 in human congenital obstructive uropathy. *Pediatr Res* 1990; **27**: 103–107.

45. Milot A, Lambert R, Cusson JR, Lebel M, Schiffrin EL, Larochelle P. Prostaglandins preserve renal function in unilateral renal artery stenosis. *Am J Hyperten* 1992; **5**: (5); (Part II), 70A, I08.

46. Sharma AK, Mauer SM, Kim Y, Michael AF. Interstitial fibrosis in obstructive uropathy. *Kidney Int* 1993; **44**: 774–788.

47. Tripp Y, Lambert R, Homsy YL. The 'boosted' renogram. Presented at the Society for Fetal Urology, 13th Semi-Annual Meeting, Dallas, Texas, 21 October, 1994.

48. MacNeily AE. Pediatric ureteropelvic junction obstruction – an update. *Can J Urol* 1995; **2**: 133–143.

49. Whitaker RH. Methods of assessing obstruction in dilated ureters. *Br J Urol* 1973; **45**: 15–18.

50. Gordon I, Dhillon HK, Gatanash H et al. Antenatal diagnosis of pelvic hydronephrosis: assessment of renal function and drainage as a guide to management. *J Nucl Med* 1991; **32**: 1649–1654.

51. Josephson S. Suspected pyelo-ureteral junction obstruction in the fetus: when to do what? I. A clinical update. *Eur Urol* 1990; **18**: 267–275.

52. Lupton EW, Testa HJ. The obstructive diuretic renogram: an appraisal of the significance. *J Urol* 1992; **147**: 981–983.

53. Blyth B, Snyder HM, Duckett JW. Antenatal diagnosis and subsequent management of hydronephrosis. *J Urol* 1993; **149**: 693–698.

54. Madden NP, Thomas DF, Gordon AC et al. Antenatally detected pelviureteric junction obstruction. Is non-operation safe? *Br J Urol* 1991; **68**: 305–310.

55. Cartwright PL, Duckett JW, Keating MA et al. Managing apparent ureteropelvic junction obstruction in the newborn. *J Urol* 1992; **148**: 1224.

56. Claesson G, Josephson S, Robertson B. Experimental partial ureteric obstruction in newborn rats. IV. Do the morphological effects progress continuously? *J Urol* 1983; **130**: 1217–1220.

57. King LR, Hatcher PA. Natural history of fetal and neonatal hydronephrosis. *Urology* 1990; **35**: 433–438.

58. Mandell J, Peters CA, Allred E, Estroff JA, Benacerraf BR. Does fetal renal 'compensatory hypertrophy' really occur in humans? Yes! In: *Section on Urology, Program for Scientific Sessions, 1992 Annual Meeting AAP, San Francisco*, 1992; **39**: 66 (abstract).

12

A rational approach to imaging newborns and infants with idiopathic hydronephrosis or hydroureteronephrosis

M. Maizels

Easily 'seeing' the urinary tract by ultrasound has improved the clinical practice of paediatric urology [1,2]. Ultrasound has also changed the 'why' and 'when' children present for care. In the past, they would present largely in childhood to evaluate symptoms or signs which derive from congenital malformations: urine infection (vesicoureteral reflux), voiding problems (ureterocele) or haematuria (renal obstruction). Nowadays, many patients are neonates, who are well and healthy, and present to pursue a possibly abnormal ultrasound. The issue in hand is whether the dilated urinary tracts which are now 'silent' in the newborn are actually 'time bombs' which are set to later 'explode' in childhood when they will cause pain, infection or haematuria. Or, are the dilated tracts merely 'props' of bombs which will remain silent. Debate in the literature does not answer the issue. It is likely that a clear answer will not be attained until several specific aspects of the issue are resolved. For example, we need better knowledge of the natural history of the asymptomatic infant with hydronephrosis. Also, we need a consensus among clinical researchers which establishes commonality in test methods and in criteria to determine when test results are different enough from the predicted normal to be 'abnormal'. Clinical trials need to be done to address these aspects. Their results will ultimately establish standards to scientifically guide the practice of postnatal hydronephrosis and will deter current practices based upon personal biases. This chapter includes a review

of the pertinent literature along with *my* personal bias. The Society for Fetal Urology guidelines for postnatal imaging are presented. The next chapter presents the pros and cons of surgery or observation for infants with renographic obstruction.

Prenatal ultrasound and coordinating pre- and postnatal care

The orderly management of fetuses with a uropathy requires the mother's obstetrician to closely coordinate the information coming from a team of specialists. The obstetric sonographer dissects the anatomy of the urinary tract and makes a diagnosis as to the possible causes of the dilatation. The surgeon and paediatrician educate the family regarding prognosis and organize newborn testing. This coordination 'dedramatizes' the problem [3]. As about one-half of the families who carry a fetus likely to have a birth defect are swayed by professional advice regarding completion of the pregnancy, most families appreciate advice from an ethicist, social worker or psychiatrist [4]. When there is consideration to terminate the pregnancy, the geneticist will determine if there is a genetic basis for the condition. Children with Down syndrome may show important hydronephrosis more often than the general population [5]. A syndrome of sonographic findings may implicate Down

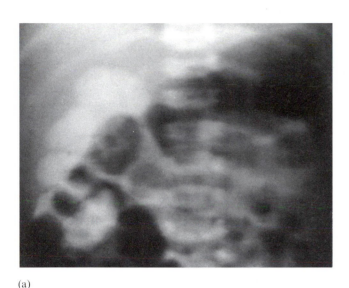

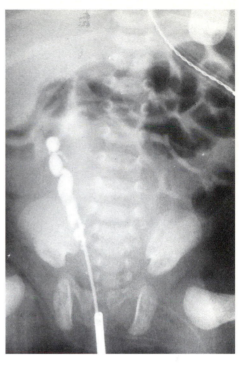

(a)   (b)

Figure 12.1 Newborn care is provided smoothly when a uropathy is seen prenatally. The prenatal sonogram showed a multicystic kidney and contralateral hydronephrosis. (a) An excretory urogram (EU) was done to follow-up HN Gr 4. The right kidney shows marked pelvocaliectasis and there is no visualization of the left kidney. (b) A retrograde pyelogram done prior to pyeloplasty shows a beaded ureter with an abrupt cut off just below the UPJ junction. A stricture of the UPJ was repaired.

syndrome in an otherwise well fetus [6]. Termination should also be planned so that there is tissue which is satisfactory to make an organ diagnosis. The pathological diagnosis should be used to determine the accuracy of the working clinical diagnosis. This coordination is important [3,7], even if it is hard to set up [8].

Thereby, when a routine maternal sonogram identifies a severe malformation, a clinical management is outlined before birth and executed smoothly for the newborn (Figure 12.1). This organization avoids the frantic phone calls, emergency room visits and morbidity which were common in the past when uropathies were identified only after the infant had become sick (Figure 12.2).

Thomas argues that prenatal diagnosis may not be as important as is popularly believed. He found that for almost 20% of newborns with a prenatally diagnosed uropathy, there was evident clinical information to indicate that there was an underlying uropathy, and

that postnatal testing showed that only 20% of the newborns with prenatally diagnosed hydronephrosis had a problem whose detection was of definite value (e.g. bilateral renal disease or an affected solitary kidney) [8,9]. Review of our patient series shows that 35 (34%) of 103 babies with a prenatally identified uropathy benefited from this examination in as much as the prenatal sonogram: showed significantly important bilateral renal disease; identified a solitarily functioning kidney; and expedited the care of newborns with posterior urethral valves. Or, also of importance, the test permitted the family to prepare themselves to deal with a pregnancy which contained a serious defect (e.g. spina bifida).

Postnatal evaluation

Controversy regarding infants with hydronephrosis involves how the urinary tract

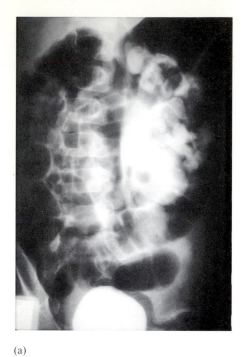

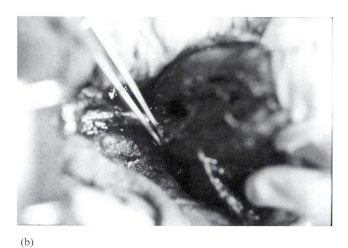

(a)   (b)

Figure 12.2 Morbidity was common when uropathies were identified only after the child became sick. This toddler fell from monkey bars at school. (a) Abdominal pain and microhaematuria prompted performing the EU, which shows extravasation of urine from a kidney which has been obstructed by congenital UPJ obstruction. (b) At surgery to drain the urinoma, the perforation in the pelvis is shown. When UPJ obstruction is recognized early, repair can be done promptly before illness strikes.

should be tested to diagnose obstruction, and when does the asymptomatic infant with renal obstruction need surgery. Since 1980, when McAlister et al. discussed the enigma of the natural history of unoperated partial UPJ obstruction [10], there is still no data to deal with this. Several authors conclude this issue can be addressed satisfactorily by a controlled prospective study which randomizes the treatment to observation or surgery [11]. Given this controversy in management, at least it should be possible to standardize the tests that newborns with nephroureteral dilatation undergo.

Clinical evaluation – history and physical examination

The routine history and physical examination should not be overlooked in the excitement to 'run' straight to testing. Even though, for neonates, the physical examination is routinely normal. When physical examination shows the hydronephrosis imaged by ultrasound is palpable, the time schedule for urological testing should be accelerated so it is done within the first few days of life (Figures 12.3, 12.4). For boys who have a buried penis or if there is an external ear deformity, an anomalous upper urinary tract may be found (Figure 12.5) [12].

For infants, the history of an unpredictable voiding interval, namely, when nappies are wet variably between 2 and 8 hours, this may be consistent with the intermittent nature of UPJ obstruction, especially when it is bilateral (Figure 12.6).

From our series, about 3% of pregnancies with prenatally detected hydronephrosis have a family history of surgically important hydronephrosis.

The laboratory examination should include the routine urine analysis and culture. I have detected urine infection even in the newborn. When hydronephrosis is bilateral or involves a solitarily functioning kidney, azotaemia and hyperkalaemic acidosis should be checked for. Azotaemia may be diagnosed after about 1 week old, when the period of effect of the mother upon the newborn's renal function is

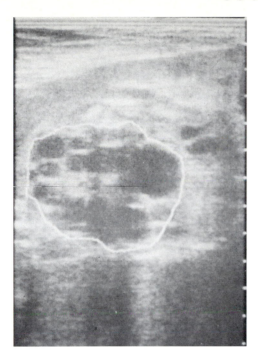

Figure 12.3 A multicystic kidney which is bulky and palpable may *rarely* interfere with respiration and require urgent nephrectomy. Fetal ultrasound (29 weeks gestation) shows multicystic kidney (delimited on image) which was so bulky it impaired respiration of the newborn. A nephrectomy was required. Later, a UPJ obstruction of the opposite kidney was repaired (not shown).

past. For term babies with normal renal function, the serum creatinine commonly falls to 0.4 mg% by 1 week old. When there is prematurity, the serum creatinine should reach this level by 36 weeks after conception.

It is worth being cautious when dealing with the association of renal and cardiac anomalies. Newborns with hydronephrosis may surprisingly develop congestive heart failure. This can be seen if a newborn with hydronephrosis also has a *large* cardiac ventricular septal defect. This is because, during the newborn period, the associated murmur may be so quiet that it is difficult to auscult; the condition may not be discovered until the next few months, when the infant surprisingly develops congestive heart failure.

The value of antimicrobials as prophylaxis against urinary tract infections (UTIs) in cases of hydronephrosis without reflux has not been investigated. Ransley prescribes antiseptics as prophylaxis against UTIs in cases of hydrone-

phrosis (whether it is obstructed or not) [11]. Yet, Arnold does not, and he has not noted documented UTIs [13]. Anecdotal clinical experience has shown that UTIs with sepsis may appear after 3 months old [14]; however, the frequency of this problem is unclear. Dispensing antibiotics may be less important if the urine is sampled frequently to check for infection.

Definitions of terms in paediatrics: hydronephrosis, pelviectasis, and obstruction

It is likely that the lack of widely accepted working definitions for terms dealing with infant hydronephrosis has led to clinical misunderstandings and controversy among researchers. The following term definitions apply to cases of 'well babies' with nephroureteral dilatation, where: the cause of the dilatation is unknown (e.g. not urethral valves, ureterocele, ureteral reflux), the urinary tract is otherwise normal and there has not yet been urological surgery. Thereby, *idiopathic hydronephrosis* of infancy is referred to as hydronephrosis and the megaureter seen in *idiopathic hydroureteronephrosis* of infancy is referred to as hydroureteronephrosis (HUN). The terms ureteropelvic junction (UPJ) obstruction, obstructive megaureter, or non-obstructive, non-refluxing megaureter are left to deal with those cases where the infants *have become* symptomatic (e.g. UTI, haematuria, pain) from their hydronephrosis or HUN. It is particularly important to differentiate pelviectasis, or an extrarenal pelvis, from hydronephrosis. Herein, *pelviectasis*, as imaged by ultrasound, is pelvic dilatation without caliceal dilatation; *hydronephrosis* is pelvic dilatation with uniformly dilated calices (with or without cortical thinning). Furthermore, as imaged by intravenous pyelography (IVP), in cases of pelviectasis, the renal papillae have sharp tips and the forniceal angles are acute, while in cases of hydronephrosis, the renal papillae and forniceal angles are blunted.

The premises behind these definitions include the supposition that for pelviectasis, the dilated pelvis is a variant of normal development and is unlikely to be associated with clinical symptoms (except perhaps that stasis may later

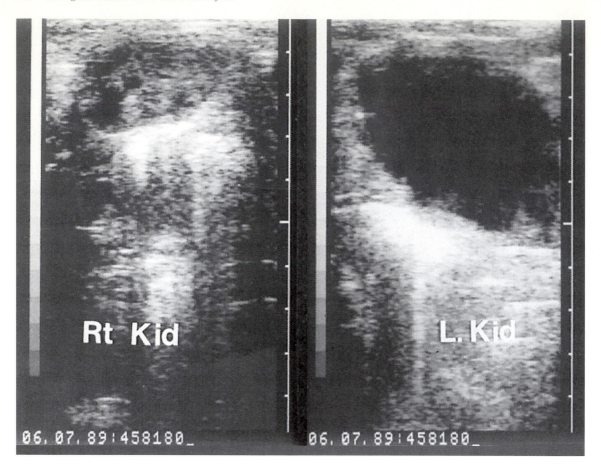

(a)

initiate stone formation). Clinical experience is the evidence for the innocent nature of pelviectasis. However, for hydronephrosis, it is supposed that the pelvis and calyces dilate as a consequence of distal obstruction acting upon a normally developed pelvicalyceal system. Furthermore, it is supposed that the obstruction causes the papillae to become blunted and the forniceal angles to become obtuse. Occasionally, a normal renal compound papillae may drain into a compound calix, most commonly in the upper pole of the kidney. When this normal situation is examined by sonography, it resembles a pathologically dilated calix. But, the normal sharp papillae can be seen by IVP (see 'Pitfalls in sonography' below and Figure 12.13).

Furthermore, a commonly accepted working clinical definition of *obstruction* has not been reached. It is agreed that renal obstruction can be diagnosed empirically using retrospective observations. That is, obstruction must have been present if, over time, there has been *progressive* loss of renal function (as monitored by isotope scanning), particularly if it is associated with impaired pelvic drainage or illness (e.g. UTI) [15–17]. This definition is too restrictive for clinical use as it does not allow for treatment before the kidney is damaged. Furthermore, this definition may not find laboratory support. As in induced partial renal obstruction, the increased intrapelvic pressure may lower the glomerular filtration rate. This reduction is not progressive, despite persistent obstruction [18].

As there are many parameters which are used to assess and therefore diagnose obstruction, it may be that the diagnosis of obstruction, or not, could come to be made depending on which parameters are used [19,20]. Further-

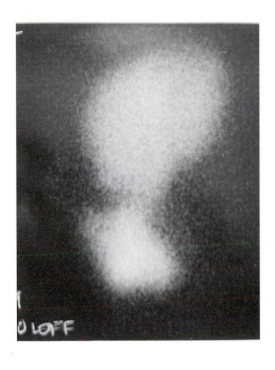

(b)

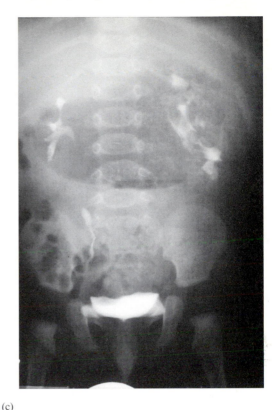

(c)

Figure 12.4 An obstructed kidney which is palpable is unlikely to resolve and is best treated expeditiously by upper tract drainage. A prenatal sonogram showed hydroureteronephrosis. (a) Office ultrasound shows marked hydronephrosis (HN Gr 4, see below) of the left kidney which was palpable. The right is normal. (b) The renal scan shows the extreme dilatation of the kidney (upper). The bladder is seen (lower). (c) After drainage of the obstructed megaureter by loop ureterostomy as a neonate, the EU shows symmetrical visualization of both kidneys.

more, the diagnosis of obstructed or free drainage may be ambiguous [3], defined liberally, or strictly [17]. I believe a definition of renal obstruction in asymptomatic infants with hydronephrosis should consider the points below.

Natural history of hydronephrosis

It is unknown when, if ever, infants with asymptomatic hydronephrosis would have eventually developed clinical problems. It is possible that the dilated newborn kidney is actually *recovering* from previous transient obstruction, *in utero*, and the parameters which cite obstruction (e.g. dilatation, reduced function, etc.) are actually resolving, rather than progressing. For example, Arnold has shown obstructed hydronephrosis resolve by 3 years with preservation of symmetrical function [13]. While other cases of 'resolution' of

obstruction are better explained by renal maturation in a non-obstructed kidney with an extra renal pelvis [16,21].

Clinical impact

Monitoring of patients' clinical status is reported scantly. For example, in adults with UPJ obstruction, Bratt noted over a 5-year follow-up that bacteriuria resolved in those having pyeloplasty, while stones developed in those having observation [22]. There is little documentation for paediatric hydronephrosis in the outcomes after surgery of failure to thrive, UTI, haematuria or pain versus the outcomes of these issues in cases treated non-operatively. Pain and haematuria seem to emerge after 1 year old [23]. If the reduction in renal function and drainage are reversible at almost any time, is it justifiable to repair hydronephrosis to avert UTIs or flank pain in

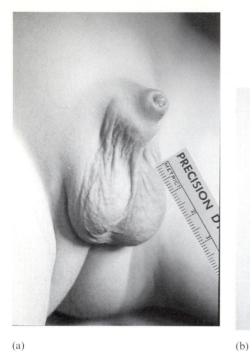

(a)

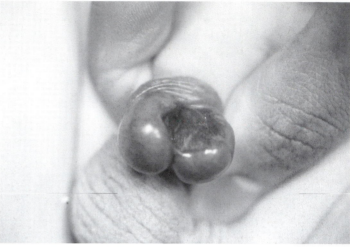

(b)

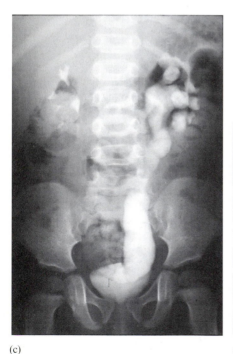

(c)

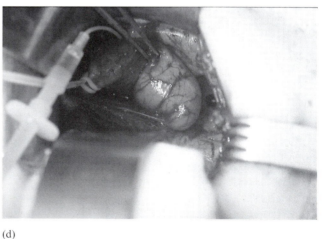

(d)

Figure 12.5 The newborn examination may show anomalies of the penis or external ear (not shown), which may warrant evaluation of the upper urinary tract. (a) As this 3-year-old boy who presented for repair of an inguinal hernia also showed a penoscrotal web which concealed the penis, and office ultrasound was done. This showed a megaureter. (b) As the prepuce was tightly phimotic, it could only be retracted under general anaesthesia. Now pubic epispadias is noted. (c) The EU shows pelvocaliectasis and a megaureter. (d) At surgery saline, which was instilled into the distal ureter, failed to drain and caused the intraluminal pressure to be more than 20 cm H_2O [116].

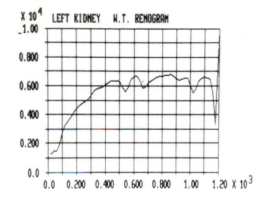

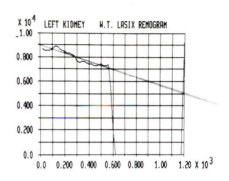

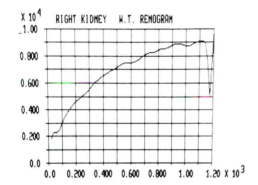

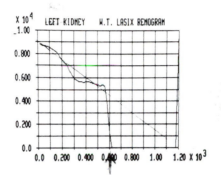

(a)

(b)

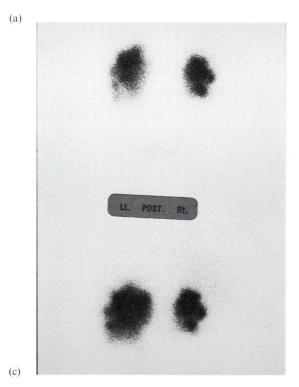

(c)

Figure 12.6 Bilateral UPJ obstruction may cause the voiding pattern to be unpredictable. This is consistent with the intermittent nature of UPJ obstruction. This neonate wet nappies variably and unpredictably at intervals between 2 and 8 hours. The renogram phase of the WTR (a) shows good function with stasis in each kidney. The diuretic phase of the WTR (b) shows non-exponential drainage consistent with obstruction. The renal scan images before (top) and after furosemide (bottom) show the drainage is poor. After both UPJ obstructions were repaired, the voiding pattern become regular.

infancy [24], stone formation, hypertension, haematuria or failure to thrive? Or, should repair be done only after the symptoms or signs appear? [14] It is not readily known if surgery can reverse reduced renal function.

Global renal function

This may be monitored as glomerular filtration rate (by direct collection of urine or by scan) or a specific function such as concentrating ability. Is there progressive loss of these functions, or is the new appearance of a fixed low urine specific gravity an indication for repair? [25] Is the failure of reduced renal function in a neonate to mature and normalize during infancy a sign of obstruction? [26]

What parameters will predict if an observed loss of function is reversible after successful reconstructive surgery? Does the presence of compensatory hypertrophy in the opposite kidney limit postoperative recovery or function? Could the obstructed kidney have shown better recovery of function after surgery if the repair had been performed before compensatory hypertrophy appeared?

Drainage function

How poorly does the dilated segment need to drain before it is considered obstructed? Should this be monitored by direct instillation of a marker into the pelvis or by noting the physiological washout of marker. Can a pyeloplasty be successful and therefore not be improved drainage? For example, does the histological finding of mural fibrosis in the pyeloplasty specimen correlate with persistent poor drainage after surgery despite a now patent tract?

In the absence of good answers to these questions, I believe a working diagnosis of obstruction can be established by assessing the: function of the kidney, ability of the pelvis to drain its contained urine by diuretic renography, and grade of hydronephrosis by sonography. Should repair be done, the accuracy of the diagnosis should be confirmed by assessing the histological status of the pelvic wall for a pathological response to obstruction (i.e. muscular hypertrophy) [27,28]. The methods for grading hydronephrosis and scan dilated kidneys are presented below, followed by the criteria for diagnosing obstruction.

Postnatal imaging

Timing of tests

The plan for postnatal testing is based mostly on the newborn physical examination and ultrasound. An abnormal physical examination (prune belly syndrome, palpable kidneys/ bladder) or a urine infection prompts urgent testing, as does a newborn ultrasound which shows a bladder or kidney(s) which is so dilated that it should be palpable, or one which shows a pathognomic lesion (i.e. ureterocele). If hydronephrosis is bilateral or affects a solitarily functioning kidney, acidosis, hyperkalaemia and azotaemia are checked. If these renal functions are reduced, testing is done urgently. As these situations are uncommon, most newborns should simply have urological testing scheduled to be done after they are 1 month old. This would include a Welltempered Renogram, an ultrasound and voiding cystourethrogram (see below). In the interim, the newborn should receive a suppressive dose of an antimicrobial. In the author's experience, this dosage avoids the urine infection which may be seen when prophylaxis is not given.

Postnatal sonography

Postnatal sonography is done to 'dissect' the anatomy of the upper and lower urinary tract. For some conditions, such as renal duplication with ectopic ureter or ureterocele, the multicystic kidney, or renal calculi the images are classic (Figure 12.7). However, most cases of nephroureteral dilatation are idiopathic (e.g. there are no urethral valves or vesicoureteral reflux). In these instances, we are left only the renal position, parenchymal thickness, renal enlargement, or dilatation of the calices, pelvis or ureter need to be checked. There has been little research to set guidelines to discriminate between normal and pathological images of kidneys in infants with hydronephrosis or HUN, and so previously it has not been possible to predict which sonograms of 'idiopathic' hydronephrosis or HUN are likely to be associated with clinical problems and which are likely to be innocent.

It is common that renal pelvic dilatation is categorized only as mild, moderate or severe

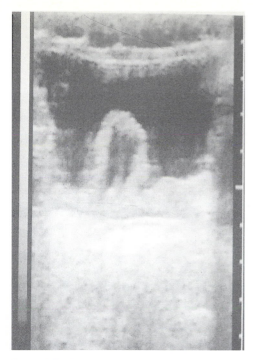

Figure 12.7 Sonogram images may be pathognomic. Clinical ultrasound showing a ureterocele.

by subjective impression. Borre et al. introduced quantitative measures (e.g. pelvic diameter, parenchyma thickness, and ratio of the thicknesses of the parenchyma/renal sinus) to grade hydronephrosis in adults, but this classification has not been validated [29].

Society for fetal urology grading of hydronephrosis and ureter dilatation

Realizing that sonographic images of hydronephrosis have not been strictly classified, a workshop of the Society for Fetal Urology (SFU) was held to reach consensus guidelines. This discussion of grading of hydronephrosis and ureter dilation is a synopsis of the workshop [30] (Figure 12.8, Table 12.1).

Rationale for grading of hydronephrosis

As background, it is accepted that the central renal complex which marks the renal sinus is normally brightly echogenic with an admixture of sonolucent areas. This appearance is due to

Table 12.1 Society For Fetal Urology Grading of idiopathic nephroureteral dilatation in infants [30]

Grade of hydronephrosis (HN Gr)

| HN Gr | Renal image | |
	Central renal complex	*Renal parenchymal thickness*
Grade 0	Intact	Normal
Grade 1	Slight splitting	Normal
Grade 2	Evident splitting, complex confined within renal border	Normal
Grade 3*	Wide splitting, pelvis dilated outside renal border, *and* calices *uniformly* dilated	Normal
Grade 4	Further dilatation of pelvis and calices (calices may appear convex)	Thin

* An extrarenal pelvis extends outside the renal border, yet, as the calices are not dilated, the HN is Gr 2. When the major calices are imaged but are not dilated, the HN is also Gr 2.

Grade of ureteral dilatation (UD Gr)

UD Gr	*Diameter of ureter*
Grade 1	<7 mm
Grade 2	7–10 mm
Grade 3	>10 mm

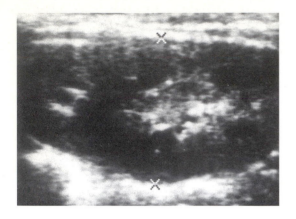

(a)

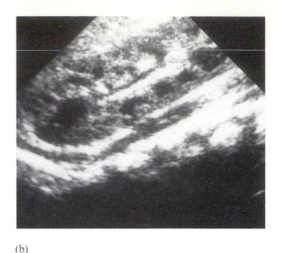

(b)

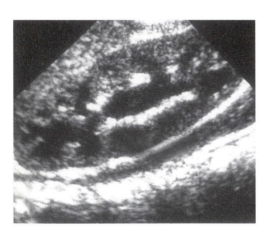

(c)

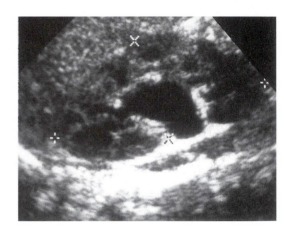

(d)

the contained echogenic renal sinus fat, sono-lucent renal pelvic urine and hilar blood. As the renal collecting system fills with urine, the accumulated urine splits and dilates the echo-genic central renal complex which now appears sonolucent. The rationale for grading hydrone-phrosis is based upon judging the degree of splitting of the complex, which is viewed to represent the degree of pelvicaliceal dilatation, and assessing the thickness of the mantle of renal parenchyma which covers the calices. Thereby, the dilatations are graded HN Gr 0–4 (Figure 12.8, Table 12.1).

Such grading relies mainly on evaluating the extent of caliceal dilatation, rather than mainly on measuring the anteroposterior diameter of the renal pelvis [31,32]. This reliance is because of clinical experience. First, isolated pelvic dilatation without caliceal dilatation (excluding vesicoureteral reflux) has not been shown to be pathological. Next, caliceal dilatation is likely to be caused by an obstructive uropathy (except when there is vesicoureteral reflux or the rare condition of megacalicosis). Finally, longitudinal examinations show that pelvic dilatation does not progress and the calices remain non-dilated when there is no obstruc-tion, and that caliceal dilatation progresses and the mantle of parenchyma ultimately becomes thin when there is obstruction. Perez et al. also recognized the importance of differ-entiating between the ultrasound appearance of pelviectasis in an extrarenal pelvis and pel-viectasis with UPJ obstruction [33].

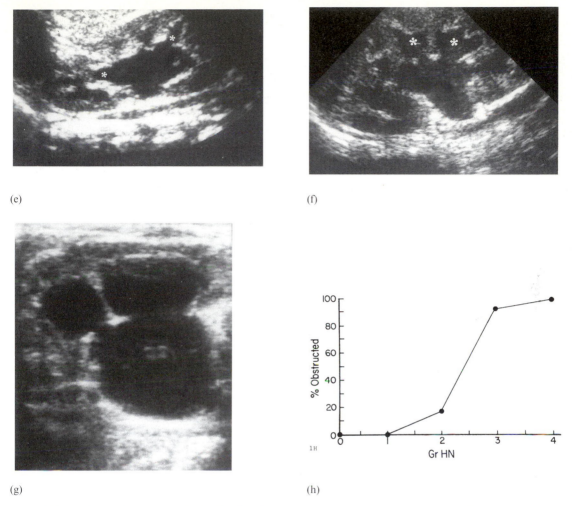

(e)   (f)

(g)   (h)

Figure 12.8 Grading of hydronephrosis. (a) Grade 0. Non-dilated kidney in a 1-month-old boy with a contralateral multicystic kidney. (× marks anterior or posterior border of kidney.) (b) Grade 1. Non-dilated kidney in a 1-month-old boy with contralateral UPJ obstruction. The central renal complex is slightly split. (c) Grade 2. Non-dilated kidney in a 1-month-old boy with contralateral UPJ obstruction. There is now more splitting of the central renal complex. Infundibula or calices are not apparent and the pelvis is confined within the renal parenchyma. The variants of Grade 2 hydronephrosis include: (d) Grade 2 – extrarenal pelvis. Dilated kidney identified prenatally in a 1-month-old boy. The renal pelvis extends beyond the renal parenchyma, but dilated calices are not seen. (e) Grade 2 – non-dilated calices. Dilated kidney identified prenatally in a 1-month-old boy. The renal pelvis extends beyond the renal parenchyma, two calices (*) are seen which drain into the pelvis, but are not dilated. (f) Grade 3 – Dilated kidney shown to have obstructive hydronephrosis by diuresis renography. Same findings as Grade 2 but now the calices (*) are uniformly dilated. The parenchyma does not appear thin. (g) Grade 4 – dilated kidney shown to have obstructive hydronephrosis by diuresis renography. Same findings as Grade 3 but pelvis and calices are now even more dilated, and the parenchyma appears thin (less than half of the contralateral side). (h) Correlation of Grade of hydronephrosis with obstruction. (All images are made along the long axis of the kidney, with the patient either supine or prone.)

Rationale for grading of ureteral dilatation

The grading of ureteral dilatation is based upon an established definition of a megaureter as being a ureter which is more than 7 mm wide [34]. The diameter of the retrovesical segment of the ureter (measured on transverse or longitudinal views) is the criterion for grading ureter dilation (UD) [30]. Thereby, the dilatation is graded UD Gr 0–3 (Figure 12.9, Table 12.1).

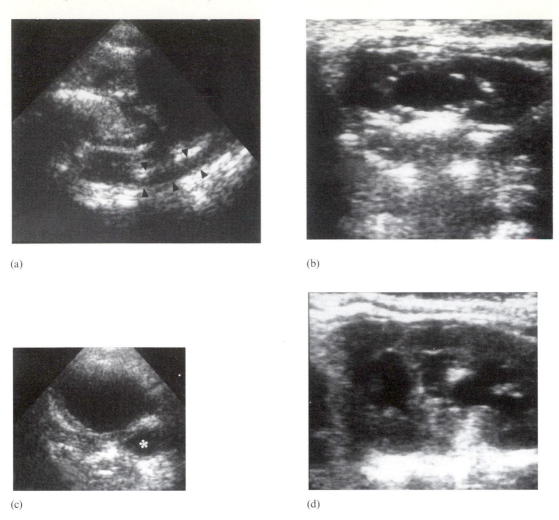

Figure 12.9 Grading of ureteral dilatation and scoring of HUN. (a) Grade 1: Ureter (right) diameter (*) measures 3 mm. As the kidney (left) shows HN Gr 2, HUN score = 3. This is a case of an infant girl with non-obstructing non-refluxing megaureter. (b) Grade 2: (right) ureter diameter (*) measures 8 mm. As the kidney (left) shows HN Gr 3, HUN score = 5. Obstructed HUN was noted by diuresis renography. At reimplantation a UVJ stricture was seen. (c) Grade 3: (right) ureter diameter (*) measures 12 mm. As the kidney (left) shows HN Gr 4, the HUN score = 7. Obstructed HUN was noted by diuresis renography. A valve of the pelvic ureter was found at ureteral reimplantation. (d) Correlation of HUN score with obstruction. (Ureter images are made as longitudinal or transverse views.)

Grade of hydronephrosis and ureter dilatation correlate with the diagnosis of obstruction

A recent review from our institution involved examining the records of 103 infants who had hydronephrosis or HUN found before 1 year old [30]. The data was examined in order to determine if grading of hydronephrosis had clinical meaning.

Hydronephrosis

There were 76 infants with hydronephrosis which involved 97 kidneys. Clinical obstruction was diagnosed in 56 (74%) of the 76 children, which involved 61 (63%) of the 97 hydronephrotic kidneys; clinical obstruction was not noted in the remainder. Obstruction was present at the UPJ or, less commonly, in the midureter. In the 61 kidneys with obstruction the mean grade was HN Gr 3.4 ± 0.7 (SD); in the 36 kidneys without obstruction the mean grade was HN Gr 1.6 ± 0.8 (p < 0.05 by t test).

It was determined that grading of hydronephrosis correlates with a diagnosis of clinical obstruction. When the hydronephrosis grade to predict obstruction was set at HN Gr ≥ 3 (i.e. pelvicaliceal dilatation is present), the sensitivity and specificity indices were 88 and 95%, respectively (Figure 12.8(h)). Namely, for sensitivity of infants who were ultimately diagnosed to have obstructed hydronephrosis, 70 (88%) of 78 ultrasound exams showed HN Gr ≥ 3. Similarly, for specificity of infants who were ultimately shown to have non-obstructed hydronephrosis 72 (95%) of 76 ultrasound exams showed HN Gr ≤ 2.

Hydroureteronephrosis

There were 27 children with HUN which involved 34 dilated renal units. In the 17 dilated units with obstruction, the mean grade of hydronephrosis was HN Gr 3.0 ± 0.7, and the mean grade of ureter dilatation was UD Gr 2.6 ± 0.6; in the 17 dilated units without obstruction, the mean grade of hydronephrosis was HN Gr 1.6 ± 1.2, and the mean grade of ureteral dilatation was UD Gr 1.1 ± 1.0 ($P < 0.001$ for Gr HN and Gr UD by t test). Despite this statistically significant difference in the grade of hydronephrosis and ureter dilatation between obstructed and non-obstructed HUN, the spread in values caused an overlap between these two groups which makes this significance not clinically helpful. For example, 5 (25%) of 21 exams of obstructed HUN showed HN Gr ≤ 2, and 12 (28%) of 42 exams in non-obstructed HUN showed HN Gr ≥ 3. Therefore, as the diagnosis of obstruction was not predicted well by the grade of hydronephrosis alone, the cases were evaluated with respect to both Gr HN and Gr UD as a score (HUN score = Gr HN + Gr UD) (Figure 12.9(d)). The average HUN score was 5.8 ± 1.0 in kidneys with obstructed HUN, and the average HUN score was 2.7 ± 1.9 in kidneys with non-obstructed HUN ($P < 0.001$ by t test).

It was determined that scoring HUN correlates with obstruction, as when the score to predict obstruction is set at HUN score ≥ 5, the sensitivity and specificity indices are 94 and

80%, respectively (Figure 12.9(d)). Namely, for sensitivity of kidneys which were ultimately diagnosed to have obstructed HUN, 15 (94%) of 16 ultrasound exams showed a HUN score ≥ 5. Similarly, for specificity of kidneys which were ultimately shown to have non-obstructed HUN, 28 (80%) showed a HUN score < 5.

Pitfalls in sonography

It is important in the evaluation of hydronephrosis to be sure that renal dilatation is not caused simply by a full bladder (dilatation persists after the bladder is empty). Also, repositioning a child to be erect or prone may empty a kidney which appears dilated when imaged with the child supine. Imaging a megaureter is helpful by having the bladder partly filled. Yet, if a long stricture is causing the HUN, the megaureter may not be imaged (Figure 12.10). Furthermore, it is becoming increasingly clear that it is important to assure the child is well hydrated. I administer Lasix (0.5 mg/lb (0.5 mg/0.45 kg)) orally along with encouraging fluid intake about 1 hour prior to sonography to assure that the upper urinary tract is as 'full' as it can be. Ebel also recognized the value of a stimulated furosemide diuresis prior to sonography because of the need to 'fill' a potentially dilated pelvis [35] (Figure 12.11). Pitfalls in the grading of hydronephrosis are shown (Figures 12.12, 12.13).

In-office sonography by urologists

Grading of hydronephrosis or ureter dilatation can be done conveniently using images personally made by a urologist during routine office visits. Personal and anecdotal experiences from many urologists in the USA and Europe show that office sonography can successfully check for a myriad of conditions such as hydronephrosis or megaureters, ectopic ureters or ureterocele, or an overdilated bladder [1,2].

Diuretic renography for well babies with hydronephrosis

The renogram has evolved over time to adapt to clinical needs. It was introduced initially to

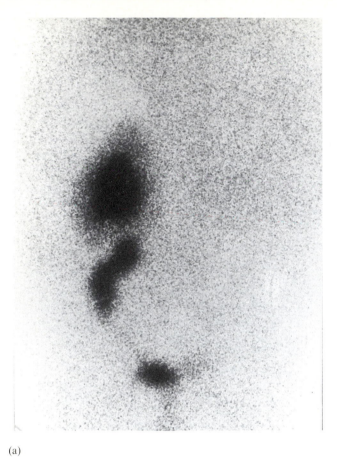

(a)

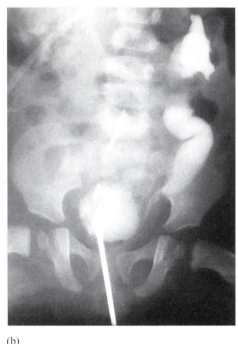

(b)

Figure 12.10 Pitfall in grading of HUN – *ureter not visualized*. A long narrowed segment of the pelvic ureter may produce proximal ureteral dilatation which cannot be detected in the pelvis behind the bladder. Renal dilatation alone may be noted. Ultrasound showed HN Gr 2. (a) The diuretic renogram shows dilatation of the left ureter far above the bladder. (b) The retrograde pyelogram shows the long stricture of the left ureter in the bony pelvis. The right ureter ends blindly.

assess renal function [36]. Later, cases of equivocal obstruction were tested by administrating a diuretic intravenously to determine if isotope static in the dilated kidney of an ill adult or child could drain [37]. Nowadays, because infants are presenting to evaluate a dilated kidney before illness strikes, renogram technology has needed to adapt to the new clinical need of assessing whether the dilated tracts of *asymptomatic* infants are obstructed. At first glance it would seem that only minor adjustments of medication dosages, collimators, and magnification hardware to techniques already established for adults or children were needed. However, heretofore, patients were tested after they became symptomatic and a dilated kidney was found. Almost all such kidneys were obstructed by renography when cases of reflux are excluded. Therefore, nowadays, given that renographic obstruction can be found in an *a*symptomatic infant, it has now become necessary to predict which cases are likely to go on to become clinically important. Questions which make this prediction controversial include: Is the obstructed pelvis/ureter of a newborn still compliant and muscular enough to show good drainage despite an anatomical obstruction? Can the obstructed segment 'grow' in calibre and over time 'resolve' obstruction? As there are more asymptomatic infants now presenting to evaluate hydronephrosis, there are now more operations being done than previously. Would some operated cases of renographically obstructed hydronephrosis have improved over time without surgery? Which ones?

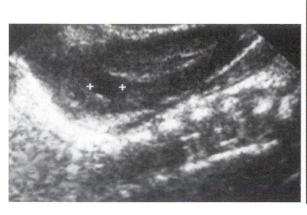

(a)

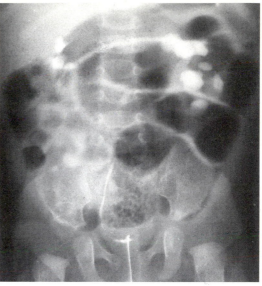

(b)

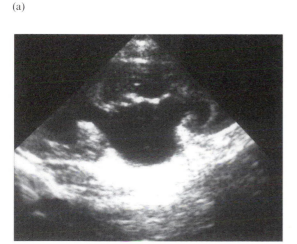

(c)

Figure 12.11 Pitfall in grading of hydronephrosis – *underhydration during sonography*. (a) Ultrasound shows only a sonolucent region in the upper pole of the kidney which was interpreted as a 'cyst' (cursors). (b) The excretory urogram shows dilatation of the left renal pelvis and calyces. (c) The postdiuretic ultrasound shows HN Gr 3. A ureteropelvic stricture was found at surgery.

Perhaps a parallel can be drawn between the clinical approach to resolution of ureteral reflux and resolution of obstruction. Children who develop symptomatic UTIs are commonly found to have high-grade reflux which they are not likely to outgrow. Yet, high-grade reflux found in asymptomatic newborns for evaluation of hydronephrosis is seen to resolve. Therefore, perhaps renographic obstruction in asymptomatic children will resolve, while such obstruction in children who develop symptoms needs to be repaired.

The 'Well Tempered Renogram' evolves from the diuretic renal scan

Much of the controversy regarding neonatal hydronephrosis stems from differences in how the diagnosis of obstruction is made. Namely, although the IVP can be useful to diagnose obstruction (see below), it is being believed, without necessarily good support, that quantitative data such as is provided by a renal scan is needed to discriminate simple dilatation

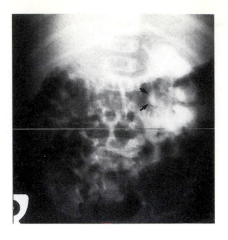

(a)   (b)

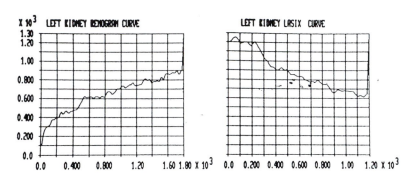

(c)

Figure 12.12 Pitfall in grading of hydronephrosis – *UPJ obstruction without a dilated extrarenal pelvis.* (a) The ultrasound at 1 month old shows dilated calyces (c) which communicate with a non-dilated pelvis (p). As the calyces are dilated this is HN Gr 3. This image could also be consistent with the syndrome of megacalicosis, a non-obstructive condition. (b) The excretory urogram shows the dilated calyces and small pelvis (arrows) and is consistent with obstruction. (c) The diuretic renogram shows obstruction. A stricture of the UPJ was seen at surgery.

(pelviectasis) from obstruction (pyelocaliceal dilatation). However, the scan criteria to diagnose obstruction remain controversial. Controversy is further fuelled by noting that clinical reports on renography use dissimilar test methods with respect to: isotope given, timing of Lasix administration, criteria to diagnose obstruction and state of bladder fullness. Such dissimilarities are likely to lead to variances in test interpretation and therefore have generated different clinical conclusions. A focus on the state of hydration at testing is illustrative. The state of hydration has not been standardized in the past. The state of hydration must influence the degree of renal pelvic distension,

as at the time of pyeloplasty children may show a renal pelvis which is only partially filled. This partial filling is likely to relate to dehydration after being kept NPO for several hours prior to induction of anaesthesia. Similarly, it is likely that pelves which are 'full' at the time of Lasix scanning will show an *un*equivocal obstructive pattern, yet those that are 'empty' secondary to underhydration will show better drainage after Lasix is given, and perhaps even show a non-obstructive pattern (as obstructive kinks unbend, they may not impede drainage as much). Therefore, there is a reciprocal relationship between pelvic fullness and flow beyond the UPJ. As it is likely

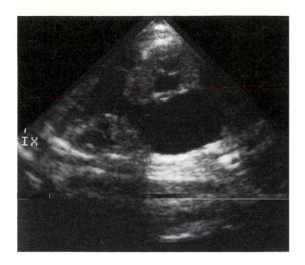

Figure 12.13 Pitfall in grading of hydronephrosis – *pelvocaliceal dilatation without obstruction; a compound papille drains in to a 'dilated' calyx.* Follow-up of prenatal hydronephrosis shows pelvocaliceal dilatation on the ultrasound. The WTR showed no obstruction (not shown). The EU shows the upper pole collecting system is 'dilated', perhaps because it drains multiple papillae.

that the children's states of hydration are not uniform prior to scanning, this may account for variable scan results [38]. Therefore, it is important to assure the children are in comparable states of good hydration at the time of testing. Suki recognized the need for standardization of these methods and initiated a standard hydration regimen prior to scanning which involved pretest oral and intravenous fluid loading [39]. Similar variabilities inherent in previous testing are likely to have existed for other factors, such as whether the bladder has been emptied by catheter or not or the dose and timing of diuretic administration. Another consideration is that the actual scan data or ultrasound images are shown infrequently in the assessment of hydronephrosis [11,40,41]. This makes comparing published results between investigators difficult.

Probably, because of these considerations and others, significant criticism of diuretic renography for asymptomatic infants with hydronephrosis emerged in the late 1980s. There were cases of 'renographic' obstruction which resolved, and, conversely, cases without renographic 'obstruction' which later developed symptoms referable to an obstructed kidney, or even loss of a previously functioning kidney. Furthermore, without a body of inde-

pendent research which focused on this question, it seemed unlikely that there would be an end to the confusion.

From this perspective, the Society for Fetal Urology conferred in 1989 with the Pediatric Nuclear Medicine Club to attempt to make renography more uniform. Test results and clinical follow-up would then be more comparable between institutions. From this conference a standardized technique to assess asymptomatic infants with hydronephrosis for obstruction was developed and is described below.

The methods which follow represent the consensus of about 40 paediatric urologists and nuclear medicine physicians. Their diverse opinions were blended, and the resultant methodology was coined the 'Well Tempered Renogram' (WTR) [42,43]. The methods for the WTR herein described are summarized from Conway [42,43].

Pretest preparation

Infants should be at least 1 month old in order to reduce the likelihood that immature renal function will significantly affect the results. Premature infants should be even older, since more time after birth is needed for their renal function to become mature enough to permit testing.

Hydration is assured for a few reasons. Nauta recognized i.v. hydration was needed to make test methods more uniform and to permit better comparison of follow-up data [23]. Furthermore, scans which are performed with i.v. hydration compare well with results of the Whitaker test [44]. Oral liquids are encouraged, and fluid (D_5.2 saline) is administered intravenously (before testing a volume of 15 ml/kg is given over 30 minutes, beginning at least 15 minutes prior to injection of isotope, and during the test a maintenance fluid volume is given at 8 ml/kg/h).

As intravenous access can be the most difficult part of the test, the bladder should not be catheterized until the venous access is attained. Furthermore, a paediatric anesthesiologist or intensive care unit (ICU) nurse can help vein catheterization. The importance of an empty bladder is emphasized by Piepsz, who noted remarkable improvements in diuretic response after the bladder spontaneously emptied [19]. Thereby, the bladder is catheterized using a balloon retention type catheter to be sure that it is empty. In this way elevated intravesical pressure does not impair emptying the upper tract, and coexistent reflux is obviated. Should an ectopic ureter be a possible cause for megaureter, then a non-ballooned catheter should be used, as the balloon of a catheter could influence test results by occluding the orifice of an ectopic ureter which is near the bladder neck. A satisfactory urine output is confirmed by monitoring the drainage from the bladder catheter. Maintaining an empty bladder is checked on the persistence scope. After these preparations, the infant is positioned supine for the test.

Method for Well Tempered Renography

Renogram phase

^{99m}Tc-Mercuroacetylglycylglycylglycine (MAG3, Mallinckrodt, Inc., St Louis, MO, USA) is the radiopharmaceutical chosen to image the kidney because it shows more rapid renal clearance and primary tubular excretion after furosemide injection than other available agents. Also, with ^{99m}Tc-MAG3 less radiation is absorbed by the infant. The ultrasound done prior to testing identifies the regions of clinical interest (i.e. dilated pelvis, upper pole dilatation of an ectopic ureter or a megaureter). These areas are identified on the computer screen and outlined as a region of interest (ROI). The activity within this 'core' which is not renal (e.g. overlying spleen or liver) is excluded by subtraction of a standard background perimeter. Hence, during the renogram phase, the regions of functioning kidney tissue and urine accumulation are identified. Analogue images (scans) are made using the gamma camera, while digital data is displayed as a time/activity curve (renogram). The renogram phase usually ends about 20 minutes after injection of ^{99m}Tc-MAG3. When there is marked hydronephrosis, the infant may be repositioned briefly in the prone position to 'mix' radioactivity better before furosemide injection.

Diuresis phase

Furosemide (1 mg/kg i.v.) is administered when the dilated upper tract is believed to be 'full'. The determination of fullness is made by checking if the renal scan images of nephro-

ureteral dilatation compare favourably with the ultrasound images. Renal scan images and renogram curves are made similar to the renogram phase of the test. The ROI delimited for assessing drainage of hydronephrosis after furosemide injection in cases of HN include the renal pelvis and collecting system, while for HUN, an additional ROI is outlined over the ureter at the ureterovesical junction. Should obstruction be suspected at the conclusion of the test, the child should be repositioned prone for about 20 minutes, to determine if this position, which makes the dilated segment more dependent, fosters improved drainage.

Data analysed

Renal function

An estimate of renal function can be attained by subjectively noting the 'intensity' of isotope on renal scan images by 2 hours after injection of ^{99m}Tc-MAG3. Reduced function can be estimated as mildly, moderately or markedly reduced. 'Fitting' the renogram curve pattern against stereotypical patterns can be used to categorize renal function as normal, immature or showing poor function (Figure 12.4). Since the adaptation of ^{99m}Tc-MAG3 as the scanning isotope, the 'immature' pattern noted with ^{99m}Tc-diethyltetrapentaacetic acid (DTPA) [45] has not been seen. The immature pattern may reflect an idiosyncrasy of the DTPA rather than being reflective of a real clinical condition. For infants, such subjective assessment of function may be less misleading than quantitative measurements derived by computer (e.g. glomerular filtration rate, estimated renal plasma flow) which have not been widely adapted. Percentage differential renal function for a kidney is the ratio of total counts for that kidney ROI (subtracted for background activity) which is measured by 2 hours after ^{99m}Tc-MAG3 injection (i.e. prior to the appearance of calices or pelvis which is usually 60–90 minutes after injection), divided by the sum of such counts for both kidneys. Monitoring the parenchymal transit time or measuring cortical function is not addressed by WTR.

Drainage of isotope

An estimate of drainage can be attained by subjectively categorizing the diuresis renogram curve generated as one of several agreed upon stereotypical patterns which are believed to reflect: normal drainage, stasis without obstruction, stasis with obstruction or indeterminate (Figure 12.5). Alternatively, drainage of isotope can be measured. The time to clear 50% of the retained isotope is a commonly reported parameter. However, there are multiple ways of assessing this, as either from the times after: injection of diuretic, expected action of diuretic or first evidence of drainage after injection. As an exponential clearance of isotope is the best indicator of free drainage, any clearance which is not exponential in nature could be obstructed. Therefore, a computer program could be used to determine whether or not there is exponential clearance. However, automatic computer programs which calculate $t_{1/2}$ have not been validated.

Determination of renographic obstruction

Diagnosis of renographic obstruction does not rely on assessing the value of a single parameter (i.e. only $t_{1/2}$); rather, a global interpretation is done which synthesizes the meaning of: function data, degree of hydronephrosis, ease of drainage and comparisons with previous testings. More specifically, the renographic diagnosis of UPJ obstruction is based on multiple criteria which are here listed in order of importance:

1. The quantitative diuretic response, namely, the $t_{1/2}$ measured from the time of diuretic injection [46].
2. The qualitative diuretic response pattern (a non-exponential response means obstruction) [47].
3. The subjective evidence of renal function loss as based upon the initial image appearance <2 minutes (reduced uptake on the involved side; not applicable in cases of bilateral hydronephrosis).
4. The configuration of the first and second phases of the renogram curve (decreased height and prolongation of the second phase is consistent with decreased perfusion and function, and therefore with obstruction).
5. The renogram pattern (a prolonged third phase is consistent with obstruction) [37].
6. The percent differential renal function (reduce % function may be consistent with

obstruction) (not applicable in bilateral cases).
7. The subjective degree of hydronephrosis assessed on scintigraphic images (not ultrasound images) (marked hydronephrosis may be consistent with obstruction).
8. The 20-minute to peak ratio which is a reflection of the profile of the renogram curve which reflects drainage during the third phase (ratio >90% implies poor washout on the renogram curve and may be consistent with obstruction).

Ultrasound partnered with the well-tempered renogram

As diuretic renography primarily gives function data, but surgeons are more interested in finding 'anatomical' causes for dilatation, it was believed that adding an examination of anatomy at the time of WTR would be likely to be helpful in understanding the nature of the hydronephrosis or HUN. Furthermore, such additional information could help to explain the discrepancy between finding no obstruction by diuretic renography and in the same case finding obstruction by radiographic tests. Gonzalez believed the most likely explanation for such discrepancy is that these are cases where the pelvis has compensated for the obstruction [48]. This is particularly likely if the kidney responds well to diuretic, and the renal pelvis is capable of vigorous peristalsis. In such a circumstance, the isotope can be rapidly washed out of the collecting system if high pressures proximal to the obstruction are generated. Gonzalez pessimistically views the scan as a good means to follow-up but not to diagnose cases 'needful' of surgery. Similarly, Lupton explains that if the pelvic wall is compliant, a dilated pelvis may show an obstructive pattern by renography and a non-obstructed pressure gradient by manometry at the time of antegrade nephrostogram [20].

The author's histological observations in pyeloplasty specimens are consistent with these views [28]. It was found that the renal pelvis obtained from pyeloplasty carried out for UPJ obstruction showed significant hypertrophy of l. muscularis, and it is plausible that rapid drainage of urine beyond the UPJ, as seen in a non-obstructed renogram curve (and scan) in infants, occurs consequent to intermittent, increased intrapelvic pressure. This pressure then causes the pelvicaliceal system to dilate. Left uncorrected, ultimately there will be progressive dilatation and parenchymal thinning and/or intra- and interfascicular fibrosis of the muscle bundles of the l. muscularis of the pelvis. A kidney which initially shows a non-obstructive renogram curve pattern may undergo such progressive changes and evolve an obstructive pattern. Monitoring the ultrasound images of the kidney after Lasix administration as part of the renogram permits this likelihood to be assessed.

Substitution of the excretory urogram with an ultrasound just after the time of renal scanning and Lasix administration, to glean the impact of diuretic on the grade of hydronephrosis or score of HUN, is now used in this laboratory. It was believed this would help to detect instances of 'physiological obstruction' despite a 'good' washout. Since 1991, all infants evaluated for hydronephrosis/hydroureteronephrosis underwent a WTR, which was partnered with an ultrasound directly after Lasix injection. The findings of the WTR (obstruction or not) were compared against the findings of the post-Lasix sonogram (pelvicaliceal dilatation or not). When the dilated kidney was examined by noting the results of the WTR alone, there was an overall accuracy of 85% (sensitivity 90% and specificity 81%). The overall accuracy was improved when the dilated kidney was examined by noting the results of the WTR along with the partnered post-Lasix ultrasound. When the tests agreed, there was an overall accuracy of 92% (sensitivity of 93% and specificity 91%). When the partnered WTR and ultrasound did not agree, further testing was done. This showed the ultrasound led to correct diagnosis more often than the WTR alone [49].

Voiding cystourethrogram

The voiding cystourethrogram (VCUG) will determine if a birth defect is causing the nephroureteral dilatation. It is uncommon for well babies with prenatally detected hydronephrosis to show abnormalities by VCUG. This differs from testing which is done when babies become ill. Here the VCUG commonly shows the classical findings of reflux, ureterocele or posterior urethral valves. These conditions are treated conventionally, as their management is not controversial.

Excretory urogram

In the late 1980s the view developed that the renal scan and not the EU should be the primary tool to diagnose obstruction. Yet, the IVP can help diagnose UPJ obstruction when the pathognomic findings of obstruction are seen: delayed appearance of 'dilute' contrast in the collecting system, papillae which are blunted or effaced uniformly, calices which are uniformly dilated, and retention of contrast in the pelvis even on a radiograph which is taken while the child is prone (kidney pelvis becomes more dependent than supine) (Figure 12.11(b)). The IVP should be done with the bladder drained by catheter. Bernstein et al. give a balanced view of the usefulness of the IVP and scan to diagnose UPJ obstruction [50].

Cystoscopy, antegrade or retrograde pyeloureterogram

Examinations performed under anaesthesia may show diverse findings. Cystoscopy may show posterior urethral valves and/or ureteral reflux which are not identified during an 'awake' cystogram. It is unusual to need to resort to percutaneous puncture of the kidney in order to directly instill a marker into the ureteropyelocalyceal system to guide clinical management (Figure 12.5). Determining if reduced renal function can be reversed by prolonged nephrostomy is usually unrewarding. A diagnostic brief percutaneous nephrostomy is helpful:

1. To resolve a discrepancy between the findings of sonography and scintigraphy.
2. When it is necessary to make a diagnosis in the newborn.
3. As part of a therapeutic nephrostomy in order to better show the anatomy.
4. To better examine for the possibility of tandem obstructions (ipsilateral UPJ and UVJ obstruction) [51].
5. To be more confident about the diagnosis of obstruction prior to anticipated surgery

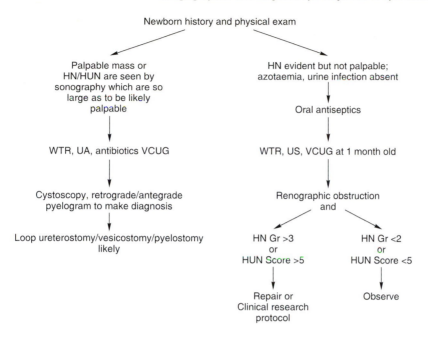

Figure 12.14 Algorithm for postnatal imaging of prenatally detected HU/HUN. There is no defined obstructive lesion (e.g. urethral valves, ureterocele, ectopic ureter are dealt with after the child is a few days or weeks old).

(solitary kidney with small pelvis and large calices) (Figures 12.1, 12.10).

Occasionally, only during cystoscopic examination will it be noted that an 'obstructed' megaureter is caused by a faecal impaction.

Determination of clinical obstruction

It is important to distinguish between *physiological*, *renographic* and *clinical* obstruction. For example, physiological obstruction refers to dysfunction of the kidney related to obstruction (e.g. hypertension, reduced concentrating ability). The diuretic renogram is performed to inform the clinician about the status of renal function and to determine the drainage status of the dilated renal unit. Therefore, renographic obstruction refers to identifying pathological delays in urine drainage which account for hydronephrosis. While clinical obstruction refers to the synthesis by the clinician of *all* clinical data in order to determine if clinical problems are likely to result, should the 'obstruction' not be corrected [52].

Exceptions to diagnosing obstruction

Obstruction need not be present when the percentage differential function is reduced and does not normalize if the kidney is hypoplastic. Kidneys with tubular disorders may not show drainage response after Lasix administration [52]. Pelvicaliceal dilatation typical of obstructive uropathy may also be seen in a non-obstructed 'compound' calix which drains compound papilla (Figure 12.12 compare with Figure 12.8(e)).

Conclusion

The clinician is responsible for determining which cases of nephroureteral dilatation in asymptomatic infants require intervention. Standardizing renographic test methodology and more objective grading of hydronephrosis permits making better intrapatient and interinstitution comparisons (Figure 12.14). In this manner, the natural history of obstructed and non-obstructed hydronephrosis will ultimately be determined. Registration of cases of asymptomatic infant hydronephrosis and prospective randomized clinical trials of surgery, or observation in the management of renographically obstructed hydronephrosis, are needed to ascertain which, if any, cases need repair.

Therefore, from this background, routine (US, WTR, VCUG, EU) or specialized (ante- or retrograde pyelogram, cystoscopy) testing should identify if there is an anatomical cause of the nephroureteral dilatation (e.g. uretero- cele, ureteral reflux). When such a cause is not seen, clinically important obstruction is likely when there is renographic obstruction and HN Gr ≥ 3 or a HUN score ≥ 5. The likelihood that such 'significant' obstructions will even- tually become clinical problems needs to be addressed by a clinical trial, to compare the outcome of surgery versus no surgery in their management. Similarly, longitudinal follow-up is needed to show that cases diagnosed as no obstruction will show resolution of hydrone- phrosis, preservation of function and main- tenance of good drainage (Figure 12.5). Furthermore, should pyeloplasty be carried out, histological examination to confirm obstructive changes in the pelvis should be done [27,28].

References

1. Maizels M, Zaontz MR, Houlihan DL, Firlit CF. In office ultrasonography (IOUS) to image the kidneys and bladders of children. *J Urol* 1987; **138**: 1031.
2. Maizels M, Zaontz M. The urosound: in-office ultra- sonography to screen infants and children for urinary obstruction. *Urol Clin North Am* 1990; **17**: 429.
3. Guys JM, Borella F, Monfort G. Ureteropelvic junc- tion obstruction: prenatal diagnosis and neonatal sur- gery in 47 cases. *J Pediatr Surg* 1988; **23**: 156.
4. Minogue J, Silver R. When does a statistical fact become an ethical imperative. *Am J Obstet Gynecol* 1987; **157**: 229.
5. Benacerraf BR, Cnann A, Gelman R, Laboda LA, Frigoletto FD Jr. Can sonographers reliably identify anatomic features associated with Down syndrome in fetuses? *Radiology* 1989; **172**: 377.
6. Riley L, Frigoletto FD Jr, Benacerraf BR. The impli- cations of sonographically identified cervical changes in patients not necessarily at risk for preterm birth. *J Ultrasound Med* 1992; **11**: 75.
7. Elder JS, Duckett J. Management of the fetus and neonate with hydronephrosis detected by prenatal ultrasonography. *Pediatr Ann* 1988; **17**: 19.
8. Thomas DFM, Gordon AC. Management of pre- natally diagnosed uropathies. *Arch Dis Child* 1989; **64**: 58.
9. Thomas DFM, Agrawal M, Laidin AZ, Eckstein HB. Pelviureteric obstruction in infancy and childhood. *Br J Urol* 1982; **54**: 204.
10. McAlister WH, Manley CB, Siegel MJ. Asymptomatic progression of partial ureteropelvic obstruction in children. *J Urol* 1980; **123**: 267.
11. Ransley PG, Dhillon HK, Gordan I, Duffy PG, Dillon MJ, Barratt TM. The postnatal management of hydronephrosis diagnosed by prenatal ultrasound. *J Urol* 1990; **144**: 584.
12. Maizels M. Surgical correction of the concealed penis. In: Horton CE, Elder JS (eds) *Reconstructive Surgery of the External Genitalia*. Boston, MA: Little Brown and Co (in press).
13. Arnold AJ, Rickwood AM. Natural history of pel- viureteric obstruction detected by prenatal son- ography. *Br J Urol* 1990; **65**: 91.
14. MacNeily AE, Maizels M, Kaplan WE, Firlit CF, Conway JJ. Does 'early' pyeloplasty really avert loss of renal function: a retrospective review. *J Urol* (sub- mitted).
15. Homsy YL, Williot P, Danais S. Transitional neonatal hydronephrosis: fact or fantasy? *J Urol* 1986; **136**: 339.
16. Homsy YL, Saad F, Laerge I, Williot P, Pison C. Transitional hydronephrosis of the newborn and infant. *J Urol* 1990; **144**: 579.
17. Gordon I, Dhillon HK, Gatanash H, Peters AM. Antenatal diagnosis of pelvic hydronephrosis: assess- ment of renal function and drainage as a guide to management. *J Nucl Med* 1991; **32**: 1649.
18. Josephson S. Experimental obstructive hydronephrosis in newborn rats. *J Urol* 1983; **129**: 396.
19. Piepsz A, Hall M, Ham HR, Verboven M, Collier F. Prospective management of neonates with pelvi- ureteric junction stenosis. *Scand J Urol Nephrol* 1989; **23**: 31.
20. Lupton EWL, Richards D, Testa HJ et al. A com- parison of diuresis renography, the Whitaker test and renal pelvic morphology in idiopathic hydronephrosis. *Br J Urol* 1985; **57**: 119.
21. Johnson HW, Gleave M, Coleman GU, Nadel HR, Raffel J, Weckworth PF. Neonatal renomegaly. *J Urol* 1987; **138**: 1023.
22. Bratt CG, Aurell M, Nisson S. Renal function in patients with hydronephrosis. *Br J Urol* 1977; **49**: 249.
23. Nauta J, Pot DJ, Mooij PPM, Nijman JM, Wolff ED. Forced hydration prior to renography in children with hydronephrosis. An evaluation. *Br J Urol* 1991; **68**: 93.
24. Dowling KJ, Harmon EP, Ortenberg J, Polanco E, Evans BB. Ureteropelvic Junction Obstruction: The effect of pyeloplasty on renal function. *J Urol* 1988; **140**: 1227.
25. Kekomaki M, Wehle M, Walker RD. The growing rabbit with solitary, partially-obstructed kidney. Analysis of an experimental model with reference to the renal concentrating ability. *J Urol* 1985; **133**: 870.

26. Dejter SW Jr, Eggli DF, Gibbons MD. Delayed management of neonatal hydronephrosis. *J Urol* 1988; **140**: (5 Pt 2), 1305.

27. dell'Agnola CA, Carmassi LM, Merlo D, Tadini B. Duration and severity of congenital hydronephrosis as a cause of smooth muscle deterioration in pyeloureteral junction obstruction. *Z Kinderchir* 1990; **45**: 286.

28. Starr NT, Maizels M, Chou P, Brannigan R, Shapiro E. Microanatomy and morphometry of the hydronephrotic 'obstructed' renal pelvis in asymtomatic infants. *J Urol* 1992; **148**: 519.

29. Boore GE, Borre DG, Pereira H, Duval AA, Corona R. New quantified echographic features of normal kidney. Hydronephrosis classification. *Rontgen-Bl* 1990; **43**: 519.

30. Maizels M, Reisman EM, Flom LS, Nelson J, Fernbach S, Firlit CF. Grading nephroureteral dilatation detected in the first year of life – correlation with obstruction. *J Urol* 1992; **148**: 609.

31. Grignon A, Filion R, Filiatrault D et al. Urinary tract dilatation in utero: classification and clinical applications. *Radiology* 1986; **160**: 645.

32. Grignon A, Filiatrault D, Homsy Y et al. Ureteropelvic junction stenosis: antenatal ultrasonographic diagnosis, postnatal investigation and follow-up. *Radiology* 1986; **160**: 649.

33. Perez KM, Friedman RM, King LR. The case of relief of ureteropelvic junction obstruction in neonates and young children at time of diagnosis. *Urology* 1991; **38**: 195.

34. Stephens FD. *Congenital Malformation of the Urinary Tract*. New York: Praeger, 1983; chap 14, p 223.

35. Ebel KD, Bliesener JA, Gharib M. Imaging of ureteropelvic junction obstruction with stimulated diuresis. *Pediatr Radiol* 1988; **18**: 54.

36. Rado JP, Bano C, Tako J, Szende L. Renographic studies during furosemide diuresis in partial ureteral obstruction. *Radiol Clin Biol* 1969; **38**: 132.

37. O'Reilly PH. Diuresis renography 8 years later: an update. *J Urol* 1986; **136**: 993.

38. Koff SA. Pathophysiology of ureteropelvic junction obstruction. Clinical and experimental observations. *Urol Clin North Am* 1990; **17**: 263.

39. Sukhai RN, Kooy PPM, Wolff ED, Scholtmeijer RJ. Predictive value of ^{99m}Tc-DTPA renography studies under conditions of maximal diuresis for the functional outcome of reconstructive surgery in children with obstructive uropathy. *Br J Urol* 1986; **58**: 596.

40. Wasnick RM. Neonatal UPJ obstruction: current controversies. *Dialogues Pediatr Urol* 1991; **14**: 1.

41. Dejter SW Jr, Gibbons MD. The fate of infant kidneys with fetal hydronephrosis but initially normal postnatal sonography. *J Urol* 1989; **142**: (2 Pt 2), 661.

42. Conway JJ. 'Well tempered' diuresis renography: its historical development, physiological and technical pitfalls, and standardized technique protocol. *Semin Nucl Med* 1992; **22**: 74.

43. Conway JJ. The 'well tempered' diuretic renogram: a standard method to examine the asymptomatic neonate with hydronephrosis or hydroureteronephrosis. *J Nucl Med* 1992; **33**: 2047–2051.

44. Kass EJ, Majd M, Belman AB. Comparison of the diuretic renogram and the pressure perfusion study in children. *J Urol* 1985; **134**: 92.

45. Koff SA, McDowell GC, Byard M. Diuretic radionuclide assessment of obstruction in the infant: guidelines for successful interpretation. *J Urol* 1988; **140**: (5 Pt 2), 1167.

46. Krueger RP, Ash JM, Silver MM et al. Primary hydronephrosis. Assessment of diuretic renography, pelvis perfusion, operative findings, and renal and ureteral histology. *Urol Clin North Am* 1980; **7**: 231.

47. Zechman W. An experimental approach to explain some misinterpretations of diuresis renography. *Nucl Med Commun* 1988; **9**: 283.

48. Reinberg Y, Gonzalez R. Upper urinary tract obstruction in children: current controversies in diagnosis. *Pediatr Clin North Am* 1987; **34**: 1291.

49. Maizels M, Fernbach S, Conway JJ. Ultrasonography partnered with diuretic renography assesses infant hydronephrosis better than diuretic renography alone. Abstract Section of Urology AAP, San Francisco October 1992. *J Urol* (submitted).

50. Bernstein GT, Mandell J, Lebowitz RL, Bauer SB, Colodny AH, Retik AB. Ureteropelvic junction obstruction. *J Urol* 1988; **140**: 1216.

51. Bockrath J, Maizels M, Firlit CF. Benign bladder neck polyp causing tandem obstruction of the urinary tract in a patient with Beckwith–Weidemann syndrome. *J Urol* 1982; **128**: 1309.

52. Maizels M, King LR, Firlit CF. Conway J. Troubleshooting the diuretic renogram. *Urology* 1986; **28**: 355.

13

Controversies in the management of prenatally detected hydronephrosis in the well infant

M. Maizels

This discussion focuses on the approach in managing the baby who is well yet shows renographic obstruction and hydronephrosis. It does not address the management of babies who have become ill from renal obstruction, as the importance of treating their problems (e.g. urinary tract infection (UTI), azotaemia, palpable masses, dyspnoea, urinary retention or ascites) is not questioned.

Is the baby ill or can an anatomical lesion which is causing the obstruction be found?

Management of newborns with prenatally detected hydronephrosis can be decided after a diagnosis is clearly made. Is the dilatation caused by a lesion (e.g. urethral valves, ureterocele) which can be imaged by routine radiological testing? Or, is it not possible to identify a responsible lesion (i.e. idiopathic hydronephrosis or hydroureteronephrosis (HUN), see Chapter 12 for definitions). For the *minority* of neonates, testing will show a discrete lesion, and this should be corrected when the medical condition permits. Posterior urethral valves are ablated as a newborn after biochemical abnormalities and/or infection are stabilized. A ureterocele which obstructs voiding and causes hydronephrosis should be managed quickly. An upper pole which is obstructed by an ectopic ureter may be repaired or excised

after a few weeks old while the newborn is receiving antiseptics [1].

For the *majority* of neonates with prenatal hydronephrosis, idiopathic hydronephrosis is the condition most frequently diagnosed postnatally, as the cause for the dilatation is not evident. However, surgeons may be slow to operate because the children are well and particularly because it is unproven that the renographic obstruction will cause a problem. Thereby, the inability to reliably predict the natural history of this disorder has sparked controversy.

Why there is controversy

In general there is consensus as to 'when' and 'why' ureters should be reimplanted, testicles should be pexed in the scrotum or hypospadias should be repaired. A similar consensus on the guidelines for managing well babies with hydronephrosis has not been reached, largely because: (1) the natural history of the disorder is unknown, (2) the meaning of tests results is not agreed and (3) the role of surgery is undefined.

1. Natural history

It is unknown which cases of renographic obstructed hydronephrosis have clinical meaning and which do not. Thereby, even though it is possible to more objectively diagnose reno-graphic obstruction and to grade hydro-nephrosis (see previous chapter) it is still undocumented under what conditions cases of renographic obstruction with 'significant' hydro-nephrosis (HN Gr $\geq$ 3) can resolve. Perhaps, with the baby's inherent growth, the lumen of the ureter will enlarge or obstructive ureter kinks will straighten. Can cases with obstruction and hydronephrosis persist or pro-gress, and yet the children still have enough 'biological reserve' so as not to show clinical problems? Or, in which cases will the infant's biological reserves be overwhelmed. Could this lead to irreversible loss of function or to mor-bidity related to urine infection, pain, haema-turia or retarded growth? Is it a valid medical concern that a carrier may not give health or life insurance because the course of hydrone-phrosis of infancy is unpredictable?

2. What do the test results mean?

Confusion developed because there was a lack of agreement in interpreting diuresis renogram tests and a recognition that ultrasound images may not be reproducible because they are operator dependent. This confusion rightly sparked a 'wait and see' approach. This seemed particularly valid, as most newborns are so healthy that it is difficult for parents to imagine that their baby might need surgery. Homsy notes that the decision to intervene surgically is more complex for asymptomatic infants, in view of reports which show spon-taneous resolution of dilatation [2]. It may be that literature reports which show hydrone-phrosis or obstruction can resolve while func-tion is preserved are likely to be depicting cases of pelviectasis (clinically not obstructive) rather than pelvicaliectasis (clinically obstruc-tive). Namely, it is likely that images presented which are intended to show spontaneous reso-lution of dilatation more realistically represent a kidney with a non-obstructed extrarenal pelvis. This view is supported by the organized report of Johnson et al. [3], who noted resolu-tion in cases of mild pyelocaliectasis. Based upon the images shown, these cases of appar-ent caliceal dilatation are likely to reflect a compound papilla with reciprocal dilatation of the calix.

3. What is the role of surgery?

Neither the role of surgery nor the criteria for successful surgery have been defined. Piepsz et al. [4] describes two assumptions which under-lie the strategy to manage postnatal hydrone-phrosis: (i) renal obstruction without surgical correction will progressively destroy the kidney, and (ii) surgery will correct the destruc-tion. Certainly, improved drainage by the Well Tempered Renogram (WTR) and down-grading of hydronephrosis are desired. How-ever, for poorly functioning kidneys, can sur-gery also be a success if there is no change in the function, drainage and grade of hydrone-phrosis, yet a postoperative antegrade pyelo-gram shows the UPJ is now patent? Perhaps the renal medulla is so thin that there is an obligatory nephrogenic diuresis and, therefore, the kidney cannot respond to an administered diuretic. Has the pelvis become so fibrotic, perhaps from chronic intravasation of urine, that mural cicatrix obviates better drainage postoperatively even though the UPJ is now patent? Furthermore, if scintigraphic and sono-graphic improvements are expected after surgery, when should they appear post-operatively?

Arnold and Rickwood nicely capsulize their changed attitudes regarding the management of newborns with obstructed hydronephrosis [5]. Initially, they did surgery for newborn UPJ obstruction without delay because they were conditioned to do so by the usual clinical experience with children and adults who pre-sented because of symptoms. The authors 'mellowed' their approach and deferred surgery to 3 months old. When renography was intro-duced, they realized the measured kidney func-tion by scan was normal or even better than that function perceived by IVP. For them the question became not whether to do early or late pyeloplasty, but whether to do any pyelo-plasty. They point out that the upper tracts are not inert drainage pipes, but as tissues which grow and adapt, they may permit improved drainage over time. These authors concur with Piepsz and defer pyeloplasty in obstructed kidneys with >40% differential function. They find that without surgery 40% of 18 kidneys show resolving obstruction, and 72% of 18 kidneys show resolving hydrone-phrosis [5].

Currently, management involving whether or not to proceed to surgery is based upon biases of individual practitioners, which have been formulated by experience in treating symptomatic children with this condition. This application of experience in treating symptomatic children to treating asymptomatic neonates may not be founded. Clinical data will be needed to make such applications relevant [6,7].

Until there are hard answers to such issues, the management of hydronephrosis/hydroureteronephrosis will remain clouded and controversial. Recognizing that a lack of data prevents a scientific basis for the management of such infants, this chapter will focus on reasons to 'jump' into surgery without a long observation period. Dr Homsy (Chapter 11) focuses on reasons for an observation period. A compromise position will then be reached.

Surgery for well babies with obstructed hydronephrosis

The traditional indications for reconstructive surgery – clinical symptoms (e.g. UTI, pain) along with radiological tests which show obstruction – are not able to be applied to the asymptomatic baby with hydronephrosis. It is not yet established which test parameters (e.g. thin parenchyma on ultrasound, reduced function or delayed drainage on scan, or identifying a 'kink/stricture' on antegrade pyelogram) will correlate with the eventual loss of renal function and/or development of clinical symptoms. Meaningful answers to this question will require data derived from longitudinal follow-up. The follow-up period is likely to be at least a decade, as in the era before prenatal ultrasound diagnosis, children eventually become symptomatic largely prior to adolescence. Current reports of series which show stable function in the face of ongoing obstruction for perhaps up to 5 years, show that many of the children will develop symptoms referable to obstruction over longer follow-up period. For example, Homsy et al. reported deterioration with obstruction by the fourth year of follow-up [2].

Clinical research to justify management

Justifying the management of hydronephrosis should be based on clinical research. This is mainly for three reasons:

1. The focus of existing animal research is to compare recovery of renal function in newborn laboratory animals with induced obstruction versus adult animals with induced obstruction. The more clinically pertinent comparison of recovery of function in newborns with induced obstruction which has been reversed after brief obstruction versus reversal after prolonged obstruction has not been carried out [8–10].
2. Laboratory research examines the effects on induced mechanical obstruction (e.g. suture or clip of ureter causing partial or complete obstruction) which are never expected to resolve. This significantly differs from the clinical situation, in which the lesion causing obstruction and hydronephrosis may 'heal' spontaneously. Therefore, function and HN Gr may normalize without surgery. For example, kinks, folds and twists, common in fetuses at 20 weeks' gestation, become less pronounced later in gestation [11]. Perhaps these configurations of the ureter restrict drainage and cause fetal hydronephrosis which persists as a newborn. Then, with the growth of infancy the folds may straighten, and drainage becomes prompt again, or the folds may remain as fixed valves which require repair [11,12]. This view is consistent with English's observations that young infants uniformly show gross histological abnormalities of the pyeloplasty specimen, while only more than half of the specimens from children over 5 years old show only moderate change [13]. Furthermore, clear-cut obstructed hydronephrosis of the newborn has been shown to resolve [5].
3. Clinical UTI may emerge which may be detrimental to recovery after surgery [14]. Yet, laboratory research in this field does not monitor urine for infection.

Justifiers and their accuracy

Justification to do surgery or not requires the longitudinal success of these two types of management to be compared. As the measures

of renal status would be assessed longitudin-
ally, the accuracy and reproducibility of the
monitoring of renal function (e.g. percent differential function, $t_{1/2}$, glomerular filtration
rate) and grading of hydronephrosis needs to
be established. Furthermore, it is necessary to
determine what parameters will be monitored
in order to determine if surgery was helpful.
Changes are considered significant if there is a
variance of 10% from normal or between tests.
However, it is unproven if measurements of
$t_{1/2}$ or percentage function are accurate to this
level. For renal function, percentage differential function is reported accurate to ±4% [15],
but this needs validation. The data types which
are used to calculate percent differential function vary. Ransley et al. [16] uses a slope of the
renogram curve between 80 and 160 seconds,
but about 10 other measures have been used
[17]. We have used total scintillation counts
by 1 minute after isotope injection (subtracted
for background) [17]. For hydronephrosis, is
pelvic width the only factor which needs to be
monitored [16], or should an assessment also
be made of the calices and parenchymal thickness? [18] Furthermore, as indications for surgery are not scientifically founded, some carry
out surgery based upon the status of renal
function almost regardless of the grade of
hydronephrosis [16,19,20]. For others, only the
single kidney glomerular filtration rate (GFR)
indicates the need for surgery [4]. According to
Nauta, as kidneys with good function which
show obstruction all have surgery, it is hard to
compare the value of surgery versus the value
of observation [20]. However, improvements in
EU and DTPA scans can be seen in 79% of
operated cases. Renal deterioration has been
seen in two (5%) of units shown on initial testing not to be obstructive up to 3 years follow-
up [6]. A better assessment of the value of
surgery is a clinical trial which incorporates
prospective random allocation to surgery or
not [21] (see below Society for Fetal Urology –
SFU – protocol).

Justification for repairing an obstructed kidney in a well baby

1. Children having repair of an obstructed
   kidney with HN Gr ≥ 3 appear to do better
   when surgery is done before rather than
   after symptoms or signs appear. In Guys'
   [22] experience, children who had surgery
   by a few months old, postoperatively
   showed a lower incidence of pyelonephritis,
   better drainage and less hydronephrosis
   than a comparable group of repairs done on
   children who presented later after conventional symptoms emerged.
2. Early repair may be associated with a better
   surgical result. Perez et al. [23] argue that
   recurrent obstruction was not seen in the
   22 kidneys having surgery before 3 months
   old, while 11% of 36 kidneys showed recurrent obstruction when the initial operation
   was done later. Using cases reported in the
   literature, a poor outcome was noted more
   often when an observation period delayed
   repair.
3. Early surgery may avert pathological
   changes in the UPJ complex and make a
   good surgical outcome more likely. dell'
   Agnola showed that secondary nephrectomy
   was only done for cases with severe hypotrophy and fibrosis of pelvis and ureter
   specimens at primary pyeloplasty [24]. These
   changes were particularly likely when the
   dilatation was noted before 32 weeks' gestation and were more common when surgery
   was done at 1 month old. The duration of
   obstruction (from prenatal detection to
   surgery) correlated directly with the pathological appearance of the pelvis and ureter
   [24]. However, these pathological conditions
   remain to be correlated with outcome of
   renal function, drainage or development of
   symptoms. Although UPJ obstruction is
   more common in boys than girls, it is
   curious to note that girls more often show
   more hydronephrosis and are detected
   earlier prenatally than boys. This observation may account for a higher frequency of
   renal deterioration in girls than boys [24].

Surgery may not enhance renal function, as
the improvements noted may be coincidental
with normal renal maturation. For example,
enhanced effective renal plasma flow [14] or
percentage differential function [23] are seen to
increase after pyeloplasty prior to 2 years (particularly if there has not been antecedent UTI).
However, could this observation be simply a
consequence of natural maturation? Can percentage differential function improve with age
in the face of renographic obstruction? This
is likely if the observations of Koff can be

validated. Namely, he observed an increase in renal function of all renographically obstructed kidneys without surgery [25]. On the other hand, Ransley shows that as the duration of follow-up of good functioning kidneys with hydronephrosis is extended, most cases require surgery before 3 years old [16]. Furthermore, 8 (60%) of 13 kidneys which underwent surgery after an observation showed reduction in percentage function which did not completely recover. It is likely that Ransley is watching the spectrum in the evolution of clinically silent obstructive hydronephrosis becoming symptomatic. Repair is then done after the 'bomb' has exploded [16]. From the same group, Gordon et al. reported that percentage differential function is improved after surgery only when it is reduced (<40%) preoperatively [26]. Of a cohort of children whose unilateral hydronephrosis merited evaluation by renography (not controlled for Grade HN), it appears that about a half ultimately had surgery by 5 years follow-up, mostly because of decreasing or reduced function [26]. It is likely that when patients are subgrouped to evaluate only those with HN Gr ≥ 3, most will be found to require surgery [18].

Indications for surgery

The indications for surgery commonly include the 'unequivocal' diagnosis of obstruction by renography and EU [6,27]. In some reports, it is not clear what guidelines were used to diagnose obstruction [6]. Piepsz is specific in his guidelines for surgery. Initially, when the glomerular filtration rate (GFR) was recued to less than half the opposite side was done. Later, surgery was done when there was no drainage of radionuclide from the pelvis after diuretic administration, even if the GFR was normal [28].

A sentiment is developing that reliance on renal function alone, as monitored by GFR or percentage differential function, is a sufficient criterion to guide the need for surgery. The premise that renal function, not obstruction, is paramount is the focus of management by Dejter et al. [19] Therefore, asymptomatic children with good functioning kidneys that show obstructed drainage should be observed as long as function is preserved [19]. Wasnick summarizes the views of several paediatric urologists to conclude that the focus of the

renal scan is changing from simply assessing drainage parameters of the kidney pelvis/ureter to emphasizing the importance of renal function (GFR, percentage differential function) [29]. This view is shared by others [5], and is underscored by the reports of Gordon [26] and Ransley [16]. In this series reduced (<40% differential function) or decreasing (a change in >10% differential function) was the indication for surgery, irrespective of the drainage status of the kidney. Piepsz et al. [28] report they have not seen the situation where a low GFR was associated with good washout on the scan. The author has seen this phenomenon (Figure 13.1).

The author's practice is to offer treatment when tests show obstruction (Figure 13.2). This strategy is based upon the premise that uncorrected obstruction ultimately leads to clinical morbidity, if not also loss of renal function. To wait for loss of function to be shown before intervening surgically may be unwise [6]. However, as there is controversy, cases with unilateral obstructed hydronephrosis (HN Gr ≥ 3) are randomized prospectively according to an ongoing protocol (see below).

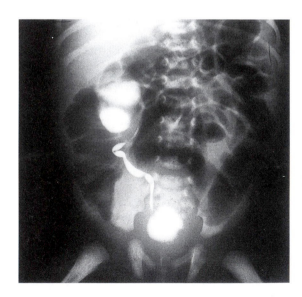

Figure 13.1 A preoperative retrograde pyelogram can guide the choice of the surgical incision. A neonate with palpable kidney; the renal scan shows obstruction. The condition could involve repairing a long strictured segment of the UPJ. The retrograde view shows the stricture *is* long, and repair was done via a flank exposure rather than a lumbotomy. The flank exposure would assure better visualization and thereby mobilization of the lower ureter to facilitate successful repair.

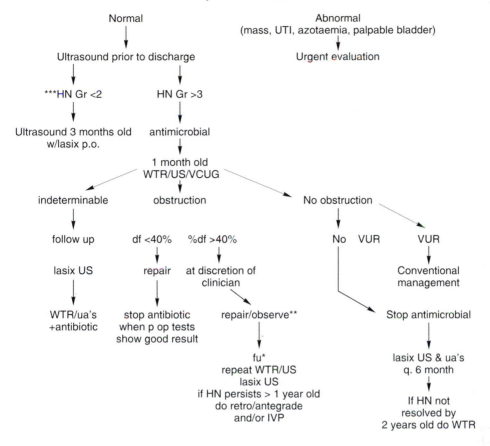

Physical examination

Normal

Abnormal
(mass, UTI, azotaemia, palpable bladder)

Ultrasound prior to discharge

Urgent evaluation

***HN Gr <2   HN Gr >3

Ultrasound 3 months old   antimicrobial
w/lasix p.o.

1 month old
WTR/US/VCUG

indeterminable   obstruction   No obstruction

follow up   df <40%   %df >40%   No   VUR   VUR

lasix US   repair   at discretion of   Conventional
clinician   management

WTR/ua's   stop antibiotic   repair/observe**   Stop antimicrobial
+antibiotic   when p op tests
show good result

fu*   lasix US & ua's
repeat WTR/US   q. 6 month
lasix US
if HN persists > 1 year old   If HN not
do retro/antegrade   resolved by
and/or IVP   2 years old do WTR

*   Repair if on follow up: HN does not resolve before 2 years old, function is reduced by 10%,
       clinical symptoms appear, UTI emerges, kidney becomes palpable
**   These patients are potential subjects for ongoing prospective study of SFU.
***   Advise that fetal dilatation could have been due to ureteral reflux. Do VCUG at discretion
       of clinician or monthly \uas every year.

Figure 13.2 Algorithm for postnatal management of unilateral fetal hydronephrosis.

Consistent follow-up is necessary when it is elected to observe the asymptomatic neonate with obstructed hydronephrosis and 'good' renal function. Lost-to-follow-up rates are under 25% [29]. Perhaps the parents chose to believe the child was well and did not return [29].

Surgery

When it is elected to repair obstructed hydronephrosis, the choice of incision and repair to be used depends on the specific anatomical findings. A preoperative retrograde pyelogram can show the level of obstruction and guide the choice of incision (flank or posterior lumbotomy) (Figure 13.1). For high-insertion anomalies of the ureter and UPJ, a dismembered pyeloplasty with modest reduction in the redundancy of the pelvis is done. For mid- or upper ureteral strictures, resection of the obstructed segment and uretero-ureterostomy is done (Figure 13.3). Debate regarding the need to stent the repair or not seems to conclude that stenting is uncommonly needed or advantageous. Reasons to stent include: an anastomosis which is technically difficult to do, perhaps because the distal ureter is atretic;

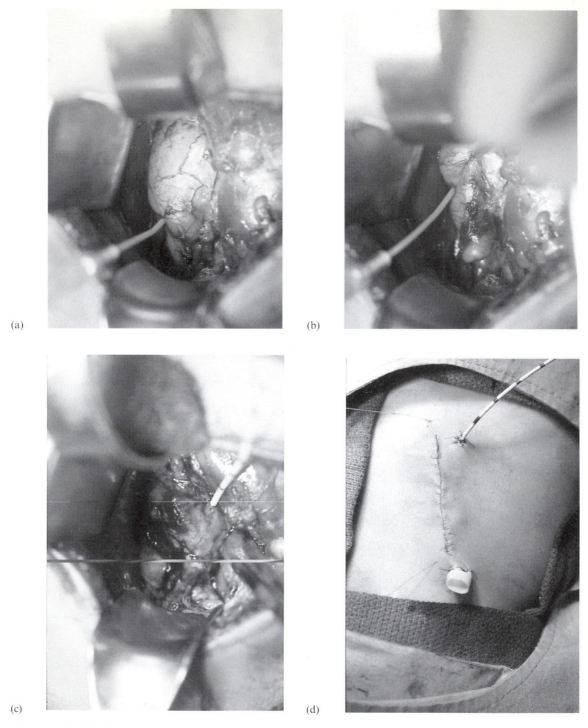

Figure 13.3 Surgical findings in a typical case of obstructed hydronephrosis. Via a dorsal lumbotomy, the right kidney shows: (a) renal pelvis is full; (b) instillation of saline into the pelvis via the intravenous catheter better delineates the stricture site and shows the pressure gradient is >25 cmH₂O; (c) the obstructed segment has been removed and the pelvis and upper ureter are now aligned in a dependent manner (the repair is stented with a KISS catheter exiting the pelvis analogous to a vesicostomy tube); (d) lumobotomy closure with Penrose drain and KISS catheter (graduations are in centimetres).

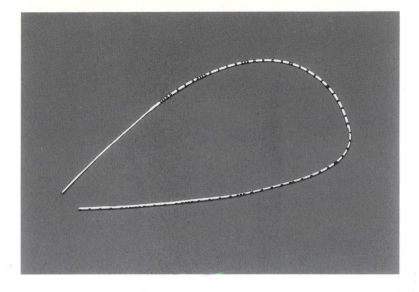

(a)

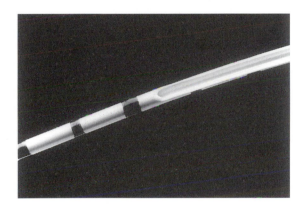

(b)

Figure 13.4 KISS catheter. (a) Trocar tip (upper) can be passed retrograde from the dilated pelvis to provide a nephrostomy tube, or the trocar tip can be cut off and the soft catheter passed retrograde out the dilated pelvis to provide a pyelostomy tube. (b) Junction of hollow segment of catheter (left) and trough segment (right). The junction is positioned to be just inside the dilated pelvis, so the trough can drain urine both in the pelvis and ureter. The trough configuration minimizes the likelihood that drainage will be impaired by blood clot and similar material (Cook Urological, Spencer, IND, USA).

because the kidney and pelvis are so dilated the repair site is mobile and kinking of the repair postoperatively is likely to cause obstruction; and nephrogenic diabetes insipidus (caused by renal medullary thinning) may outpour dilute urine, overcome the drainage ability of the repair, and extravasation and copious flank drainage follow. To overcome these real or potential problems, a stenting catheter could be used. Wasnick routinely stents with a 3Fr whistle-tipped catheter passed endoscopically prior to pyeloplasty [29], while Gonzalez seldom stents the repair. However, such repairs are still associated with a 15% extravasation rate [30]. Poor experiences with stenting of paediatric pyeloplasty prob-

ably relate in good measure to occlusion of the side holes of the stenting catheter. Conversion of a side-holed catheter to one which drains fluid via a 'trough' (KISS catheter) seems to avoid many of the previous bad experiences with stenting at pyeloplasty [31] (Figure 13.4). The catheter provides external drainage until Penrose drainage is scant. This is usually on the first postoperative day. Now the KISS catheter is plugged, and this establishes internal drainage. The catheter is removed in the clinic about 1 week after surgery. This form of internal drainage permits the ureteropyelostomy anastomosis to 'seal'. When the renal pelvis is large and floppy and the parenchyma is thin (HN Gr 4), the KISS catheter permits

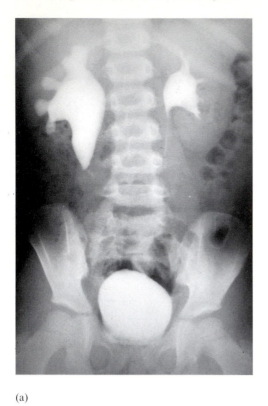

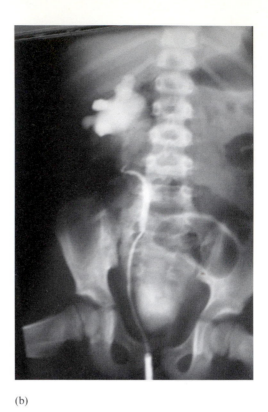

(a)   (b)

Figure 13.5 Obstruction associated with an extrarenal pelvis in a 6-year-old boy with recurrent attacks of abdominal pain. (a) IVP shows right HN Gr 3 with pelvicaliceal dilatation. (b) Retrograde pyelogram shows a stricture segment. After repair, the pain episodes resolved.

the ureter and pelvis to remain aligned and avoids postoperative kinks.

Longitudinal studies are needed – protocol of SFU

The need for clinical or experimental data to evaluate the benefits of neonatal versus infant pyeloplasty for congenital UPJ obstruction has often been cited by paediatric nephrologists [21] and urologists [32] for more than a decade.

Thomas argues that as some cases of UPJ obstruction resolve in infancy, he defers surgery until a kidney which had shown 'good' function (>40% differential) loses function irrespective of whether there is free or obstructed drainage [7]. From this vantage Thomas concludes that the strategy of surgery for UPJ obstruction 'may be misguided. At worst . . . it will lead to the deferment of sur-

gery, in the knowledge that function is most unlikely to deteriorate rapidly. At best it will save some children from undergoing an unnecessary major operation.' If this position is to be followed, it is important to improve the accuracy of the monitoring of differential renal function which is recognized to be accurate only to a level of ±10. Furthermore, if one is to operate because there is loss of function, it is unknown if function can be recouped by successful surgery. This position of operating when there is reduced function may undervalue the experience in cases of hydronephrosis which showed deterioration of function after surgery was withheld. For example, isolated cases of prenatally detected hydronephrosis may initially show a non-obstructive renogram curve (and scan) and later show an obstructive pattern by 1 year old [33]. Macalister reported a case of an initial IVP which showed only an extrarenal pelvis with no obstruction; by 4 years later, the IVP showed obstruction, still with the child asymptomatic. Similarly, Macalister showed by 3 months after surgery an IVP with normalization of UPJ obstruction, but by 9 months after surgery there was asymptomatic progression of obstruction by an intrinsic stricture necessitating nephrectomy [7]. Noe and Macgill noted the UPJ showed a narrowed lumen which histologically contains fibrous tissue. Based upon this observation, they speculate that as renal maturity improves during infancy, there is enhanced urine output. If the fibrosis noted in the UPJ does not permit normal growth of the UPJ, the larger volumes of urine made by the more 'mature' kidney would be likely to cause progression in the pelvicaliceal dilatation and cause 'obstruction' to be unmasked [3]. Adults who are symptomatic from pain may show a normal IVP. However, follow-up IVP years later will show UPJ obstruction which, when repaired, corrects the pain [34].

Clearly, several decades of follow-up are necessary before realistic conclusions can be drawn. Children with prenatal diagnosis of hydronephrosis need follow-up at least with a hydrated ultrasound (see Chapter 12) until caliceal dilatation is no longer evident. The appropriate duration of follow-up for children with an extrarenal pelvis is not known, but it is likely that the majority will not develop problems and a minority will, in later years, show symptoms referable to a slowly progressive obstructive phenomenon, perhaps related to kinks (Figure 13.5). By analogy, just as follow-up into childhood of congenital solitary functioning kidney showed it to be a benign condition [35], longer follow-up into adulthood is showing hyperfiltration renal injury. Perhaps cases of obstructed hydronephrosis with good function are deemed not to warrant surgery in infancy, but follow-up to childhood and adolescence may show clinical morbidity, perhaps loss of function.

Gordon indicates that if a planned long-term follow-up study shows the majority of cases of newborn obstructed hydronephrosis ultimately develop clinical problems (UTI, pain, stone), then prophylactic pyeloplasty will be justified as the treatment of choice to avert these clinical problems [26].

Since 1992, in America the Society for Fetal Urology has organized a national clinical trial involving paediatric urologists, nuclear medicine physicians and radiologists, which pro-

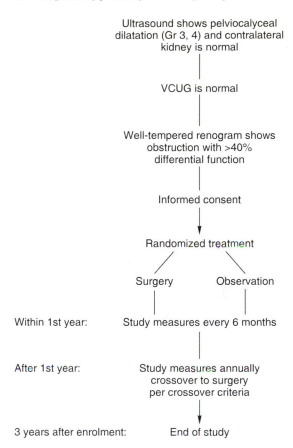

Figure 13.6 Society for Fetal Urology: study protocol flow diagram.

spectively compares the outcome of cases of renographic obstruction and HN Gr $\geq$ 3 which are randomly allocated to observation versus pyeloplasty. The management chart is shown in Figure 13.6. Data from this protocol in the following years will hopefully provide answers to our questions.

References

1. Smith F, Ritchie EL, Maizels M, Huseh W, Kaplan, WE, Firlit CF. Surgery for duplex kidneys with ectopic ureters: ipsilateral ureteroureterostomy versus polar nephrectomy. *J Urol* 1989; **142**: (2 Pt 2), 532.
2. Homsy YL, Saad F, Laerge I, Williot P, Pison C. Transitional hydronephrosis of the newborn and infant. *J Urol* 1990; **144**: 579.
3. Johnson HW, Gleave M, Coleman GU, Nadel HR, Raffel J, Weckworth PF. Neonatal renomegaly. *J Urol* 1987; **138**: 1023.

4. Piepsz A, Ham HR, Hall M, Verboven M, Collier F. Long-term follow up of separate glomerular filtration rate in partially obstructed kidneys. *Contrib Nephrol* 1990; **79**: 137.

5. Arnold AJ, Rickwood AM. Natural history of pelviureteric obstruction detected by prenatal sonography. *Br J Urol* 1990; **65**: 91.

6. Najmaldin AS, Burge DM, Atwell JD. Outcome of antenatally diagnosed pelviureteric junction hydro-nephrosis. *Br J Urol* 1991; **67**: 96.

7. Thomas DFM, Gordon AC. Management of pre-natally diagnosed uropathies. *Arch Dis Child* 1989; **64**: 58.

8. Chevalier RL, Gomez RA, Jones CE. Developmental determinants of recovery after relief of partial ureteral obstruction. *Kidney Int* 1988; **33**: 775.

9. Chevalier RL. Renal response to ureteral obstruction in early development. *Nephron* 1990; **56**: 113.

10. Chevalier RL, Dahr SE. The case for early relief of obstruction. *J Urol* 1988; **140**: 1305.

11. Leiter E. Persistent fetal ureter. *J Urol* 1979; **122**: 251.

12. Maizels M, Stephens FD. Valves of the ureter as a cause of primary obstruction of the ureter. *J Urol* 1980; **123**: 742.

13. English PJ, Testa HT, Gosling JA, Cohen SJ. Idiopathic hydronephrosis in childhood – a compari-son between diuresis renography and upper urinary tract morphology. *Br J Urol* 1982; **54**: 603.

14. Dowling KJ, Harmon EP, Ortenberg J, Polanco E, Evans BB. Ureteropelvic junction obstruction: the effect of pyeloplasty on renal function. *J Urol* 1988; **140**: 1227.

15. Pieretti R, Gilday D, Jeffs R. Differential kidney scan in pediatric urology. *Urology* 1974; **4**: 665.

16. Ransley PG, Dhillon HK, Gordan I, Duffy PG, Dillon MJ, Barratt TM. The postnatal management of hydronephrosis diagnosed by prenatal ultrasound. *J Urol* 1990; **144**: 584.

17. MacNeily AE, Maizels M, Kaplan WE, Firlit CF, Conway JJ. Does 'early' pyeloplasty really avert loss of renal function: a retrospective review *J Urol* 1993; **150**: 769.

18. Maizels M, Reisman EM, Flom LS, Nelson H, Fern-bach S, Firlit CF. Grading nephroureteral dilatation detected in the first year of life – correlation with obstruction. *J Urol* 1992; **148**: 609.

19. Dejter SW, Eggli DF, Gibbons MD. Urinary tract obstruction. *J Urol* 1988; **140**: 1305.

20. Nauta J, Pot DJ, Mooij PPM, Nijman JM, Wolff ED. Forced hydration prior to renography in children with hydronephrosis: an evaluation. *Br J Urol* 1991; **68**: 93.

21. Stewart CL, Jose PA. Transitional nephrology. *Urol Clin North Am* 1985; **12**: 143.

22. Guys JJ, Borella F and Monfort G. Ureteropelvic junction obstruction in the neonate. *J Urol* 1988; **23**: 156–157.

23. Perez KM, Friedman RM, King LR. The case of relief of ureteropelvic junction obstruction in neonates and young children at time of diagnosis. *Urology* 1991; **38**: 195.

24. dell'Agnola CA, Carmassi LM, Merlo D, Tadini B. Duration and severity of congenital hydronephrosis as a cause of smooth muscle deterioration in pyelo-ureteral junction obstruction. *Z Kinderchir* 1990; **45**: 286.

25. Koff SA, Campbell K. Nonoperative management of unilateral neonatal hydronephrosis. *J Urol* 1992; **148**: (2 Pt 2), 525.

26. Gordon I, Dhillon HK, Gatanash H, Peters AM. Antenatal diagnosis of pelvic hydronephrosis: assess-ment of renal function and drainage as a guide to management. *J Nucl Med* 1991; **32**: 1649.

27. Homsy YL, Williot P, Danais S. Transitional neo-natal hydronephrosis: fact or fiction? *J Urol* 1986; **136**: 339.

28. Piepsz A, Hall M, Ham HR, Verboven M, Collier F. Prospective management of neonates with pelviure-teric junction stenosis. *Scand J Urol Nephrol* 1989; **23**: 31.

29. Wasnick RM. Neonatal UPJ obstruction: current controversies. *Dialog Pediatr Urol* 1991; **14**: 1.

30. Nguyen DH, Aliabadi H, Ercole CJ, Gonzalez R. Nonintubated Anderson–Hynes repair of uretero-pelvic junction obstruction with hydronephrosis: an evaluation. *J Urol* 1989; **142**: 704.

31. Ritchie EL, Maizels M, Zaontz MR, Kaplan WE, Firlit CF. Experience with the internal splint-stent (KISS) catheter for internal urinary diversion after pyeloplasty. *Urology* (accepted).

32. McAlister WH, Manley CB, Siegel MJ. Asympto-matic progression of partial ureteropelvic obstruction in children. *J Urol* 1980; **123**: 267.

33. Noe HN, MaGill HL. Progression of mild uretero-pelvic junction obstruction in infancy. *Urology* 1987; **30**: 348.

34. Jacobs JA, Berger BW, Goldman SM, Robbins MA, Young JD. Ureteropelvic obstruction in adults with previously normal pyelograms: a report of 5 cases. *J Urol* 1979; **121**: 242.

35. Argueso LR, Ritchey ML, Boyle ET Jr, Milliner DS, Bergstralh EJ, Kramer SA. Prognosis of children with solitary kidney after unilateral nephrectomy. *J Urol* 1992; **148**: (2 Pt 2), 747.

14

Posterior urethral valves and other congenital anomalies of the urethra

P.D.E. Mouriquand and D.F.M. Thomas

Introduction

Congenital anomalies of the human urethra date from the first 4 months of pregnancy and involve the complex interaction of several embryological structures [1–3]. The urogenital sinus (UGS), the urogenital membrane (UGM) – the anterior portion of the cloacal membrane, the distal part of the wolffian system (WS) and the glanular ectodermal plug (GEP) constitute the four principal components of the male urethra. General aspects of the normal development of the male urethra are considered elsewhere in Chapter 2. The embryological basis of posterior urethral valves is not fully understood but is believed to occur at the site where a number of components of the lower urinary tract undergo a complex interaction. The portion of the posterior urethra above the veru montanum derives from the urological zone of the UGS, whereas the posterior urethra below the veru montanum arises from the superior portion of the genital zone of the UGS. The distal part of the pelvic segment of the UGS is destined to form the membranous urethra. The formation of the posterior urethra (prostatic urethra) occurs during the third month of gestation. The complexity of embryological development of the urethra accounts for the relative frequency and variety of congenital anomalies that can affect it (Figure 14.1). It has been observed that embryologically the most vulnerable parts of the urinary tract are located at the junction between different embryological structures. For example, the calicotubular junction, the pelviureteric junction, the ureterovesical junction and the vesicourethral junction.

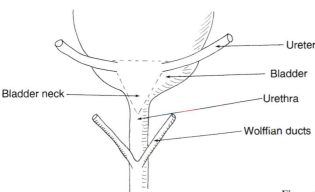

(a)

Figure 14.1 (a) Principal embryological components of the posterior urethra (8 weeks' gestation).

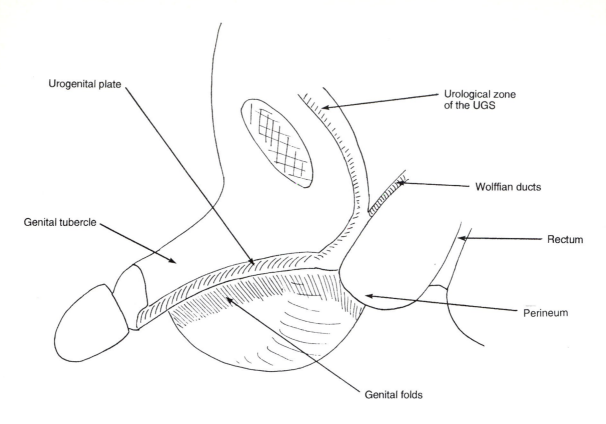

(b)

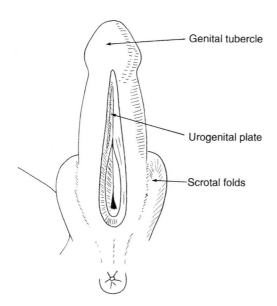

(c)

Figure 14.1 (*continued*) (b), (c) Embryological components of the anterior urethra (11 weeks' gestation).

Myogenesis and the maturation of the detrusor and urethral musculature are complex processes, possibly representing the development of two distinct muscular systems [4,5]. Continuity of the histological connections between the urethra and the bladder and trigonal musculature is not complete before 26 weeks of pregnancy. Since it seems unlikely that the fetal urethra functions as an inert conduit, the relatively late development of urethral and bladder musculature raises questions about the functional role of the fetal urethra. In particular, there are unanswered questions about the route and mechanism whereby fetal urine is voided for the first half of gestation. The phenomenon of transient dilatation of the fetal urinary tract occasionally observed on serial prenatal ultrasound scans may represent self-limiting infravesical obstruction.

Congenital lesions of the posterior urethra

Posterior urethral valves

Definition and incidence

Posterior urethral valves are confined to males, although a rare comparable form of urethral obstruction has been described in females. The condition is generally diagnosed in infancy (or on the basis of prenatal ultrasound), but it may present in later childhood or adult life. The reported incidence lies between 1 in 4000 and 1 in 25 000 [6–8].

The first description of the disorder is attributed to Morgagni [9] in the eighteenth century and subsequently to Langenbeck [10] in 1802. However, in 1919 Young [11] published the first classification in which three anatomical types were defined. The Type I valve of the Young classification is the most common form and probably represents a pathological pattern of fusion of the urethrovaginal folds (wolffian structures). In contrast, the Type III valve described in the Young classification is probably due to the persistence of the urogenital membrane. Doubt exists about the existence of Young's Type II valve. The Type I valve is probably the outcome of events around the seventh week of pregnancy, whilst the Type III anomaly arises around the eleventh week of pregnancy. Young's classification has recently

been challenged and it has been argued that some of the differences in the appearances of the valve membrane that form the basis of the Young classification are artefactual, reflecting techniques used for post-mortem dissection and damage to the membrane caused by the passage of instruments or catheters per urethrum. On the basis of their observations in boys whose bladders were drained suprapubically, Dewan et al. [12] have suggested that the Type I and Type III valves represent a single entity and that the characteristics of the valve membrane can be summarized as follows: the membrane is usually attached posteriorly immediately below the level of the verumontanum with a pin hole meatus posteriorly adjacent to the verumontanum. The anterior anchorage of the membrane can be very distal and extend beyond the region of the external sphincter. Paramedian, parallel reinforcements and distal ballooning are also common features.

Pathophysiology of posterior urethral valves

Nature and timing of infravesical obstruction
Considering that the embryological events that give rise to the formation of the urethral valve membrane occur between the seventh and eleventh week of pregnancy, it is surprising that upper tract dilatation is often not apparent on ultrasound until 25–27 weeks or even later in pregnancy. The detailed dissection studies of Gonzales [2] suggest that despite patency of the urethra, histological continuity of the external sphincter, bladder neck and detrusor is not fully established before 26 weeks of gestation. It seems highly unlikely, therefore, that the fetal bladder empties by a process that mirrors normal voiding. Indeed, there is some doubt about the route whereby the filtrate (urine) produced by the primitive fetal kidney finds its way into the amniotic fluid. In the primitive urinary tract there may be significant direct diffusion from the lumen of the collecting system and bladder which, it is believed, does not possess an impermeable lining of transitional epithelium at that stage [13,14]. The urachus could also represent a transitory, physiological conduit between 19 and 26 weeks. This hypothesis is supported by the observation that in male infants with prune belly syndrome (a condition in which gross

urinary tract dilatation is believed to be due to self-limiting urethral obstruction), the urachus is often patent. However, if the urachus does sometimes serve as a 'safety valve' providing transient decompression of the obstructed lower urinary tract in fetuses with posterior urethral valves, this mechanism must be limited to the early stages of pregnancy. Patent urachus is not encountered in term (or indeed premature) infants with posterior urethral valves. Furthermore, dissections of human fetuses indicate that the urachus is rarely patent after 22 weeks of pregnancy and when present it forms a connection between the dome of the bladder and the placental structures rather than a direct route of drainage into the amniotic cavity.

Anatomical changes secondary to posterior urethral valve obstruction

The anatomical effects of obstruction by posterior urethral valves are mainly represented by dilatation and elongation of the posterior urethra, thickening of the bladder neck (which can be widely open or very narrow) and hypertrophy of the detrusor muscle – which often results in gross trabeculation. The posterior bladder neck is often prominent, creating another potential level of outflow obstruction. In approximately 50% of cases there is secondary vesicoureteric reflux (VUR), often resulting in marked dilatation of the ureter and renal collecting systems. Detrusor hypertrophy can result in secondary obstruction at the level of the ureterovesical junction, although the magnitude of this risk was probably overestimated in the past. The aetiology of the renal dysplasia associated with posterior urethral valves is probably multifactorial in origin, with factors including high pressure VUR, outflow obstruction and a primary defect of renal embryogenesis.

Experimentally and clinically, it seems that the timing of the obstructive insult plays a key role in determining the pattern of renal damage. Early obstruction results in dysplasia [15,16], whereas obstruction in later pregnancy reduces the appearances of hydronephrosis [17]. Some studies have suggested that vesicoureteric reflux, bladder diverticula and urinary extravasation can provide some safeguard against renal dysplasia by constituting a 'pop-off' mechanism to relieve pressure on the developing upper tracts [18,19]. In particular, the existence of gross unilateral VUR is often associated with good preservation of function in the non-refluxing contralateral kidney. However, the protective effect of unilateral VUR has been challenged by the findings of Parkhouse et al. [20], who did not document a long-term benefit associated with unilateral VUR in a study of 114 boys with posterior urethral valves undertaken at the Hospital for Sick Children, Great Ormond Street.

Functional changes associated with posterior urethral valves

Abnormalities of bladder function occur as a consequence of infravesical obstruction by posterior urethral valves. Variable urodynamic bladder profiles have been reported in boys with the condition, but it is sometimes difficult to establish whether these urodynamic disorders are the consequence of the underlying congenital disorder or its subsequent treatment. Urodynamic profiles classically described in patients with bladder outflow obstruction include myogenic failure, hyperreflexia, bladder hypertonia and non-compliance [21–23]. Significant overlap may exist between these categories. Holmdahl et al. [24] have reported that most 'valve' bladders are hypercontractile at the time of presentation and have a reduced functional capacity.

Urinary incontinence was noted in 33% of boys with posterior urethral valves in a follow-up study of 114 boys with posterior valves treated at the Hospital for Sick Children, Great Ormond Street between 1966 and 1975 [20]. Mollard has documented incontinence in 22% of 77 patients on follow-up (unpublished data). Although some incontinence may be related to damage to the striated sphincter complex incurred during instrumentation and endourethral surgery, this has become a relatively uncommon cause of incontinence following the introduction of specialized paediatric endoscopic equipment. Nowadays the presence of urinary incontinence is more likely to signify an underlying disorder of bladder and renal functions (hyperdiuresis due to concentrating tubular disorders).

The follow-up study reported by Parkhouse et al. [20] identified incontinence as an important prognostic predictor of eventual functional outcome. Of the boys who were dry under the age of 5 years, only 4% subsequently developed renal failure. In contrast, 46% of boys with incontinence persisting after 5 years of age, subsequently developed renal failure. Similar findings have been reported by Connor [25]. These and other studies support the view that disordered function in the 'valves' bladder contributes to ongoing upper tract damage and the subsequent likelihood of chronic renal failure.

Renal function and posterior urethral valves

Although the fetal kidney contributes to the maintenance of a normal fetal environment by the production of amniotic fluid, its role as an excretory organ is very limited. In effect, the fetus is dialysed via the placenta, a fact that explains the observation that even anephric infants have levels of plasma creatinine and electrolytes that mirror those in the maternal circulation at the time of birth.

The nature and timing of the pressure insult to the developing renal parenchyma *in utero* is unclear, but nevertheless it seems likely that there are two mechanisms, i.e. renal dysplasia, determined at an early period in gestation (hence the failure of *in utero* bladder shunting to prevent renal failure associated with dysplasia) [26] and an on-going pressure-related insult exacerbated by the presence of high-pressure VUR.

Renal failure is a common feature of posterior urethral valves and a degree of renal impairment is present in 40–50% of cases at the time of diagnosis [27,28]. The long-term outcome for renal function is poor, with approximately a third of patients ultimately destined to develop some degree of renal failure [20]. The North American Paediatric Renal Transplant Co-operative Study of 2819 renal transplants in children from 0 to 17 years, noted that males accounted for 69% of transplant recipients under 1 year of age and 66% of those between the ages of 2 and 5 years. Obstructive uropathy was the single most important indication for renal transplantation in boys under 5 years of age. Obstructive uropathy and renal dysplasia continue to figure prominently in the indications for transplantation in boys throughout the paediatric age range [29].

Sexual function

Woodhouse [30] reported that 9 out of 21 men treated in infancy for posterior urethral valves had impaired, i.e. slow or dry, ejaculation. However, retrograde ejaculation was rare (1 out of 21 patients) and semen counts were within the fertile range.

Diagnosis of posterior urethral valves

Prenatal diagnosis

Following the advent of obstetric ultrasound a proportion of cases of posterior urethral valves are now identified prenatally. It is important to note, however, that the interpretation of abnormal ultrasound findings is often difficult and the distinction between posterior urethral valves and other causes of dilatation may not be evident until further investigations are undertaken in early postnatal life. Even with modern ultrasonic equipment the reported detection rate varies considerably from centre to centre. Between 16 and 55% of cases [6,31,32] of posterior urethral valves are detectable before 24 weeks of gestation. One study designed to examine the relationship between gestational age at detection and subsequent functional outcome found that the presence of dilatation before 24 weeks carried a significantly greater risk of neonatal death and chronic renal failure.

The diagnosis of posterior urethral valves is suspected in a fetus with a thick-walled bladder and bilateral dilatation of the upper urinary tract, regardless of whether this is associated with oligohydramnios. Ultrasound can also detect structural anomalies such as increased echogenecity of the kidneys and the absence of normal corticomedullary differentiation – which appears to be a predictor of renal impairment. Extravasation of urine is sometimes detected prenatally and, as indicated previously, has been identified as a favourable predictive factor. Prenatal ultrasound identifies cases at the more severe end of the spectrum and the available evidence [6] suggests that the prognosis for renal function is worse in prenatally detected cases. Overall there is little evidence to indicate that prenatal detection and earlier treatment are reflected in improved clinical outcome. Within the prenatally detected group (which constitute more than 50% of cases in some centres) is a subgroup of infants with obstructive uropathy of mild to moderate severity. It is possible that prenatal detection, early intervention and prevention of infection in this group may have some benefit for renal function, but long-term studies will be needed to establish whether this is the case.

Clinical presentation

Neonatal period

Any manifestations of severe metabolic disorder resulting from renal failure (hyperchloraemic acidosis; hyperkalaemia), respiratory distress (including spontaneous pneumothorax or pneumomediastinum) and urinary tract infection (plus septicaemia, meningitis) demand urgent resuscitative measures. On clinical examination the kidneys and bladder are often readily palpable. In severely affected cases the features of Potter's syndrome may be present, including evidence of intrauterine growth deficiency, pulmonary hypoplasia, limb moulding defects, e.g. talipes equinovarus, and characteristic Potter's facies.

Infancy and early childhood

Urinary symptoms are more common, e.g. poor stream, dysuria, haematuria, urinary tract infection, sometimes associated with systemic sepsis, e.g. septicaemia, meningitis. Renal failure may be present.

Later childhood

Urinary incontinence, urgency, dysuria and other voiding symptoms.

Investigations

Ultrasound imaging of the urinary tract

This is the initial investigation. Characteristic findings include dilatation of the upper urinary tract, abnormal echogenicity of the renal parenchyma, increased bladder wall thickness, bladder diverticula and dilatation of the posterior urethra.

Perineal ultrasound, with a 7.5-mHz probe, is being developed for the investigation of urethral anomalies. With miniaturization of ultrasound probes, transrectal ultrasound may be a promising development for the investigation of older children.

Micturating cystourethrogram

MCU remains the key investigation for the detection of posterior urethral valves and associated anomalies (Figure 14.2). The passage of a transurethral catheter can damage the anatomy of the valve membrane and some paediatric urologists prefer to perform suprapubic MCUs. The distinction between Type I and Type III valves (if this distinction exists [12]) is of no practical relevance, since the treatment is identical.

Isotope studies

Isotope studies are essential to assess the functional outcome of intrauterine obstruction by posterior urethral valves. Intravenous urography is no longer performed routinely, since it has largely been superseded by ultrasound and isotope imaging.

Urodynamic studies

Urodynamic studies (see above) play no role in the initial diagnosis but are useful in follow-up, particularly for the investigation of urinary incontinence.

Treatment

The role of fetal surgery is considered elsewhere, but from a paediatric urologist's perspective the indications for fetal intervention are few. Worsening oligohydramnios accompanied by increasing bilateral upper tract dilatation and deteriorating biochemical parameters represent the most legitimate indication. Intervention consists of the insertion of a double J stent under ultrasound guidance. When inserted into the fetal bladder or dilated kidney, the stent permits decompression of the urinary tract by draining urine into the amniotic cavity in the hope of protecting development of the fetal kidney and allowing

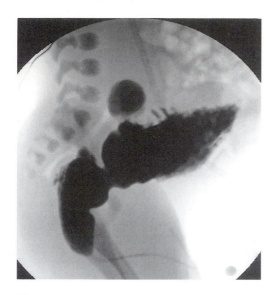

(a)

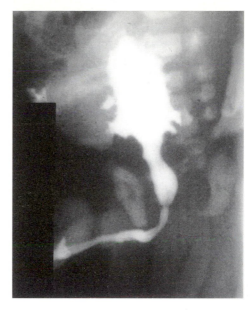

(b)

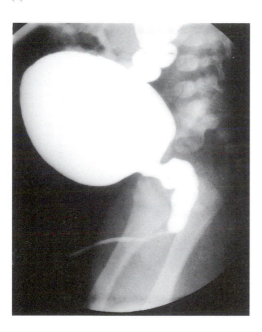

(c)

Figure 14.2 Micturating cystourethrogram (MCU). Spectrum of radiological findings in three infants with posterior urethral valves. (a) MCU in 32-week gestation preterm infant with gross upper tract dilatation detected prenatally on second-trimester ultrasound scan. MCU reveals massive dilatation of the posterior urethra with hypertrophy of the bladder neck, trabeculation and diverticulum formation. (b) Moderate trabeculation and sacculation (thick-walled bladder on ultrasound). The posterior urethra is dilated above the level of valvular obstruction. (c) Dilated posterior urethra with unilateral grade V vesicoureteric reflux but smooth-walled bladder. Posterior urethral valves not detected prenatally. This infant presented with a urinary infection of mild severity in the first 3 months of postnatal life.

maturation of the fetal lungs by restoring an adequate volume of amniotic fluid. Although some anecdotal evidence indicates that *in utero* shunting may be beneficial in preventing pulmonary hypoplasia, there is as yet no convincing evidence that it is capable of reversing renal dysplasia to improve the prognosis for renal function.

The severely ill child

Drainage of the infected upper tract may be indicated, ideally by percutaneous nephrostomy. The role of temporary ureterostomy (terminal or loop) in this situation is very limited since this may not guarantee effective drainage and carries the risk of ureteric damage. Following relief of obstruction, post-obstructive diuresis may demand careful monitoring of electrolyte and fluid balance.

Ablation of the valve membrane
(Figure 14.3)

This can be undertaken within a few days of birth or as soon as resuscitation has been completed. A number of techniques have been devised but following the introduction of neonatal and paediatric cystourethroscopes with instrumentation channels, most paediatric urologists favour ablation of the valve tissue under direct vision – either with a high frequency or a bug-bee electrode or resectoscope loop. Care must be taken to avoid damage to the external sphincter, as this can result in incontinence.

Neodymium-YAG laser

Use of the neodymium-YAG laser has been described [33,34]. A 600-μm fibre is advanced through the side channel of a paediatric cystourethroscope and the valve tissue vapourized under vision.

Percutaneous antegrade valve ablation [35,36]

This approach avoids urethral instrumentation and the possible risk of urethral stricture. Suprapubic puncture is performed and the neonatal resectoscope is introduced via this route and advanced antegradely through the bladder neck to visualize the valve membrane from above.

Urethral valve hook

Originally devised by Innes Williams et al. in 1973 [27], the hook concept was refined in the 1980s by Whitaker and Sherwood [37]. The insulated hook is passed up the urethra under X-ray control, the valve tissue engaged by traction on the hook and ablated by a diathermy current passing through the non-insulated inner curve of the hook.

Fogarty balloon catheter [38]

As with the hook technique, the Fogarty balloon is passed per urethrum under X-ray

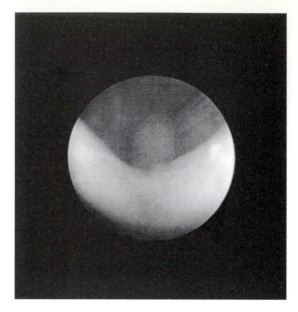

(a)

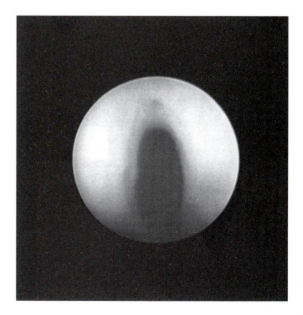

(b)

Figure 14.3 Endoscopic appearances of the intact (type I) valve membrane in an infant who had not been catheterized urethrally prior to urethroscopy. (a) Lateral cusps of valve membrane appear as the cystourethroscope is withdrawn through the posterior urethra. The veru montanum remains visible on the posterior wall of the dilated posterior urethra. (b) Occlusion of the urethral lumen by the intact type I valve membrane.

control. Once positioned in the region of the valve membrane, the balloon is inflated and withdrawn distally to rupture the valve membrane.

Whichever technique is chosen, X-ray screening should be available and postoperative catheter drainage of the bladder is advisable. Although perineal urethrotomy was previously employed to allow direct access to the posterior urethra, this approach is outdated, although a possible indication still exists in countries which do not have access to modern endoscopic or radiological equipment [39].

Postoperative management

The risk of postobstructive diuresis with loss of sodium and potassium, coupled with the risk of urinary tract infection after urethral instrumentation, demand careful supervision in the early postoperative period.

Subsequent management

Following ablation of the urethral valve tissue, there is generally progressive improvement in bladder and upper tract function. However, upper tract dilatation may resolve slowly over several years [28]. VUR ceases in around 50% of cases [40], particularly in renal units in which function is preserved. Nephroureterectomy may be indicated when gross reflux is associated with a non-functioning kidney. Although nephroureterectomy was previously undertaken routinely in this situation, some authors have advocated preservation of asymptomatic refluxing units for possible use in bladder augmentation (ureterocystoplasty). Ureteric reimplantation should be avoided in view of the technical difficulties encountered in the trabeculated bladder and the relatively high failure rate. Furthermore, antireflux surgery in this situation does not appear to carry any benefit for eventual renal function [20].

Surgery of the bladder neck should be avoided if possible. True secondary bladder neck obstruction is rare and bladder neck surgery is generally unnecessary and potentially hazardous. Persistent upper tract dilatation without VUR may very occasionally reflect a genuine degree of obstruction at the ureterovesical junction. In the past, however, this risk was almost certainly overestimated and re-implantation to correct the perceived obstruction at this level almost certainly carries more risks than it is designed to resolve. In most instances persisting upper tract dilatation reflects the legacy of a severe obstructive insult *in utero* and on-going bladder dysfunction in postnatal life. In infancy and early childhood, cutaneous vesicostomy has been employed in some centres to ensure more effective lower tract emptying. Although, the benefits of vesicostomy have been called into question, there is little hard evidence that the formation and closure of vesicostomy in infancy may contribute to bladder dysfunction in later childhood.

Bladder augmentation

The possible role of bladder augmentation in the management of poorly compliant unstable 'valves' bladders is being examined in a number of centres. Although this is a theoretically attractive concept, both for the correction of urinary incontinence and the preservation of upper tract function the results of bladder augmentation, either conventional ileocystoplasty or ureterocystoplasty [41], will need to be carefully assessed over a number of years. A major disadvantage is the possible cessation of normal voiding, requiring intermittent catheterization to empty the bladder in around a third of cases [42]. Boys with normal urethral sensation may be understandably reluctant to embark on intermittent urethral catheterization and the creation of a continent catheterizable stoma (Mitrofanoff procedure) may prove necessary.

Urinary incontinence has been reported in between 14 and 38% [20,40] of patients in some studies. Urinary incontinence associated with treatment for posterior urethral valves has a tendency to improve with puberty, presumably as a result of prostatic development and increased outflow resistance. In the past urinary incontinence usually resulted from postinstrumentation damage to the striated sphincter complex. Nowadays this mechanism is less common and when urinary incontinence occurs it generally reflects a severe pattern of detrusor dysfunction. Urinary tract diversion has not been shown to influence the progression of renal failure or growth velocity in children with posterior urethral valves [43].

Ultimately a degree of renal impairment can be demonstrated in almost 50% of children with this condition.

Four factors have been identified as predictors of poor long-term outcome: presentation before the age of 1 year, bilateral VUR, proteinuria and daytime incontinence after the age of 5 years [20].

Other congenital lesions of the posterior urethra

Polyp of the posterior urethra

Congenital posterior urethral polyps, benign lesions arising from the veromontanum, are generally found in young male infants [44]. However, similar polyps do arise, rarely, within the female urethra (Figure 14.4). Symptoms and signs include dysuria, haematuria and obstructed voiding. The diagnosis is usually made by contrast voiding cystourothrography. Treatment is endoscopic in most cases, i.e. endoscopic resection of the polyp and its fibrovascular stalk [45]. Large polyps are best removed transvesically. No recurrence has been recorded in the paediatric population [46].

Mullerian tract anomalies

So-called cysts of the posterior urethra or prostatic utricle are usually derived from some persistent component of the mullerian ducts. They can be associated with prune belly syndrome, hypospadias or other virilization defects [47]. Many are asymptomatic findings but when symptoms occur these include dysuria, epididymitis, haematuria and haemospermia [48]. A midline cystic structure at the base of the prostate may be evident on digital rectal examination. The diagnosis is made with a combination of ultrasound, micturating cystourethrography and urethroscopy. The most common variant consists of a short, blind-ending pouch opening on the veromontanum. In many cases no treatment is necessary but where indicated surgery includes transurethral endoscopic unroofing – to facilitate drainage into the urethra. For large mullerian remnants a suprapubic transtrigonal approach is preferred.

Urethral duplication in males

These are rare anomalies. As recently as 1986 only 150 cases were documented in the literature. Several classifications have been devised, but the one suggested by Effmann et al. [49] has been adopted most widely:

- Type 1 – blind-ending, incomplete urethral duplication.
- Types 2A, 2A i, 2A ii, 2B – different patterns of complete duplication.
- Type 3 – urethral duplication forming part of a more complex form of partial or complete caudal duplication.

Williams and Kenawi [50] and Woodhouse and Williams [51] divide urethral duplications into those occurring in a frontal plane (complete or abortive) or a sagittal plane (epispadiac, hypospadiac, 'Y' duplication, etc.). The embryological derivation of these anomalies is confusing and poorly understood (Figure 14.5).

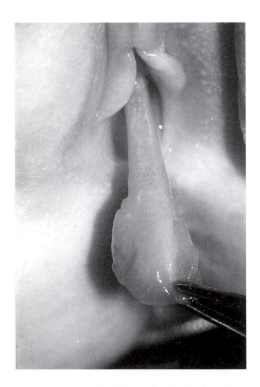

Figure 14.4 Large benign urethral polyp in a female infant.

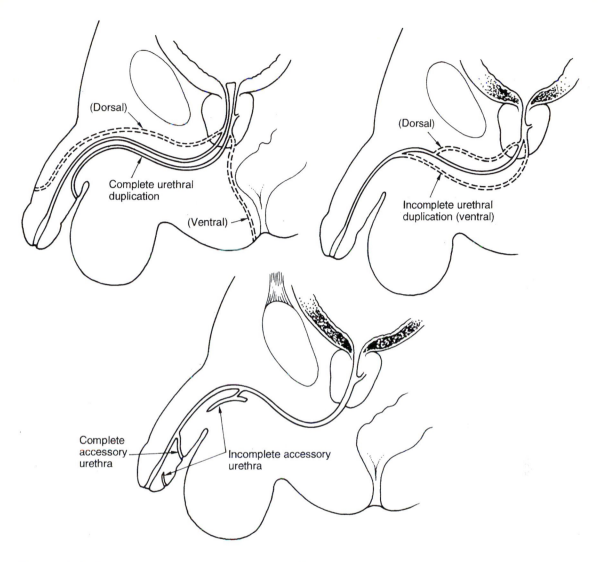

Figure 14.5 The broad anatomical spectrum of urethral duplication anomalies.

Patients with urethral duplication may be asymptomatic or can present with a double stream, urinary incontinence, urinary tract infections or outflow obstruction. Obstructive symptoms usually relate to stenosis at the level of the urethral junction, whereas incontinence is due to the existence of an accessory urethra bypassing the normal sphincteric anatomy. Physical examination usually reveals the presence of two external meatuses as the only visual abnormality. More complex forms associated with anomalies of the genitalia include epispadias, penile chordee or ambiguous genitalia. Investigations consist of micturating cystourethrography, retrograde contrast urethrography and urethroscopy. Treatment may not be necessary if the patient is asymptomatic. Where symptoms are present, the operative procedure is tailored to the extent and pattern of the anatomical abnormality.

Urethral duplication in females

These are extremely rare anomalies. Although urethral duplication can occur in association with an otherwise normal bladder, it may also be a manifestation of bladder duplication, 'covered' bladder exstrophy and genital anomalies, e.g. clitoral hypertrophy.

Congenital anomalies of the anterior urethra

Megalourethra

Megalourethra is a rare anomaly which may be associated with severe urological abnormalities including prune belly syndrome. It is likely that megalourethra represents a spectrum of defects resulting from the failure of differentiation of the mesoderm in the urethral folds and failure of migrating spongiosium tissue from the inner genital folds [52,53]. The anomaly is readily evident on clinical examination. When not associated with lethal co-existing anomalies, megalourethra can give rise to symptoms, e.g. postmicturition dribbling and erectile deformity. Supravesical diversion is suggested as the primary form of treatment if the upper tract is grossly dilated [54]. Reduction urethroplasty can be performed at a later date if necessary.

Anterior urethral diverticulum

This may result from a localized deficiency of the corpus spongiosum or as a cystic dilatation of normal or accessory urethral glands [55]. Small diverticula may not cause obstruction but in larger diverticula the distal lip acts as a flap valve occluding the urethra during voiding. Treatment is by endoscopic resection or open surgical excision. Anterior urethral valves probably form part of the same embryological spectrum as anterior urethral diverticula and their treatment is similar. Valves of the fossa navicularis have also been described.

Cowper's duct syringocele

The main Cowper's glands are paired and lie posterolateral to the membranous urethra and caudal to the external urethral sphincter. The two ducts run a submucosal course to open into the floor of the bulbar urethra [56,57]. Accessory glands are located in the depth of the corpus spongiosum of the bulb. Some cases of apparent urethral obstruction *in utero*, for which no obvious cause can be identified post-natally (Figure 14.6), may have resulted from

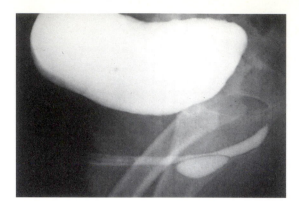

Figure 14.6 Micturating cystourethrogram demonstrating the remnants of Cowper's duct cyst (syringocele).

the transient presence of obstructing syringoceles derived from Cowper's duct. Occasionally remnants of syringoceles can be identified post-natally. When a syringocele persists in post-natal life treatment consists of endoscopic uncapping.

Skene's duct cysts

This is a rare lesion consisting of a cystic mass in the perimeatal region [56]. The aetiology of the ductal obstruction is unknown but several glands may be involved. Differential diagnosis includes Gardiner's cyst, urethral prolapse and prolapsed ectopic ureterocele. Treatment consists of marsupialization or simple needle aspiration.

Urethral atresia, agenesis and 'congenital' urethral stricture

Complete congenital occlusion of the urethra (urethral atresia or agenesis) is incompatible with survival [8,57]. Fetal anuria gives rise to oligohydramnios and pulmonary hypoplasia, whilst the profound obstructive insult to the fetal urinary tract results in renal dysplasia of lethal severity. When the condition occurs in female fetuses it is usually found in association with an atretic bladder. Survival can only occur in those cases in which urethral atresia forms part of the complex of anomalies, which includes a congenital fistula decompressing the urinary tract [58]. Partial congenital urethral atresia has been described in infants of both sexes in association with the high variety of rectal atresia. It is reported that congenital strictures may occur at the junction between the bulbar and membranous urethra [59,60]. Familial cases have been published [61,62], but since most examples have been diagnosed during adult life, it is doubtful whether this anomaly is truly congenital in aetiology.

Congenital meatal stenosis

This is an extremely rare anomaly [63], even in males with hypospadias. When present congenital meatal obstruction is generally associated with other anomalies, e.g. rectal atresia. The concept of urethral stenosis as a cause of recurrent urinary infection and voiding dysfunction in girls is now largely discredited [64,65].

References

1. Gonzales J, Gonzales M, Mary JY. Size and weight study of human kidney growth velocity during the last three months of pregnancy. *Eur Urol* 1980; **6**: 37–44.
2. Gonzales J. Relation Structure et Fonction dans le Développement de l'Appareil Urinaire du Foetus. *J Urol (Paris)* 1985; **91**: 108–117.
3. Altemus AR, Hutchins GM. Development of the human anterior urethra. *J Urol* 1991; **146**: 1085–1093.
4. Droes J Th PM. Observations on the musculature of the urinary bladder and the urethra in the human fetus. *Br J Urol* 1974; **46**: 179–185.
5. Brockis JG. The development of the trigone of the bladder with a report of a case of ectopic ureter. *Br J Urol* 1952; **24**: 192–200.
6. Hutton KAR, Thomas DFM, Arthur RJ et al. Prenatally detected posterior urethral valves: is gestational age at detection a predictor of outcome? *J Urol* 1994; **152**: 698–701.
7. Atwell JD. Posterior urethral valves in the British Isles: a multicenter BAPS review. *J Pediatr Surg* 1983; **18**: 70–74.
8. Kaplan GW, Scherz HL (1992) *Infravesical Obstruction in Clinical Pediatric Urology*, 3rd edn. Philadelphia: WB Saunders, pp 821–864.
9. Morgagni JB. Adversaria Anatomica Omnia. *J Cominus* 1719; Part 1, Article 10, p 5.
10. Langenbeck B. *Mémoire sur la Lithotomie*, 1937. Cited by Campbell MF In: *Pediatric Urology*. Philadelphia: WB Saunders.
11. Young HH, Frontz WA, Baldwin JC. Congenital obstructions of the posterior urethra. *J Urol* 1919; **3**: 289–365.
12. Dewan PA, Zappala SM, Ransley PG et al. Endoscopic reappraisal of the morphology of congenital obstruction of the posterior urethra. *Br J Urol* 1992; **70**: 439–444.
13. Ruano-Gil D, Coca-Payeras A, Tejedo-Mateu A. Obstruction and normal recanalization of the ureter in the human embryo: its relation to congenital ureteric obstruction. *Eur Urol* 1975; **1**: 287–293.
14. Alcaraz A, Vinaixa F, Tejedo-Mateu A et al. Obstruction and recanalization of the ureter during embryonic development. *J Urol* 1991; **145**: 410–416.
15. Henneberry MO, Stephens FD. Renal hypoplasia and dysplasia in infants with posterior urethral valves. *J Urol* 1980; **123**: 912–915.
16. Bellinger MF, Comstock CH, Gross D, Zaino R. Fetal posterior urethral valves and renal dysplasia at 15 weeks gestational age. *J Urol* 1987; **128**: 1238–1239.
17. Beck AD. The effect of intra-uterine urinary obstruction upon the development of the fetal kidney. *J Urol* 1971; **105**: 784–789.
18. Rittenberg MH, Hulbert WC, Snyder HM et al. Protective factors in posterior urethral valves. *J Urol* 1988; **140**: 993–996.
19. Greenfield SP, Hensle TW, Berdon WE et al. Urinary extravasation in the newborn male with posterior urethral valves. *J Pediatr Surg* 1982; **17**: 751–756.
20. Parkhouse HF, Barrett TM, Dillon HS et al. Long-term outcome of boys with posterior urethral valves. *Br J Urol* 1988; **62**: 59–62.
21. Campaiola JM, Perlmutter AD, Steinhardt GF. Non-compliant bladder resulting from posterior urethral valves. *J Urol* 1985; **134**: 708–710.
22. Lortat-Jacob S, Dietrich JC, Nihoul-Fékété C. Séquelles Vésicales des Valves de l'Urèthre Postérieur. Etude Urodynamique de 14 cas. Implications Thérapeutiques. Lecture – Congrès de Chirurgie Pédiatrique – Paris, 1990.
23. Peters CA, Bolkier M, Bauer SB et al. The urodynamic consequences of posterior urethral valves. *J Urol* 1990; **144**: 122–126.
24. Holmdahl G, Sillen U, Bachelord M et al. The changing urodynamic pattern in valves bladder during infancy. *J Urol* 1988; **153**: 463–467.
25. Connor JP, Burbige KA. Long-term urinary incontinence and renal function in neonates with posterior urethral valves. *J Urol* 1990; **144**: 1209–1211.
26. Sholder AJ, Maizels M, Depp R et al. Caution in antenatal intervention. *J Urol* 1988; **139**: 1026–1029.
27. Williams DI, Whitaker RH, Barratt TM et al. Urethral valves. *Br J Urol* 1973; **45**: 200–210.
28. Scott JES. Management of congenital posterior urethral valves. *Br J Urol* 1985; **57**: 71–77.
29. Avner ED, Chavers B, Sullivan EK, Tejani A. Renal transplantation and chronic dialysis in children and adolescents: the 1993 annual report of the North American Pediatric Renal Transplant Co-operative Study. *Pediatr Nephrol* 1995; **9**: 61–73.
30. Woodhouse CRJ, Reilly JM, Bahadur G. Sexual function and fertility in patients treated for posterior urethral valves. *J Urol* 1989; **142**: 586–588.

31. Dineen MD, Dhillon HK, Word HC et al. Antenatal diagnosis of PUV. *Br J Urol* 1993; **72**: 364–369.

32. Mouriquand P, Mollard P, Ransley PG. Dilemmes soulevés par le Diagnostic Anténatal des Uropathies Obstructives et leurs Traitements. *Pédiatrie* 1989; **44**: 357–363.

33. Ehrlich RM, Shanberg A. Neomydium Yag laser ablation of posterior urethral valves. *Dialog Pediatr Urol* 1988; **11**: 4–5.

34. Biewald W, Schier F. Laser treatment of posterior urethral valves in neonates. *Br J Urol* 1992; **69**: 425–427.

35. Zaontz MR, Gibbons MD. An antegrade technique for ablation of posterior urethral valves. *J Urol* 1984; **132**: 982.

36. Datta NS. Percutaneous transvesical antegrade ablation of posterior urethral valves. *Urology* 1987; **30**: 561–564.

37. Whitaker RH, Sherwood T. An improved hook for destroying posterior urethral valves. *J Urol* 1986; **135**: 531–532.

38. Diamond DA, Ransley PG. Fogarty balloon catheter ablation of neonatal posterior valves. *J Urol (Paris)* 1987; **93**: 43–46.

39. Garg SK, Lawrie JH. The perineal urethrotomy approach to posterior urethral valves. *J Urol* 1983; **130**: 1146–1149.

40. Mollard P. In: *Précis d'Urologie de l'Enfant*. Paris: Masson, 1984; pp 264–294.

41. Hitchcock RJI, Duffy PG, Malone PS. Ureterocystoplasty: the 'bladder' augmentation of choice. *Br J Urol* 1994; **73**: 575–579.

42. Kajbafzadeh AM, Quinn FMJ, Duffy PG, Ransley PG. Augmentation cystoplasty in boys with posterior urethral valves (PUV). Data presented to British Association of Urological Surgeons Annual Meeting, Brighton, 1995.

43. Reinberg Y, Gonzales R, Fryd D et al. The outcome of renal transplantation in children with posterior urethral valves. *J Urol* 1988; **140**: 1491–1493.

44. Kimche D, Lash D. Congenital polyp of the posterior urethra. *J Urol* 1982; **127**: 134.

45. Foster RS, Garrett GA. Congenital posterior urethral polyp. *J Urol* 1986, **136**: 1146–1149.

46. Kearney GP, Lebowitz RL, Retik AB. Obstructing polyps of the posterior urethra in boys: embryology and management. *J Urol* 1979; **122**: 802–804.

47. Devine CJ Jr, Gonzales-Serva L, Stecker JF Jr. Utricular configuration in hypospadias and intersex. *J Urol* 1980; **123**: 407–411.

48. Van Poppel H, Verreecken R, Degetter P, Verduyn H. Hemosperm owing to utricular cyst: embryological summary and surgical review. *J Urol* 1983; **129**: 608–609.

49. Effman EL, Lebowitz RL, Colodny AH. Duplication of the urethra. *Radiology* 1976; **119**: 179–185.

50. Williams DI, Kenawi MM. Urethral duplications in the male. *Eur Urol* 1975; **1**: 209–215.

51. Woodhouse CRJ, Williams DI. Duplications of the lower urinary tract in children. *Br J Urol* 1979; **51**: 481–487.

52. Stephens FD. *Congenital Intrinsic Lesions of the Posterior Urethra in Congenital Malformations of the Urinary Tract*. New York: Praeger, 1983; pp 95–125.

53. Lockhart JL, Reeve HR, Krueger R P et al. Megalourethra. *Urology* 1978; **12**: 51–54.

54. Mortensen PHG, Johnson HW, Coleman GU et al. Megalourethra. *J Urol* 1985; **134**: 358–361.

55. Ortlip SA, Gonzales R, Williams RD. Diverticula of the male urethra. *J Urol* 1980; **124**: 350–355.

56. Nan Hyuk L, Sang Youn K. Skene's duct cysts in female newborns. *J Pediatr Surg* 1992; **27**: 15–17.

57. Aaronson IA, Cremin BJ. *Lower Urinary Tract Obstruction in Clinical Paediatric Uroradiology*. Edinburgh: Churchill Livingstone, 1984; pp 210–232.

58. Valiki BF. Agenesis of the bladder: a case report. *J Urol* 1973; **109**: 510–511.

59. Cobb BG, Wolf SA, Ansell JS. Congenital stricture of the proximal urethral blub. *J Urol* 1968; **99**: 629–631.

60. Kelalis PP. Anterior urethra. In: Kelalis PP, King LR, Belman AB (eds) *Clinical Pediatric Urology*. Philadelphia: WB Saunders, 1976.

61. Michon P. Retrecissement 'Familial' de l'Urètre. *J Urol Nephrol (Paris)* 1978; **84**: 107–109.

62. Redman JF, Frasier LP. Apparent congenital anterior urethral strictures in brothers. *J Urol* 1979; **122**: 707.

63. Allen JS, Summers JL, Wickerson JE. Meatal calibrations in newborn boys. *J Urol* 1991; **146**: 1085–1093.

64. Graham JB, King LR, Kropp KA, Uehling DT. Significance of distal urethral narrowing in young girls. *J Urol* 1967; **97**: 1045–1049.

65. Averous M, Guiter J, Grasset D. Les Stenoses Uretrales de la Fillette: Mythe ou Réalité. *J Urol (Paris)* 1981; **87**: 67–75.

15

Vesicoureteric reflux

D.F.M. Thomas

The potential for reflux, the retrograde flow of urine, exists at two anatomical sites in the urinary tract, the vesicoureteric junction and the renal papilla, i.e. intrarenal reflux. In practice, the term 'reflux' is generally used synonymously with 'vesicoureteric' reflux. Whilst vesicoureteric reflux (VUR) is widely seen as an abnormal, essentially pathological occurrence, the reality may be less clear cut. The phenomenon of borderline competence, i.e. a ureterovesical junction which permits intermittent low-grade reflux when subjected to periodically increased intravesical pressures, as demonstrated in young experimental animals [1], almost certainly occurs in man. The potential for VUR to resolve spontaneously in postnatal life is well documented and it seems likely that this process may also occur *in utero*. It may not be valid, therefore, to regard competence of the ureterovesical junction valve mechanism as an all or none phenomenon throughout gestation and some degree of VUR may be a common, possibly even a 'physiological', feature of the developing fetal urinary tract.

Reflux, both at the level of the ureterovesical junction and the renal papilla, is important for two reasons. First, because it predisposes to infection – giving rise in turn to ill health in childhood and scarring-related morbidity in later life. Second, reflux may be associated with congenital renal damage, i.e. renal dysplasia. Although renal dysplasia and the anatomical abnormality of the ureterovesical junction may both represent the outcome of an underlying fault with the embryological development

of the ureteric bud, the possibility of physical, i.e. 'waterhammer', damage to the fetal kidney cannot be entirely discounted.

Aetiology of vesicoureteric reflux

Abnormal anatomy

In simple terms the normal ureterovesical junction is thought to function as a passive flap valve. Rising intravesical pressure, particularly during voiding, causes the walls of the intramural and submucosal portion of the ureter to close and coapt against the underlying detrusor, thus preventing reflux. The competence of the valve mechanism is conferred by the length of intramural and submucosal ureter. This explanation is consistent with the observation that ureteric orifices sited in an abnormally lateral position on the trigone are more prone to reflux. Similarly, in complete ureteric duplication, the lower pole system is more prone to reflux because of its shorter submucosal tunnel than the upper pole ureter.

Bladder dysfunction

The presence or absence of reflux depends on a balance of factors, i.e. the competence of the valve mechanism and the hydrostatic pressure of the urine to which it is subjected. In recent years the concept of borderline competence and the role of bladder dysfunction in the aetiology of VUR has attracted increasing attention. The role of high resting and voiding intravesical pressures is seen most clearly in cases of secondary VUR associated with bladder outflow obstruction and neuropathic bladder. VUR, usually high grade, is present in 50% of boys with posterior urethral valves at the time of presentation. More than half these ureters cease to reflux once the urethral obstruction has been relieved and bladder pressures revert to more normal levels (Figure 15.1). Secondary VUR is also a phenomenon of the poorly compliant or unstable neuropathic bladder.

Although primary VUR (i.e. reflux occurring in an anatomically normal and normally innervated bladder) has been historically regarded as a structural anatomical abnormality, it is becoming clear that this view is oversimplistic. Abnormal bladder dynamics and elevated intravesical pressures also appear to make an important contribution to 'primary VUR'. Koff and Lapides [2] documented a 50%

incidence of VUR in children (predominantly girls) with urodynamically documented forms of bladder dysfunction such as sphincter detrusor dyssynergia and unstable detrusor contractions. Likewise, Van Gool and his colleagues [3] have also highlighted the importance of dysfunctional voiding in the aetiology of low-grade VUR in girls. Typically VUR in girls tends to be low grade, presents later in childhood and is often associated with voiding disorders. In contrast, VUR in boys is characterized by earlier clinical presentation and a higher grade of reflux. Gross primary VUR in male infants has previously been cited as arguably the most convincing example of the role of abnormal anatomy, i.e. a congenitally determined abnormality of the vesicoureteric junction (Figure 15.2). However, the findings of recent studies have challenged this view by raising the intriguing possibility that even in this form of VUR, bladder dysfunction plays a key aetiological role. Video urodynamics in a small group of male infants with primary VUR

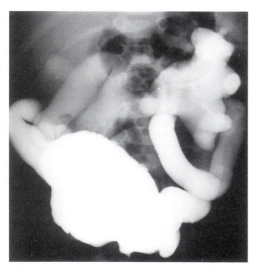
(a)

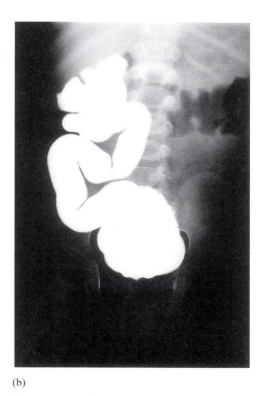
(b)

Figure 15.1 (a) Voiding cystourethrogram at presentation in a 4-month-old male infant with clinically presenting posterior urethral valves. Bilateral grade V VUR. (b) Follow up VCU 6 months after endoscopic urethral valve ablation. Persisting right VUR. The left VUR, however, has resolved completely following relief of infravesical obstruction.

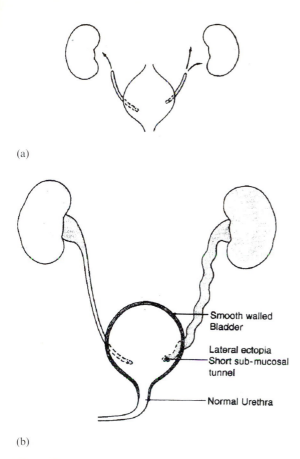

(a)

(b)

Figure 15.2 (a) Defective development of the ureteric bud resulting in abnormality of the uterovesical junction and the potential for renal dysplasia associated with faulty interaction between the ureteric bud and developing metanephric mesenchyme. (b) Postnatal characteristics of the bladder in primary VUR attributed to defective ureteric bud development.

performed between 3 and 9 months of age by Hjalmas and his colleagues [4] revealed unexpectedly high intravesical pressures, i.e. 100–234 cmH₂O on voiding. Yeung and associates [5], studying 28 infants with primary VUR at a mean age of 5.9 months, documented a range of urodynamic abnormalities, notably detrusor instability and inadequate bladder emptying. Follow-up studies by both groups of authors have revealed a tendency for bladder function to revert to normal, with resolution of hypercontractility and increasing functional bladder capacity [5,6].

The term 'transient urodynamic dysfunction of infancy' has been coined by Chandra and associates [7] who, like the previous authors,

have identified self-limiting abnormalities of detrusor function in a high percentage of male infants with primary VUR. Yeung [5] observed that reflux was most likely to resolve spontaneously in those infants whose bladder function reverted to normal. In an earlier study (not involving urodynamics), Yeung and his associates noted that 24 out of 63 boys with prenatally detected primary VUR had a bladder wall thickness measured by ultrasound of over 3.5 mm [8]. In contrast, in a group of 21 girls with prenatally detected primary VUR, none had a bladder wall thickness greater than 3.5 mm. This difference was highly significant ($p < 0.01$).

The increased bladder wall thickness coupled with urodynamic evidence of bladder dysfunction have been interpreted by Yeung and others as possible evidence that so-called 'primary' VUR in male infants is, in fact, a secondary phenomenon resulting from transient bladder outflow obstruction in fetal life (Figure 15.3). Evidence of transient urethral obstruction can occasionally be inferred from the finding of minor urethral anomalies e.g. Cowper's duct cyst on postnatal voiding cystourethrography. In the majority of male infants with primary VUR, however, the radiological appearances of the urethra are normal. This observation may not be incompatible with the concept of transient urethral obstruction. Detailed post mortem anatomical studies undertaken by Homsy's group have highlighted important morphological changes in the striated urethral sphincter occurring in late fetal and early postnatal life. These authors have postulated that abnormal maturation of the external urethral sphincter could result in a form of functional (as opposed to fixed anatomical) urethral obstruction of a self-limiting nature. The high intravesical pressures and abnormalities of detrusor function thus generated could, in turn, result in vesicoureteric reflux [9]. Although many of the issues raised by these studies remain unresolved, it is clear that even in males with seemingly 'straightforward' primary VUR, the interrelationship between anatomy and function is more complex than was previously believed.

Aetiology of intrarenal reflux

The detailed experimental studies of Hodson [10], Ransley and Risdon [11] have greatly

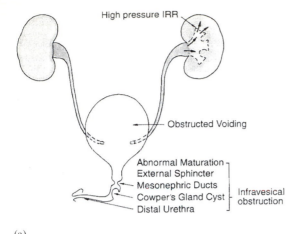

(a)

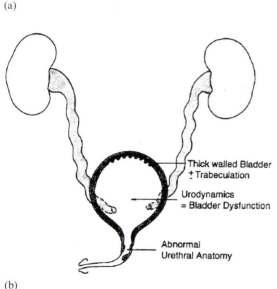

(b)

Figure 15.3 (a) Suggested mechanisms of transient infravesical obstruction and bladder dysfunction resulting in apparent 'primary' high-grade VUR in male infants. (b) Postnatal radiological clues to the previous existence of transient infravesical obstruction.

advanced our understanding of the pathogenesis of reflux nephropathy. In essence, it is believed that the normal conical configuration of the renal papilla, which is traversed obliquely by the collecting ducts, confers a second level of protection against the reflux of urine into the renal parenchyma. Morphologically abnormal flat or 'compound' papillae, which are concentrated in the polar regions of the kidney, permit reflux of urine from the calices into the renal parenchyma. Although compound papillae are generally thought to be the result of defective embryogenesis, it is con-

ceivable that the abnormal morphology reflects effect rather than cause and is itself the outcome of a sustained hydrodynamic insult resulting from sterile VUR *in utero*.

Genetics, patterns of inheritance

This topic is covered more comprehensively in Chapter 1. Briefly, two modes of inheritance have been suggested, i.e. autosomal genes of variable penetrance or multiple genes with a cumulative effect. Workers in the USA have noted a relatively low incidence of VUR in the black population, whereas the condition is seen more commonly in fair-haired, blue-eyed children of Scandinavian lineage. The order of risk whereby VUR is transmitted from one generation to another is not known but the increased incidence of VUR in the siblings of affected children has been extensively studied. A 10-year prospective screening study undertaken by Noe [12] identified a 34% incidence of VUR in a large sibling population. The incidence of VUR is also substantially increased in the offspring of parents with known VUR. The rationale for screening siblings is considered later in this chapter.

Incidence

Our knowledge of the incidence of VUR in the general paediatric population is derived largely from voiding cystourethrogram (VCU) studies performed in the 1950s and 1960s. It is exceedingly unlikely that these studies could be repeated in healthy children in today's ethical climate. From these studies the incidence in the general paediatric population appears to lie in the range 1–2% [13–15]. The principal exception to these figures comes from the study reported by Köllerman and Ludwig [16], which reported an unparalleled 30% incidence of reflux in healthy children under 3 years of age. From the description of the radiological technique employed, however, it is likely that bladders were overfilled and that unphysiologically high intravesical pressures were produced. Köllerman and Ludwig's study probably tells us more about the existence of borderline competence than the true incidence of primary VUR.

Sex ratio

The sex ratio of 2079 children with clinically presenting VUR documented in six large studies [12,17–21] is detailed in Table 15.1. The high proportion of females in studies spanning the whole paediatric age range conceals an important exception, i.e. a reversed male to female ratio of 5 : 1 in clinically presenting reflux during the first year of life [20]. Decter et al. [17] reported that boys constituted 13.5% of their study population and that in a quarter of boys their reflux had presented clinically with infection before the age of 3 months. Although the International Reflux Study [21] included children up to the age of 11, two-thirds of the boys recruited into the study were under 2 years of age. The proportion of males in the European arm of the study (24%) was significantly higher than for the North American (10%) – a difference attributed to the statistically higher percentage of European boys who were uncircumcised. The term 'prenatal diagnosis of VUR' is a convenient shorthand for the detection by prenatal ultrasound of dilatation of the fetal urinary tract which proves, on postnatal cystography, to be due to VUR. Six studies of prenatally detected VUR (Table 15.2) [22–27] have consistently identified a male predominance. Of the 141 cases reported in six series of prenatally detected VUR, males accounted for 118 (84%). Whether this subpopulation of males with high-grade VUR detected prenatally would otherwise have been destined to present with infection in the first year or two of life, or whether a significant proportion would have remained free of infection and thus unrecognized, is an intriguing question.

Aetiology of reflux nephropathy

Functional imaging of the kidneys, with intravenous urography or, more recently, isotope renography, reveals evidence of renal damage in 20–50% of children whose VUR has been discovered following presentation with urinary infection. By this stage in the natural history, however, it becomes difficult, if not impossible, to distinguish the relative contributions of renal dysplasia and postinfective renal scarring. Much of our understanding of the aetiological mechanisms of reflux nephropathy is derived from the experimental studies of Hodson and Ransley and Risdon, who highlighted the central role of intrarenal reflux. The outcome of extensive studies in animal models can be (very) broadly summarized as follows:

1. At physiological voiding pressures reflux of sterile urine does not result in renal scarring.
2. Focal renal scarring (reflux nephropathy) occurs as a consequence of infected intrarenal reflux.
3. In the experimental situation, sterile reflux only results in renal damage at abnormally high pressures, corresponding in clinical practice to those observed in cases of posterior urethral valves or neuropathic bladder.
4. Renal damage is maximal at the time of the first (often undiagnosed) serious infection of

Table 15.1 Clinically presenting reflux: sex ratios

	Male		Female		Total no. of patients
	No.	%	No.	%	
Decter et al. 1989 (Houston) [17]	86	14	549	86	635
Skoog et al. 1987 (Washington) [18]	78	14	467	86	545
Smellie et al. 1981 (London) [19]	54	23	116	67	170
Leneghan et al. 1976 (Melbourne) [20]	35	34	67	66	102
Weiss et al. 1992 (International Reflux Study) [21]	89	20	363	80	452
Noe 1992 (Tennessee) [12]	51	18	224	82	275
Total	355	17	1724	83	2079

Table 15.2 Prenatally detected reflux: sex ratios

	Male	Female	Total
Scott 1987 [22]	6	1	7
Steele et al. 1990 [23]	14	3	17
Gordon et al. 1990 [24]	21	4	25
Anderson and Rickwood 1991 [25]	31	3	34
Sheridan et al. 1992 [26]	16	3	19
Burge et al. 1992 [27]	30	9	39
Total	118 (84%)	23 (16%)	141 (100%)

childhood, i.e. Ransley's 'big bang' hypothesis.

5. Kidneys are most vulnerable to the infective scarring process during infancy and early childhood.

Virulence of the infecting organism, coupled with its capacity for adherence, is now thought to be an important factor in the process of scar formation. Fimbriated forms of *E. coli* which have the capacity to adhere to carbohydrate receptors on the urothelial cell wall, appear to be particularly destructive.

In the experimental model described by Roberts [28], bacterial endotoxins, combined with ischaemic damage, resulted in the production of toxic free radicals, tubular destruction, microabscess formation and the eventual development of a renal scar.

Renal dysplasia

The mechanisms responsible for renal dysplasia and hypoplasia associated with VUR are far less amenable to direct study than the mechanisms of postnatal renal scarring. The most plausible explanation is derived from the hypothesis originally proposed by Stephens [29] to account for the association between ureteric ectopia and renal dysplasia. When applied to primary VUR the hypothesis is extended to propose that a ureteric bud destined to give rise to a refluxing ureter originates from an abnormal site on the mesonephric duct and extends in a cephalad direction to penetrate an abnormally peripheral part of the metanephros rather than the central zone. Whereas the interaction between a normally derived ureteric bud and the metanephros gives rise to the

orderly formation of the intrarenal collecting system and collecting ducts, when the two interact abnormally the outcome is renal dysplasia. This extrapolation of Stephens 'ureteric bud' hypothesis is consistent with the observed association between laterally placed ureteric orifices, VUR and renal dysplasia.

Although sterile VUR at physiological voiding pressures does not appear to give rise to renal damage in postnatal life, the possibility that VUR results in a hydrodynamic 'water-hammer' insult to the developing fetal kidney cannot be discounted. Furthermore, little is known of bladder pressures generated during fetal voiding.

Acquired scarring or congenital dysplasia?

Sibling studies and the prenatal ultrasound detection of VUR afford an opportunity to investigate renal function and morphology in refluxing units which have never been exposed to infection.

Sibling studies

The authoritative 10-year prospective study undertaken by Noe [12] identified VUR in 119 (34%) of 354 siblings of 275 clinically presenting index patients. The incidence of renal damage in the index patients, i.e. those presenting with infection, was 24%, compared with 13% of the siblings whose reflux had been detected by screening. Some siblings, however, had been symptomatic and others may have had previous undiagnosed urinary tract infections (UTIs). For this reason comparison between rates of renal scarring in siblings and clinically presenting index cases in the early period of childhood probably provides a more reliable picture. In the subgroup of infants and children under 18 months of age the incidence of renal damage associated with clinically presenting reflux was 25%, whereas renal damage was observed in only 7% of asymptomatic siblings with VUR.

Ten (4%) of the 275 index cases had evidence of renal failure or unilateral renal damage of sufficient severity to justify nephrectomy, whereas none of the sibling refluxers were in this category.

Prenatal ultrasound diagnosis

Although the prenatal detection of reflux might seem to offer an ideal opportunity to study the contribution made by congenital factors to reflux nephropathy, a number of drawbacks limit the value of this approach:

1. Prenatal ultrasound identifies an unrepresentative subpopulation characterized by males with high-grade reflux, rather than females who constitute the largest group in most published studies.
2. Differential renal function is derived by comparing isotope uptake in one kidney with another. A reliable estimate of differential function in an affected kidney, therefore, requires the contralateral kidney to be normal if it is to serve as a valid functional control. Since prenatally detected VUR often occurs bilaterally or is associated with coexistent pathology, this is often not the case.
3. The physical 'hard-copy' images generated by isotope renography in this age group are small and the appearances of focal or polar scarring may be difficult to interpret.

Within these limitations, we documented evidence of renal damage in 4 (17%) of 24 kidneys exposed to sterile VUR *in utero* and early postnatal life [30]. Severe loss of function associated with grade V VUR was seen in only one kidney, whereas the remaining three showed moderate global reduction of uptake with differential function between 20 and 40%. Since this study was published, however, we have encountered occasional cases in which sterile high-grade VUR *in utero* has been associated with virtual absence of function in the affected kidney. Burge et al. [27] found isotope evidence of renal damage in 7 (33%) of 21 prenatally detected refluxing units. The 60% incidence of renographic abnormalities in 55 refluxing units reported by Anderson and Rickwood [25] should be interpreted cautiously, since their series included duplication, solitary kidneys and some cases complicated by documented infection. Sheridan et al. [26] undertook a direct comparison between the DMSA findings in 17 infants with clinically presenting VUR during the first 6 months of life and 19 infants whose VUR had been detected as a result of prenatal ultrasound. DMSA evidence of renal damage was found in 68% of the clinically presenting group, as opposed to 29% in those whose reflux had been detected prenatally.

Conclusion

The renal damage found in association with VUR can be either congenital or acquired in origin (commonly a combination of both). Sibling studies and evidence derived from prenatal diagnosis suggest that postnatal infective scarring is the more important of the two mechanisms. Since the congenital component is not amenable to prevention, the best hope of reducing reflux-related renal damage lies in early detection of reflux combined with active measures to prevent urinary infection.

Screening for vesicoureteric reflux?

On the premise that reflux nephropathy has a substantial preventable, i.e. infective, component, a number of studies have been undertaken to screen asymptomatic infants in the hope of identifying VUR before infection has supervened to give rise to renal damage. The financial argument for screening is persuasive. Broyer et al. [31] identified reflux nephropathy as the underlying cause in 24% of children and young adults on end-stage renal failure programmes. The cost of treating end-stage renal failure in the USA in 1989 was estimated at $6 billion per annum (J. Gearhart, personal communication, 1992). Even if reflux nephropathy accounts for as little as 10% of end-stage renal failure, the burden on the health care budget is clearly considerable. In addition, VUR generates substantial morbidity in childhood and adult life, e.g. symptomatic UTI, hypertension, toxaemia in pregnancy, etc., which might theoretically be prevented by a successful screening programme.

Unfortunately the prospects for an effective screening programme in the general paediatric population are not encouraging. Voiding cystography, the only reliable test, is too invasive and too expensive for this purpose and no non-invasive modality has yet emerged which meets the required level of sensitivity and specificity for a screening test.

Postnatal ultrasound

Three variants have been studied, i.e. conventional real-time ultrasound, Doppler and ultrasound bubble cystography. Whilst real-time ultrasound is a valuable modality for the detection of hydronephrosis, ureteroceles, etc., VUR is regularly missed. Scott et al. [32] in Newcastle undertook a formal prospective ultrasound screening study in an unselected 'low risk' paediatric population. Unfortunately, the few cases of VUR positively identified by screening were matched by an equal number in which reflux had been missed and only came to light with infection during the subsequent follow-up phase of the study. In these cases, even when the original images were reviewed with the benefit of hindsight, ultrasound had provided no clue to the presence of reflux.

Other variants of ultrasound include bubble cystography in which air bubbles introduced into the bladder are visualized on ultrasound in the upper tracts in the presence of reflux, and the use of colour Doppler to localize laterally placed ureteric orifices. Both techniques are time consuming and neither is sufficiently sensitive to form the basis of a screening test.

Prenatal real-time ultrasound

Despite claims to the contrary [33], prenatal ultrasound as presently practised is most unlikely to constitute a feasible screening test for VUR. In the UK routine scanning of low-risk pregnancies is limited to the second trimester. At this stage in gestation lethal anomalies are usually evident but the majority of non-lethal abnormalities of the urinary tract, including VUR, are not. Even at 28 weeks' gestation, the detection rate for VUR on ultrasound is poor. Livera et al. [34] scanned 6292 pregnant women at 28 weeks' gestation. Forty-two confirmed renal abnormalities were identified, of which VUR accounted for only two. However, during the 18-month period of postnatal follow-up, five cases of unsuspected VUR came to light with urinary infection. Finally, as already indicated, prenatal ultrasound is currently detecting a subpopulation of males with VUR and there is no evidence that a systematic screening programme, even one based around scanning in later pregnancy, would detect females with low-grade VUR – the population numerically most at risk from urinary infection and reflux nephropathy.

Urinary biochemical markers

The prospect of detecting VUR by a simple urine test is appealing. The basis for this approach lies in the observation that biochemical markers of tubular damage have been identified in the urine of some patients with VUR and reflux nephropathy. Of these, the urinary enzyme *N*-acetyl BD glucosominidase (NAG) [35] has emerged as a possible marker for the presence of VUR, but unfortunately the overlap in urinary levels between children with reflux and non-refluxing controls is currently too wide to permit its use as a reliable screening test. Other markers, i.e. α_1-microglobulin and retinal binding protein, are more sensitive discriminants but their presence in the urine correlates primarily with the extent of any renal damage rather than the presence and grade of VUR. Further research is under way in a number of centres.

Clinical management of vesicoureteric reflux in the first year of life

VUR generally presents in one of three ways in infants and young children:

1. Prenatally.
2. Clinically – with urinary infection.
3. As an incidental finding during a routine investigation of other anomalies, e.g. anorectal malformations.

Clinical examination

The majority of children with primary VUR are outwardly normal with no stigmata of underlying urological disease. Exceptions include prune belly syndrome and other syndromes of which urinary tract anomalies form a part.

Diagnostic imaging
Ultrasound

Ultrasound forms the initial step in the diagnostic investigation both for prenatally detected uropathies and for children with proven urinary infections. For the investigation of prenatally detected dilatation, the initial postnatal ultrasound should be postponed to 48–72 hours of age until a more representative urinary output has been established. It is important to restate, however, that normal ultrasound appearances do not preclude the existence of VUR. Ultrasound findings suggestive of reflux include dilatation of the pelvis and calices and/or ureteric dilatation which is seen to vary in severity during the course of the ultrasound examination. Occasionally, primary VUR in males is associated with a thick bladder wall or incomplete emptying, but these findings more commonly signify outflow obstruction due to the presence of posterior urethral valves.

Voiding cystourethrography

This invasive investigation remains the definitive diagnostic modality for the assessment of VUR. The need for urethral catheterization, combined with anxieties relating to the radiation dose received by the gonads, particularly the ovaries, has considerably reduced its routine use in recent years. The precise indications for voiding cystography vary from centre to centre, but in our institution these include:

1. Ultrasound evidence of ureteric dilatation (usually associated with pelvicaliceal dilatation).
2. Bilateral pelvicaliceal dilatation in males.
3. Abnormal appearances of the bladder on ultrasound.
4. Documented symptomatic infection in the first year of life regardless of normal ultrasound appearances.

A conventional contrast study is essential to provide the necessary anatomical information on the urethra and to grade the severity of reflux (Figures 15.4, 15.5).

Grading of vesicoureteric reflux

A number of schemes have been described, but the classification devised by the International Reflux Study Committee [36] is the scheme most widely adopted by paediatric urologists (Figure 15.6). VUR detected as a result of

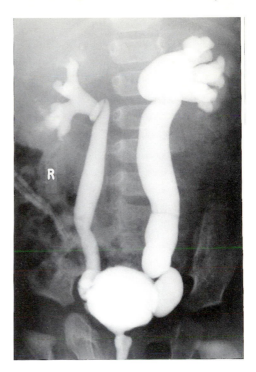

Figure 15.4 Bilateral VUR in a male infant. Prenatal detection of dilatation.

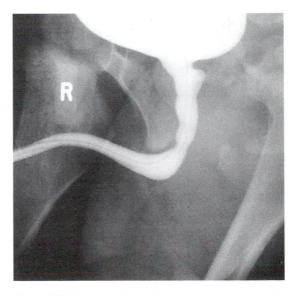

Figure 15.5 Normal infant male urethra. A conventional contrast voiding cystourethrogram remains the definitive investigation – not only to grade the severity of VUR but, more importantly, to visualize urethral anatomy and exclude the presence of infravesical obstruction.

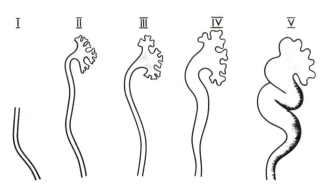

International Reflux Study Committee 1981

Figure 15.6 System of grading VUR (grades I–V) proposed by International Reflux Study Committee now widely adopted internationally:

Grade I – reflux into non-dilated distal ureter.
Grade II – reflux to level of kidney (pelvis, calices), no dilatation.
Grade III – mild to moderate dilatation but minimal blunting of calices.
Grade IV – moderate dilatation with a loss of angles of fornices; papillary impressions in calices still visible.
Grade V – gross dilatation and tortuosity; impressions of papillae no longer present.

prenatal ultrasound is characterized by much higher grades of reflux than when the condition has presented clinically with infection in later childhood. Prenatally detected VUR is characteristically high grade, with Grades III–V accounting for more than 80% of the refluxing units reported in six series of prenatally detected cases [22,23,24,25,26]. In contrast, low-grade VUR predominates in the large clinically based series. For example, the series of 844 refluxing units reported by Skoog, Belman et al. [18] documented the following distribution of grades of VUR:

Grade I – 56 ureters, 6.6%.
Grade II – 457 ureters, 54.1%.
Grade III – 267 ureters, 31.6%.
Grade IV – 48 ureters, 5.7%.
Grade V – 16 ureters, 1.9%.

Whether low-grade VUR identified as a result of infection in later childhood is truly congenital in aetiology (and has gone undetected on prenatal ultrasound), or whether it constitutes a different entity, i.e. borderline competence coupled with acquired patterns of high pressure dysfunctional voiding, is unclear.

Functional renal imaging

Static imaging with ^{99m}Tc-DMSA (Figure 15.7) is the favoured form of functional imaging for the detection of renal scarring and the measurement of differential renal function in early childhood. Dynamic imaging, e.g. with ^{99m}Tc-DTPA or ^{99m}Tc-MAG3 is preferred when the underlying pathology is obstruction rather than reflux. Intravenous urography (IVU) now plays a limited role in modern protocols for the investigation of VUR.

Clinical management
Prenatally detected vesicoureteric reflux

Although our understanding of the natural history of prenatally detected VUR is limited, the available evidence suggests that the likelihood of spontaneous resolution is at least as high, if not higher, than for clinically presenting VUR. The early outcome of a total of 142 prenatally detected refluxing units is reported by five sets of authors [22,23,24,25,26]. In Grades I and II, 63% of ureters had ceased to reflux by 3 years of age. Even for the higher Grades, i.e. III–V, a 40% spontaneous cessation rate was reported at 2–3 years of age. Of the remaining high-

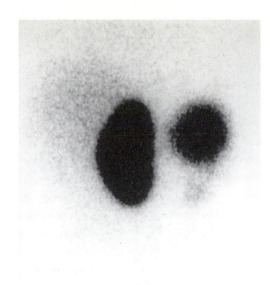

Figure 15.7 DMSA isotope study. Normal right kidney. Duplex left kidney. Reflux into lower pole moiety. Virtual absence of isotope uptake (function) in scarred/dysplastic lower pole.

grade refluxing units, approximately half continued to reflux, but at a lower grade, whilst in the remainder the severity of reflux was unchanged. These observations, indicating that 40–60% of prenatally detected refluxing ureters cease to reflux during the first 2 or 3 years of life, underpin the conservative approach to the management of prenatally detected VUR. Furthermore, the evidence from clinically based studies suggests that in boys (who account for the majority of prenatally detected cases) the incidence of symptomatic urinary infection and the risk of renal damage is low [17], even when reflux persists into later childhood. Finally, the technical difficulties associated with reimplanting wide ureters into small infant bladders and the higher failure rate of antireflux surgery in this age group provide further arguments for avoiding surgery if possible.

Conservative management consists of regular antibiotic prophylaxis, e.g. trimethoprim 1–2 mg per kg per day, given as a single night-time dose, combined with urine surveillance for infection. Regular mid stream urine checks in the asymptomatic child are less important

than the need for parents and general practitioners to ensure that a urine sample is checked promptly if the child becomes lethargic, febrile or inexplicably unwell. Annual ultrasound follow-up, however, is performed mainly to exclude the rare development of a secondary pelviureteric junction obstruction. In the absence of documented urinary infection we do not perform follow-up cystography on a systematic basis unless the information is likely to alter management. As a general rule, regular antibiotic prophylaxis is discontinued somewhere between the age of 3 and 5 years, once an effective pattern of regular voiding has been established.

Surgical intervention

Circumcision

An increasing weight of evidence, much of it admittedly anecdotal, supports the concept of 'prophylactic' circumcision in boys with prenatally detected VUR. For the moment, however, we reserve circumcision for boys with proven VUR who have experienced at least one breakthrough infection. A properly constructed prospective trial would be helpful in defining the possible role of circumcision in boys with prenatally detected VUR.

Ureteric reimplantation

The aim of surgery is to provide the refluxing ureter with a longer submucosal course, thus reconstituting the competence of the flap valve mechanism. As a working rule the ratio of submucosal tunnel length to ureteric width should be of the order of 4 : 1. Technically this aim may be difficult, if not impossible, to achieve when attempting to reimplant a widely dilated ureter (e.g. Grade IV or Grade V) into a relatively small infant's bladder using the conventional cross-trigonal (Cohen) technique. To achieve the dimensions required for a successful antireflux procedure, a Leadbetter type of ureteric reimplantation may be necessary, ideally combined with a psoas hitch. Even in skilled hands the technical difficulties of reimplanting megaureters in this age group should not be underestimated. In a series from one major specialist centre (Boston), Peters et al. [37] reported the outcome of surgery for obstructive megaureter in 42 infants operated upon at a mean age of 1.8 months. Six children (14%) developed significant anaesthetic or systemic complications and the failure rate (i.e. postoperative reflux or obstruction) of 24% was considerably higher than would normally be anticipated for ureteric reimplantation in an older age group. Although this report relates specifically to obstructed megaureter, the technical difficulties of reimplanting refluxing megaureters are very similar. Ideally, ureteric reimplantation should be avoided under 12 months of age, and certainly under the age of 6 months unless there are compelling indications.

Cutaneous vesicostomy

The creation of a stoma between the fundus of the bladder and the lower abdominal wall provides an effective way of decompressing refluxing upper tracts and ensuring adequate drainage. Potential complications include stomal stenosis and mucosal prolapse, but in a personal series of 20 cutaneous vesicostomies performed for a variety of indications only two (10%) (D.F.M. Thomas, unpublished data) required revision. Cutaneous vesicostomy has largely replaced ureterostomy in the management of severe sepsis and/or reduced renal function in infants and young children. Vesicostomy closure, a simple procedure, can be combined with ureteric reimplantation or performed in isolation in the second or third year of life.

Endoscopic correction of reflux

This innovative concept, developed and popularized by O'Donnell and Puri [38], entails the endoscopic injection of a small volume of polytetrafluoroethylene (PTFE) paste submucosally beneath the ureteric orifice. In Europe large numbers of children have undergone endoscopic correction of VUR with a reported success rate of more than 80% after one or two injections. Anxieties have been expressed, however, about the long-term safety of implanted Teflon particles following animal experiments, suggesting the potential for migration to distant sites. The introduction of biologically compatible or biodegradable materials for use in conjunction with endoscopic correction would remove many of the reservations sur-

rounding the technique. At present the equipment available for the endoscopic correction of reflux is unsuitable for instrumentation of the infant male urethra in the first year of life.

References

1. Duckett JW. Update on vesicoureteral reflux. *AUA Update Ser* 1993; Lesson 5; XII.
2. Koff SA, Lapides J, Plazza DH. Association of urinary tract infection and reflux with uninhibited bladder contractions and voluntary sphincteric obstruction. *J Urol* 1979; **122**: 373–376.
3. Van Gool JD, Hjalmas K, Tamminen-Möbius T, Olbing H. Historical clues to the complex of dysfunctional voiding, urinary tract infection and vesicoureteral reflux. *J Urol* 1992; **148**: 1699–1702.
4. Sillen U, Hjalmas K. Detrusor contractility as a Cause of Gross Bilateral Reflux in Infants. A Video Urodynamic Study. Data presented to the Urological Section of the American Academy of Pediatrics, Washington, 1993.
5. Yeung CK, Godley ML, Liu A, Duffy PG, Ransley PG. Physiological fill bladder monitoring in young infants with primary vesicoureteric reflux. Read to the Annual Meeting of European Society for Paediatric Urology, Gothenburg, April 1994.
6. Sillen U, Bachelard M, Hermanson G, Hjalmas K. Gross bilateral reflux in infants: gradual decrease of initial detrusor hypercontractility. *J Urol* 1996; **155**: 668–672.
7. Chandra M, Maddix H, McVicar M. Transient urodynamic dysfunction of infancy: relationship to urinary tract infections and vesicoureteral reflux. *J Urol* 1996; **155**: 673–677.
8. Yeung CK, Dhillon HK, Duffy PG, Ransley PG. Vesicoureteric reflux in infants with prenatally diagnosed hydronephrosis. Read to the Annual Meeting of the American Academy of Pediatrics, New Orleans, October 1991.
9. Kokoua A, Homsy Y, Lavigbe J-F et al. Maturation of the external urinary sphincter: a comparative histopographic study in humans. *J Urol* 1993; **150**: 617–622.
10. Hodson CJ, Maling TMJ, McManamon PJ. Reflux nephropathy. *Kidney Int* 1975; **8**: 50–58.
11. Ransley PG, Risdon RA, Goldy ML. High pressure sterile vesicoureteral reflux and renal scarring: an experimental study in the pig and minipig. *Contr Nephrol* 1984; **39**: 320–343.
12. Noe HN. The long term results of prospective sibling reflux screening. *J Urol* 1993; **148**: 1739–1742.
13. Lich R Jr, Howerton L Jr, Goode LFF, Davis LA. The ureterovesical junction in the newborn. *J Urol* 1964; **92**: 436–438.
14. Iannnaccone G, Panzironi PE. Ureteral reflux in normal infants. *Acta Radiol* 1955; **44**: 451–456.

15. McGovern JH, Marshall VF, Paquin A Jr. Vesicoureteral regurgitation in children. *J Urol* 1960; **83**: 122–149.

16. Köllerman MW, Ludwig H. Uber den vesicoureteralen reflux bein normalen kind in sauglings – und kleindindalter. *Z Kinderheilkund* 1967; **100**: 185–190.

17. Decter RM, Roth DR, Gonzales ET. Vesicoureteral reflux in boys. *J Urol* 1988; **140**: 1089–1091.

18. Skoog SJ, Belman AB, Majd M. A nonsurgical approach to the management of primary vesicoureteral reflux. *J Urol* 1987; **138**: 941–946.

19. Smellie JM, Edwards D, Normand ECS, Prescod N. Effect of vesicoureteric reflux on renal growth in children with urinary tract infection. *Arch Dis Child* 1981; **56**: 593–600.

20. Lenaghan D, Whitaker JG, Jensen F, Stephens FC. The natural history of reflux and long-term effects of reflux on the kidney. *J Urol* 1976; **115**: 728–730.

21. Weiss R, Tamminen-Möbius T, Koskimies O, Olbing H et al. on behalf of the International Reflux Study in Children. Characteristics at Entry of Children with Severe Primary Vesicoureteral Reflux Recruited for a Multicenter, International Therapeutic Trial Comparing Medical and Surgical Management. *J Urol* 1992; **148**: 1644–1649.

22. Scott JES. Fetal ureteric reflux. *Br J Urol* 1987; **59**: 291–296.

23. Steele BT, Robitaille P, Demaria J, Grignon A. Follow up evaluation of prenatally recognised vesicoureteral reflux. *J Pediatr* 1989; **115**: 95–96.

24. Gordon AC, Thomas DFM, Arthur RJ, Irving HC, Smith SEW. Prenatally diagnosed reflux: a follow up study. *Br J Urol* 1990; **65**: 407–412.

25. Anderson PAM, Rickwood AMK. Features of primary vesicoureteric reflux detected by prenatal sonography. *Br J Urol* 1991; **67**: 267–271.

26. Sheridan M, Jewkes F, Gough DCS. Reflux nephropathy in the 1st year of life. *Pediatr Surg Int* 1991; **6**: 214–216.

27. Burge DM, Griffiths MD, Malone PS, Atwell JD. Fetal vesicoureteral reflux: outcome following conservative postnatal management. *J Urol* 1992; **148**: 1743–1745.

28. Roberts JA. Vesicoureteral reflux and pyelonephritis in the monkey: a review. *J Urol* 1992; **148**: 1721–1725.

29. Stephens FD. The pathogenesis of renal dysplasia. In: Stephens, FD (ed.) *Congenital Malformations of the Urinary Tract*. New York: Praeger, 1983; pp 193–201, 441–462.

30. Crabbe DCG, Thomas DFM, Gordon AC, Irving HC, Arthur RJ, Smith SEW. Use of ^{99m}Tc-DMSA to study patterns of renal damage associated with prenatally detected VUR. *J Urol* 1992; **148**: 1229–1231.

31. Broyer M, Rizzonie G, Brunner FP et al. Combined report on regular dialysis and transplantation of children in Europe. *Proc EDTA* 1985; **22**: 55–79.

32. Scott JES, Lee REJ, Hunter EW et al. Ultrasound screening of newborn urinary tract. *Lancet* 1991; **338**: 1571–1573.

33. Editorial Prevention of Reflux Nephropathy. *Lancet* 1991; **338**: 1050.

34. Livera LN, Brookfield DSK, Eginton JA, Hawnaure JM. Antenatal ultrasonography to detect fetal renal abnormalities: a prospective screening programme. *Br Med J* 1989; **298**: 1421–1423.

35. Hanbury DC, Calvin J. Proteinuria and enzymuria in vesicoureteric reflux. *Br J Urol* 1992; **70**: 603–609.

36. International Reflux Study Committee. Medical versus surgical treatment of primary vesicoureteral reflux: a prospective International Reflux Study in Children. *J Urol* 1981; **125**: 277–283.

37. Peters CA, Mandell J, Lebowitz, RL et al. Congenital obstructed megaureters in early infancy: diagnosis and treatment. *J Urol* 1989; **142**: 641–645.

38. O'Donnell BJ, Puri P. Treatment of vesicoureteric reflux by endoscopic injection of Teflon. *Br Med J* 1984; **289**: 7–9.

16

Duplication and other anomalies of the kidney and ureter

P.M. Cuckow and D.F.M. Thomas

Ureteric duplication

Ureteric duplication is the commonest congenital anomaly of the upper urinary tract with a post-mortem incidence of 1 in 125 (0.8%) [1–3]. It is bilateral in 15–23% of cases and commoner in females (63%) [1,2,4,5]. The 2–4% incidence in children investigated by IVU reflects an association with complications [4,6]. Inheritance is autosomal dominant with incomplete penetrance [7] and it affects 11% of first degree relatives [8].

The nomenclature has been simplified by consensus [8]. *Duplex* kidneys have *upper* and *lower poles* with about one-third of the parenchyma forming the upper pole [4]. *Bifid ureters* unite above the bladder with a single ureteric orifice and *bifid renal pelvis* is a minor variant [9]. *Double ureters* have separate orifices. Of 95 duplications on intravenous urography (IVU), 33 (29%) were complete, 57 (52%) bifid or partial and 21 (19%) unclassified. *Lateral ectopia* (usually with lower pole ureters) and *caudal or medial ectopia* are relative to the normal orifice position on the trigone. The latter are sited at the proximal lip of the bladder neck or beyond and are found in some upper pole ureters, often called simply *ectopic ureters*. *Intravesical ureteroceles* are sited completely within the bladder. *Ectopic ureteroceles* have a portion that is permanently at the bladder neck or beyond. Figure 16.1 illustrates the range of duplication anomalies.

The embryology of ureteric duplication is discussed elsewhere. The upper pole ureter crosses the lower pole ureter to drain via the lower ureteric orifice. This is the Weigert–Meyer law [10,11]. The lower pole ureter, draining laterally on the trigone with a shorter tunnel, is prone to vesicoureteric reflux. For both, the distance from the normal orifice position has been related to the degree of dysplasia of their renal parenchyma [12].

Presentation

Antenatal scanning has increased the numbers of patients presenting with duplication by 500% or more [3,5,13–19]. Non-specific hydronephrosis or hydroureteronephrosis are seen [5,15], although more specific features may be apparent. Avni diagnosed duplication antenatally in 4 of 19 patients and saw 1 of 11 ureteroceles [5], whilst Jee (15) suspected 5 duplications antenatally in 39 patients. More recently, duplication was seen antenatally in 11 of 23 duplex ureteroceles and the ureterocele in seven [20]. Although duplication with dilatation may have a high risk of future complications, it may also have the potential to be asymptomatic [15].

Apart from antenatal diagnosis, presentation in infancy is usually due to associated reflux, ureterocele or ectopic ureter occurring singly or in combination. Urinary infection is commonest, although duplication is a great mimic in paediatric urology and must always be considered when a diagnosis is illusive [21–25]. Presentation may be quite non-specific. Acute life-threatening infection, more chronic failure

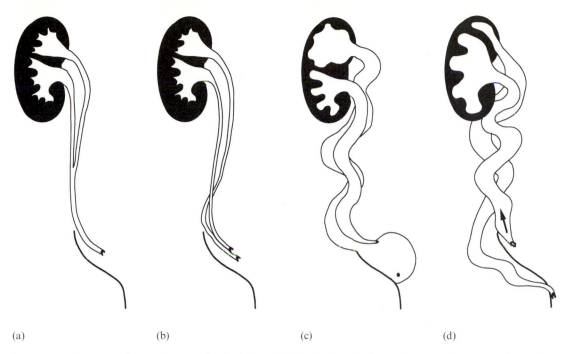

(a)   (b)   (c)   (d)

Figure 16.1 The range of anomalies associated with ureteric duplication. (a) Incomplete or partial duplication. The ureters fuse and drain through a common distal segment and a single normally sited ureteric orifice. (b) Complete duplication. The upper pole ureter drains below the lower pole ureter (the Meyer–Weigert Law). (c) Ectopic ureterocele. Normally associated with a dysplastic poorly functioning upper pole. It may be a cause of bladder outlet obstruction and threaten the remaining upper tracts. (d) Ectopic ureter. The ureter may be associated with a diminutive or even invisible upper pole. The lower pole ureter is laterally ectopic and prone to vesicoureteric reflux.

to thrive, non-specific abdominal symptoms and urinary retention are all recognized [23, 26]. Evaluation with ultrasound, micturating cystourethrography, IVU and DMSA scan usually confirms the anomaly. Occasionally it may not be discovered until cystoscopy or open bladder surgery is performed [23,27].

Vesicoureteric reflux

Vesicoureteric reflux is commoner in duplex than single systems [24,28] and is found in 70% of patients presenting with infection [4,29,30]. It involves the lower pole only in 84–90% of cases and both poles in the remainder [24,30–32]. Isolated upper pole reflux is rare and due to a refluxing ureterocele or urethrally ectopic ureter [32–35]. Bipolar reflux occurs when both orifices are laterally ectopic or with incomplete duplication [29,33]. Single system reflux occurs in 20% of patients with unilateral refluxing duplications [31,33,34].

Micturating cystourethrogram allows grading of the reflux [35]. Compared to patients with single system reflux, Peppas found higher grade reflux at presentation and scarring in 10% of renal units on IVU [32]. DMSA scanning shows parenchymal abnormalities in two-thirds of affected renal units [31] (Figure 16.2). In antenatally diagnosed uninfected patients, DMSA showed moderate or severe functional impairment in Grades IV–V but none in Grade II [15]. This may reflect lower pole dysplasia associated with lateral ectopia of the ureteric orifice [12].

Initial reports suggested little spontaneous resolution of primary duplex reflux [24,30]. Husmann showed 10% of lower pole grade II reflux resolved over 2 years, compared to 35% in single systems [25]. Ben-Ami found comparable rates of resolution (38%) in Grades I and II to matched single systems but no resolution in Grade III reflux at 1 year [36]. An uncontrolled study with median 40 months observation documented 85% resolution for Grades I and II and 35% for Grade III in lower poles, comparable to reported rates in single systems [31]. In bipolar reflux, only 1 of 6 resolved and

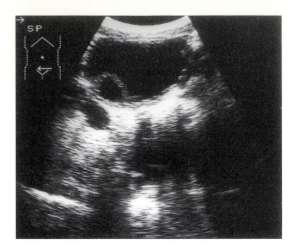

Figure 16.2 Bladder ultrasound. Transverse view of bladder demonstrating an echogenic wall of the ureterocele and its associated dilated upper pole ureter lying posteriorly.

another required surgery for breakthrough infection and none with Grade IV or V reflux [31]. The success of antibiotic prophylaxis in these studies did allow surgery to be safely deferred [25,31,32]. Indications for surgery are similar to single systems: severe reflux grade, severe renal damage, failed medical management, persisting low-grade reflux, bipolar reflux or other anomalies needing attention.

Polar nephrectomy (or total nephroureterectomy when both poles are involved) is indicated with function below 10% [31,37]. The lower ureters have a common fascial sheath and blood supply, so a short ureteric stump is left [33]. Later excision of this may be required if complications occur due to persistent reflux [31,38].

Conservative surgery is indicated for good function. Ahmed advocates ureteroureterostomy and distal ureterectomy for patients with non-refluxing ipsilateral ureters [33]. Nineteen consecutive cases were clinically successful, but asymptomatic reflux was demonstrated in six ureteric stumps. Separation and lone reimplantation of the refluxing ureter is possible, particularly when the orifices are widely apart [33,39]. Usually the ureters are dissected together through the hiatus and reimplanted within their common sheath by a Leadbetter–Politano or Cohen technique. Kistler reported one recurrence of reflux and two ureteric

stenoses in 69 duplicated ureters [34], whilst Lee had one recurrence of reflux and one ureteric stenosis from 23 cases [31]. Ureteric tapering is effective, with no complications and one instance of low-grade reflux in six patients [37], although marked dilatation often means poor function and ablative surgery is preferable [15,40]. Endoscopic injection of Teflon paste in duplex ureters abolished reflux in 66% of patients, down graded 22% and failed in 12%, whilst 100% of contralateral single reflux disappeared [41].

Ureterocele

Ureterocele is an obstructive anomaly of the terminal ureter, with a 1 in 4000 incidence and a female predominance (4–7 : 1) [1,13,15,42–45]. Seventy-five per cent occur with duplication and 60–80% are ectopic. Most single system ureteroceles are intravesical [22,42,44, 46]. Ten per cent are bilateral [22,23,26,44, 47,48]. Half of prenatally detected patients have signs postnatally, including palpable kidney, distended bladder and prolapsed ureterocele [15]. Symptoms are common in infancy and most patients present before 1 year [13,23,26,42,44,45,47–49]. Abdominal mass is reported in 10–15% of cases and bladder outflow obstruction in about 10% [23,26,43,45, 50,51].

Prolapsed ureterocele, visible in the perineum, occurs in 3.5–11% of baby girls with ureteroceles [13,23,26,44,49,50,52,53]. It causes acute or chronic infravesical obstruction, depending on its size. Mucosal congestion with necrosis and ulceration make reduction difficult and cause bleeding and sepsis [52]. Reduction is achieved by aspirating or deroofing the ureterocele, although resection may be required [52].

Ultrasound usually confirms the diagnosis, the ureterocele forming an echogenic circle inside the bladder (Figure 16.2). A dilated ureter is followed to the upper pole, often missed on IVU [26]. Micturating cystogram demonstrates the ureterocele and documents ipsilateral lower pole reflux in 50% of cases [23,28,33,50]. Reflux into the ureterocele is rare [54], but contralateral reflux occurs in 30% [50]. On micturition ureteroceles occasionally prolapse through their hiatus mimicking bladder diverticulum or bulge posteriorly, demonstrating a weakened trigone [23,28].

Obstruction of the bladder outlet by ectopic ureteroceles can be assessed [23,40]. Intravesical ureteroceles are surrounded by a clear rim of contract [28].

IVU clarifies the anatomy of the ureters and assesses potential obstruction [26,44,46] (Figure 16.3). Dilatation of the lower pole ureter is seen in around 50% of patients and is usually due to reflux [23]. Upper pole function is poor in most ectopic ureteroceles [50], but indirect evidence often indicates their presence [55]. The displaced lower pole pelvis may have the classical 'drooping flower' appearance [6]. Its upper calix is short and the parenchyma medial to it thicker than normal and its ureter, indented by its distended non-opacified fellow, can have a 'scalloped' appearance [26]. Upper pole function is often good in intravesical ureteroceles [15,26] which opacify to give a characteristic 'cobra head' appearance [28,43]. DMSA scan assesses the function of all renal units and is essential in planning surgery [42,44] (Figure 16.4).

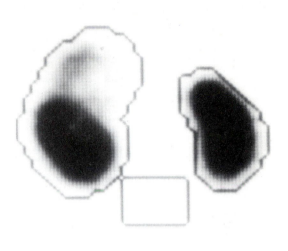

Figure 16.4 DMSA scan demonstrating virtual absence of function (less than 5% of total function) in the upper pole parenchyma of a right duplex kidney.

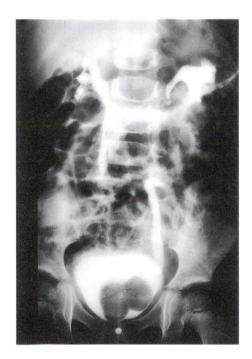

Figure 16.3 Intravenous urogram (IVU). Left duplex system. Poorly opacified (dysplastic) upper pole moiety is associated with an ectopic ureterocele – the filling defect outlined by intravesical contrast. The lower moiety of the left duplex system has the characteristic 'drooping flower' appearance and its associated ureter is moderately dilated due to the presence of lower pole vesicoureteric reflux.

Non-operative management may be appropriate in antenatally diagnosed and asymptomatic uncomplicated ureteroceles but most come to surgery [44]. Most authors agree that treatment should be individualized and based on function, the involvement of other renal units and the clinical state and age of the patient [15,23,44,49]. Consensus has moved from one-stage radical reconstruction of upper and lower urinary tracts, which is a challenging undertaking in a neonate [40]. Prophylactic antibiotics and initial decompression of the ureterocele successfully delay or avoid this difficult surgery, and its complications [50,52].

Endoscopic ureterocele incision is straightforward and can be used in septic patients [56]. Lower pole reflux often follows, probably due to its ureter losing support from the ureterocele [22,57]. Thus, bladder outlet obstruction by the collapsed ureterocele or failure of decompression may necessitate bladder surgery [13,51]. Tank decompressed 40 patients endoscopically or by open deroofing of their ureteroceles [51]. Eighteen (45%) showed improved function.

The remainder needed reconstruction; two (5%) with improved function but recurrent infections and 20 (50%) with no improvement in function. Rich described a low 2–3-mm incision with a bugbee electrode, leaving the ureterocele wall as an antireflux valve. Seven single system intravesical ureteroceles were successfully treated, with reflux appearing in one [58]. Using this technique Blyth compared intravesical and ectopic ureteroceles [59]. Ninety-three per cent of intravesical ureteroceles were decompressed, 18% developed reflux (half of which resolved) and only 7% needed further surgery. Seventy-five per cent of ectopic ureteroceles were decompressed but reflux appeared in 47% and 50% had secondary surgery. In prenatally diagnosed duplex ureteroceles, treated at a median age of 4 weeks, endoscopic incision produced reflux

in less than 10%. This was definitive in 52% and it postponed more complex surgery in the remainder [20]. There is a strong argument for the use of endoscopic incision as first line treatment [13], particularly in intravesical ureteroceles and those diagnosed antenatally (Figure 16.5).

Upper pole heminephrectomy and partial ureterectomy has been the preferred treatment for ectopic ureteroceles [23,26,44,48]. The upper pole is taken off the lower pole (Figure 16.6), its ureter carefully dissected from its fellow, divided above the common sheath and the ureterocele aspirated by catheterizing the stump [22]. Between 20 and 43% of patients need further surgery [23,24,48,60], although 9% has been reported [44]. However, this depends on the surgeon's approach to persistent reflux [22]. In infants alone results are

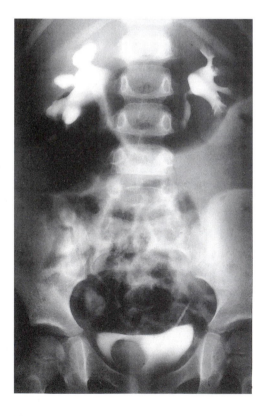 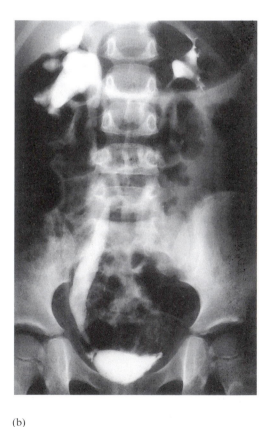

(a)   (b)

Figure 16.5 (a) Right-sided single system, orthotopic ureterocele. In early films the ureterocele is seen as a non-opacified filling defect due to the delayed passage of contrast within the dilated, obstructed upper tract. (b) At 20 minutes the ureter has opacified along its length and the ureterocele is no longer visible within the bladder as a filling defect. Despite the dilatation and obstruction caused by the ureterocele, DMSA imaging revealed symmetrical distribution of parenchymal function between the two kidneys. Treatment consisted of endoscopic incision of the ureterocele.

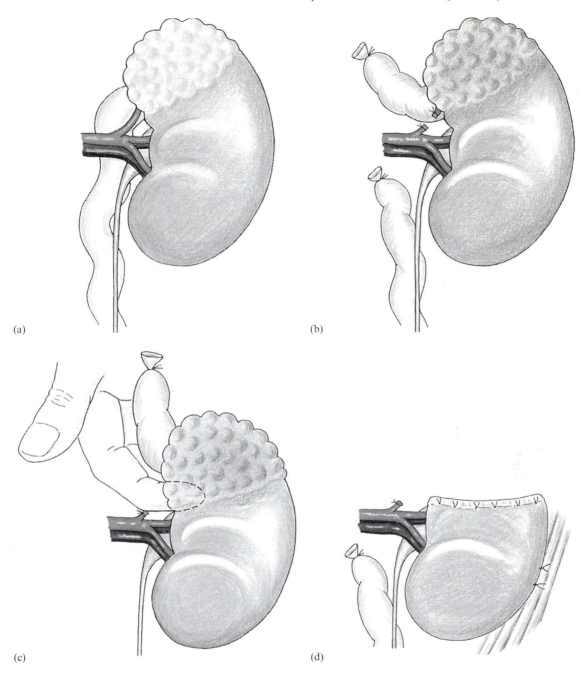

(a)

(b)

(c)

(d)

Figure 16.6 Heminephrectomy: surgical technique. (a) Surgical exposure of the kidney through a supra 12 flank incision reveals dysplastic upper pole parenchyma with a dilated upper pole ureter. In contrast, the lower pole ureter is normal in calibre and the parenchyma healthy. (b) Once the vascular anatomy has been established with certainty, the vessels serving the upper pole are ligated and divided. Division of the upper pole ureter at this stage facilitates mobilization of the upper pole parenchyma. (c) Defining the level of transection is aided by observing the line of demarcation between normally perfused lower pole cortex and ishaemic upper pole cortex following ligation of the upper pole vessels. Gentle traction on the divided upper pole ureter often reveals a hilar plane of dissection which can be opened up further by blunt dissection. (d) Excision of the upper pole parenchyma has been completed and haemostasis achieved. The lower pole moiety is fixed to prevent the risk of torsion on the vascular pedicle. Further mobilization and excision of the upper pole ureter from above is performed under vision via the loin incision. Where indicated, excision of the distal ureteric stump plus ureterocele is performed through a separate suprapubic incision.

poorer, with 50% needing bladder surgery which was nonetheless postponed a mean of 1.2 years [50]. Long ureteric stumps may need reoperation [48] and initial extravesical total ureterectomy has been definitive in 81% of cases, although more difficult [47]. Bladder outlet obstruction by the collapsed ureterocele and lower pole reflux are the commonest indications for further surgery [26,44,60]. The compromise of lower pole function through atrophy or secondary pelviureteric (PUJ) obstruction in a displaced lower pole, are reported [44,49].

The histology of most upper poles shows severe dysplasia, secondary inflammation and scarring and vindicates excision [23,26,44], including uninfected antenatally diagnosed patients [15]. Ureteropyelostomy or uretero-ureterostomy with partial ureterectomy preserve functioning parenchyma but size differences between the two ureters pose problems. Complications may occur from anastomotic strictures, retained ureteric stumps and yo-yo reflux [44,48,61]. Ureterocele excision and bipolar reimplantation is probably preferable [44].

Ureterocele excision with ureteric reimplantation (bipolar or unipolar after upper pole nephrectomy) is advocated as primary definitive treatment [40,45]. Only 14% reported by Schertz required second operation for recurrent reflux, although these were older patients [45]. Major complications of this approach include ureteric damage or incontinence due to bladder neck injury or vesicovaginal fistula [62]. Surgery is easier in older patients and prior decompression of the ureterocele and its ureter significantly reduce blood loss and operation time [53]. No distal ureterocele is left to obstruct the urethra, confirmed by passing a large catheter antegradely [45]. Hendren enucleated the ureterocele to allow repair of the trigone and bladder neck behind it [40]. Marsupialization, leaving its posterior wall *in situ*, avoids potential complications of damage to the sphincter mechanism and vesicovaginal fistula [45,63]. When reimplantation is combined with heminephrectomy, leaving a portion of the wall of upper pole ureter attached to the lower pole ureter minimizes the risk of injury [22].

Ectopic ureter

Ectopic ureter occurs in 1 in 1900 people or 0.5% of ureteric duplications [1,4,64]. Eighty per cent are female [65,66] and 8% bilateral [67]. Eighty per cent of ectopic ureters drain the upper pole of a duplication and contralateral duplication is seen in 40–50% of these [65,66,68]. Some series of single system ectopic ureters show a male predominance, and they are bilateral in 30–50% [65,69,70]. In Japan these trends are reversed; 70% of ectopic ureters are single and 80% of these are in females [71].

Presentation

Ectopic ureters commonly come to light with urinary incontinence or infection. In a series of 39 patients reported by Brannan and Henry [72], however, only six (15%) were diagnosed in infancy, all of whom were female. In females in whom the ectopic ureter drains below the continence mechanism, the classical presentation in childhood is with continuous dribbling incontinence superimposed on a background of normal intermittent voiding [72–74]. Urinary incontinence is not a feature of males, since for embryological reasons ectopic ureters invariably drain above the level of the striated sphincter mechanism [75]. Although ectopic ureters may present with 'straightforward' urinary infection, the occurrence of an unusual infection, e.g. epididymo-orchitis or infected vaginal discharge, should prompt suspicion of an ectopic ureter [66,73,76]. In the neonatal period dilated ectopic ureters may give rise to a palpable or visible abdominal mass [65,66, 70,77]. Single ectopic ureters may be associated with coexisting congenital anomalies, the commonest being anorectal malformations, tracheo-oesophageal fistula, myelomeningocele and diaphragmatic hernia [65,68,69,78,79].

Ellerker [67] documented the drainage site of 494 ectopic ureters in 366 females and 128 males. In the females, the ectopic ureter drained into the urethra in 35%, the vestibule in 34%, the vagina in 25%, the cervix or uterine cavity in 5%, Gartner's duct in 0.5% and urethral diverticulum in 0.5%. In males the site of drainage was the posterior urethra in 47% of cases, seminal vesicle in 33%, the prostatic utricle in 10%, the ejaculatory duct in 5.5% and the vas deferens in 4.5%. Infants and children with ectopic ureters continue to present clinically but an increasing number are now being diagnosed following the discovery of upper tract dilatation on antenatal ultrasound [15,18,73].

Postnatal imaging usually comprises ultrasound, isotope renography (usually DMSA) and intravenous urography – the latter to demonstrate possible duplex anatomy of non-dilated ureters. Although an ectopic upper pole ureter may be dilated, the parenchyma it drains is often dysplastic and difficult to visualize [80]. Similarly, the ureter may be narrow in its proximal portion, with dilatation limited to the distal segment. Occasionally it can prove extremely difficult to establish the existence of a poorly functioning upper pole ectopic ureter as a cause of dribbling urinary incontinence in girls [81].

Dye tests have been used to help locate ectopic ureteric orifices [82] and additional contrast studies, e.g. vaginogram, ascending ureterogram [71], may also be helpful in the hunt for an elusive ectopic orifice. Despite investigation by a range of imaging modalities, some ectopic ureters defy preoperative visualization and in this situation surgical exploration can be justified on the basis of a high index of suspicion. The management of duplex ectopia usually consists of upper polar nephrectomy combined with a limited proximal ureterectomy or total ureterectomy. As with other forms of duplication, however, the surgery should be tailored to the individual's circumstances and the pattern of duplex anatomy. Considerable caution is required when dealing with ectopic ureters traversing the region of the bladder neck and striated sphincter complex. In general, it is safer to leave a short pelvic stump of ectopic ureter draining onto the perineum rather than risk surgically induced sphincter weakness incontinence [83]. Conservative, parenchymal sparing options [84], e.g. ureteroureterostomy or common sheath reimplantation [85], are occasionally appropriate.

Single ectopic ureter

In cases of single ectopic ureter the ipsilateral trigone and bladder neck often fail to develop normally and the endoscopic appearances of a hemitrigone may be mistaken for the appearances of renal agenesis [86,87], particularly if the kidney is also ectopic [71]. Bilateral single ectopic ureters are usually associated with defi-ciency of the bladder neck and trigone and, in consequence, the prognosis for continence is poor [68,79,86].

Nephrectomy is the standard treatment of most unilateral cases but ureteric reimplantation is preferable when there is good ipsilateral renal function or an abnormality in the contralateral kidney [22,65,66,71]. Surgical management of bilateral single ectopia is difficult, since the bladder is often small and poorly developed. Satisfactory outcomes have been reported after ureteric reimplantation alone [88], but unfortunately incontinence may prove a major problem despite bladder neck reconstruction and augmentation. In the past children with bilateral single ectopic ureters often came to urinary diversion [65,66,71,79,86].

Coexisting ureteric pathology

PUJ obstruction occurs in association with duplication and has been documented in 5% of prenatally detected cases [15,89]. PUJ obstruction invariably affects the lower pole moiety of a bifid system, as the PUJ is poorly developed in the upper pole collecting system [89,90]. Prenatally detected PUJ obstruction can be managed conservatively [15] or by pyeloplasty [18]. Reduced function throughout the kidney may dictate bipolar nephrectomy [89]. Vesicoureteric junction (VUJ) obstruction has also been reported in association with duplication [91].

Yo-yo reflux

The term 'yo-yo' or 'saddle' reflux has been used to describe the presumed flow of urine between the two limbs of the Y configuration produced by incomplete duplication. Yo-yo reflux has been implicated as a possible cause of loin pain in later life and may also give rise to urinary infections. In these cases the upper pole ureter is frequently dilated and it is sometimes possible to visualize reflux of contrast between the limbs of the Y duplication on intravenous or ascending urography [4,92] or dynamic isotope scans [93]. Where surgical intervention is indicated the options include pyelopylostomy [94], i.e. joining the ureters at a higher level, or reimplantation of both ureters separately into the bladder [95].

Other rare duplication anomalies

Blind-ending ureter

If one of the ureteric buds fails to make contact with the metanephric blastema, a blind-ending duplicated ureter will result. Reviewing the literature Bauer found less than 70 reported cases, six of which had come from one group [96–98]. Symptoms relate to infection or calculi (which in turn reflect reflux or urinary stasis). Management is by excision [22,99].

Inverted Y ureter

This probably occurs when two duplicated ureteric buds fuse together before making contact with the metanephric blastema. As with complete duplication, the upper ureter may terminate ectopically [100] or in a ureterocele [101]. Distal atresia of one limb or an inverted Y has also been reported [102]. Treatment is by excision of the ectopic or troublesome ureter.

Ureteric triplication

Ureteric triplication is the result of three ureteric buds arising from the mesonephric duct [96]. It occurs more commonly in females and on the left side [103]. Triplicated ureters mostly join to form a single distal ureter, but separate upper moiety ureters may be ectopic [103]. Complications are secondary to reflux, ectopic ureter or ureterocele, and are managed in a similar fashion to duplication.

Bladder duplication

In cases of complete duplication the two bladders usually lie side by side, each with its own complete muscular wall, ipsilateral ureter, hemitrigone and duplicated urethra [104,105]. In 90% of cases the external genitalia are also duplicated and in 42% there is an associated hind gut duplication. Other genitourinary anomalies are common, as are vertebral anomalies [106]. In the rarer incomplete forms of duplication, the bladders communicate and drain via a single urethra [106,107]. Bladders divided by a septum containing muscle or just mucosa have been confused with duplication. Drainage is into a single urethra and complete septation, isolating one-half of the bladder, is associated with ipsilateral non-functioning kidney [106]. Management of these complex anomalies is aimed at unifying the bladders, reducing stasis and preserving continence.

Other anomalies

Some anomalies are compatible with normal life and rarely present in childhood [107], but are identified by antenatal ultrasound or through associated anomalies. Careful assessment and surveillance may be required to prevent future complications.

Malrotation of the kidney

This anomaly is seen in 1 in 939 post-mortems [108]. It is of little intrinsic significance but may form part of other anomalies of position and fusion.

Simple renal ectopia

Ectopic kidneys lying in the bony pelvis or low on the posterior abdominal wall are found in 1 in 900 individuals with an equal sex incidence [109]. In 10% of cases ectopia occurs bilaterally. Whereas most are sited below the pelvic brim, over the sacrum, or in the iliac fossa and iliolumbar area [110], rare instances have been reported in which an ectopic kidney has been found within the chest [111,112]. The blood supply is anomalous, axis deviation and rotation are common, and ectopic kidneys are often smaller than normal [110,113]. Most are asymptomatic and when the diagnosis is made prenatally, this usually stems from the discovery of an empty renal fossa on ultrasound [114,115]. Clinical presentation in infancy or childhood reflects the presence of complications notably PUJ obstruction, or VUR. Some asymptomatic pelvic kidneys are discovered as an incidental finding on abdominal examination. Associated anomalies of the cardiovascular, skeletal and gastrointestinal systems are not uncommon [112,113] and coexisting urological anomalies include hypospadias, cryptorchidism and urethral duplication in males, uterine and vaginal anomalies in females. Gleason reviewed 77 patients and found hydronephrosis in 56%; due to PUJ or VUJ obstruction in 52%, VUR in 26% and a redundant extrarenal pelvis in 22% [116]. The kidney's function and prognosis are determined by these problems.

Crossed renal ectopia

In this anomaly the functioning parenchyma corresponding to two kidneys lies fused on the same side of the abdomen with one of the two ureters crossing the midline. An incidence of 1 : 1000 live births has been reported [109] and the anomaly is more common in males [117,118]. Crossed renal ectopia accounts for 20–40% of ectopic kidneys [119,120]. In 90% the kidneys are fused, with two-thirds of ectopic kidneys lying inferiorly [121]. Solitary crossed ectopia is exceedingly rare [118,122].

Fifty per cent of cases have associated anomalies [109,117,118,120], with cardiovascular, skeletal, gastrointestinal and neurological systems involved.

Crossed renal ectopia may be diagnosed prenatally [114,117] or present as an asymptomatic mass during the course of abdominal palpations. When it gives rise to symptoms these usually reflect the presence of obstruction, reflux or calculi and management is individualized [119,120].

Horseshoe kidney

The commonest renal anomaly, it occurs in 0.25% of the population [108,123,124] with a male to female ratio of 2 : 1 [123,125–129]. Renal masses either side of the vertebral column are joined by a parenchymatous or fibrous isthmus at their lower poles in 95%, or more rarely at their upper poles [113,127]. Malrotation is usual and horseshoe kidneys are slightly ectopic [125]. Prenatal diagnosis is uncommon, since most horseshoe kidneys are not associated with detectable dilatation [130]. It has been estimated that only 10% of affected children present with clinical symptoms [129].

One-third of patients in clinical series have anomalies [131,132] of cardiovascular, CNS, musculoskeletal or gastrointestinal systems. Horseshoe kidney occurs in 3% of children with neural tube defects [133], 7% of patients with Turner's syndrome and 20% of cases of trisomy 18 [134]. Hypospadias and cryptorchidism are seen in 4%, with uterine and vaginal anomalies in females [132]. Duplication occurs in 10–30%, VUR in 8–32% and PUJ obstruction in 15–32% [113,125,126,129, 131,132]. Adult polycystic disease [127] and multicystic dysplasia [135,136] are described and there is an increased risk of Wilm's tumour [137].

Horseshoe kidney is found at post-mortem or during assessment of other anomalies [127]. Clinical presentation is mainly with urinary infection, although haematuria, abdominal pain, enuresis and abdominal mass are described in children [113,126,129]. All children require full urinary tract investigation and lifelong surveillance, although the kidney itself rarely causes death [126,132]. In one study, 60% of patients remained asymptomatic for 10 years [123]. Problems are caused by hydronephrosis in 8% of renal units and calculi in 12% [127]; this is commoner on the left and is due perhaps to its greater malrotation [125]. Stones recur if drainage is poor [128,129]. Pyeloplasty may be performed [113,127] and ureterocalicostomy is an option to establish good drainage [138]. Division of the isthmus is rarely, if ever, indicated [113,123,127].

Renal agenesis

Bilateral renal agenesis, Potter's syndrome, is a lethal anomaly affecting 0.3 in 1000 pregnancies. A male preponderance has been reported [5 : 1] [139]. Characteristic features include oligohydramnios, pulmonary hypoplasia, characteristic facies and moulding limb abnormalities. Death results from respiratory or renal failure [140]. Major cardiovascular, skeletal, gastrointestinal and chromosomal abnormalities are common [139,140]. The prenatal detection of severe oligohydramnios, coupled with an empty bladder and failure to identify the kidneys, offers the option of termination of pregnancy [141,142]. However, diagnostic difficulties can arise in early pregnancy as a result of poor ultrasound visualization, the late onset of oligohydramnios and difficulty in distinguishing the fetal kidneys and adrenals. Repeated ultrasound scans and other investigative modalities may be needed to establish the diagnosis with confidence [142–144].

Unilateral renal agenesis is relatively common. Mass screening of school children in Japan and Taiwan revealed an incidence of 1 in 1000 [145] and 1200 [146] respectively. It is slightly more common in males and affects the left kidney more frequently than the right [107]. Unilateral renal agenesis is being detected *in utero* [114], but cases of apparent renal agenesis in later childhood or adult life may represent the outcome of involution of a multicystic-dysplastic or hydronephrotic kidney [147,148]. The compensatory hypertrophy of the solitary contralateral kidney occurs in postnatal life but has also been noted *in utero* [149].

Cardiovascular, gastrointestinal, anorectal, musculoskeletal and chromosomal anomalies are common [150,151] and neural tube defects are recognized [133]. Structures derived from wolffian or mullarian ducts may be affected. Thus uterine, ovarian, tubal and vaginal anomalies are frequently seen in girls and cryptorchidism, hypospadias, urethral, vasal and prostatic anomalies in boys [152,153].

Whilst associated with normal life expectancy, solitary kidneys need evaluation postnatally and surveillance throughout life. Ultrasound and IVU reveal an abnormality in 90% of kidneys and reflux is demonstrated in 30% [154]. Argueso showed proteinuria in 19%, hypertension in 47%, increased filtration fraction in 54% and decreased renal function in 13% of patients evaluated at a mean age of 56 years [155]. Survival figures matched the general population, although 6 of 157 patients (4%) died of renal failure.

Supernumary kidney

This rare anomaly affects both sexes equally and is more usually left sided [156]. The supernumerary kidney is composed of hyperplastic tissue with an anomalous blood supply, lying above or below a normal kidney. Its parenchyma is separate from it and the two ureters cross, obeying the Wegert–Meyer law [157,158]. This condition is normally asymptomatic during childhood; its discovery is usually incidental [107].

References

1. Campbell MF, Harrison JH. Anomalies of the ureter. In: Campbell MF, Harrison JH (eds) *Urology* vol 2, 3rd edn. Philadelphia: WB Saunders, 1970; pp 1488, 1800.

2. Nation EF. Duplication of the kidney and ureter. A statistical study of 230 new cases. *J Urol* 1944; **51**: 456.

3. Perlmutter AD, Retik AB, Bauer SB. Anomalies of the upper urinary tract. In: Walsh PC, Gittes RF, Perlmutter AD, Stamey TA (eds) *Campbell's Urology*, vol 2, 5th edn. Philadelphia: WB Saunders, 1986; pp 1665–1759.

4. Privett JT, Jeans WD, Roylance J. The incidence and importance of renal duplication. *Clin Radiol* 1976; **27**: 521–530.

5. Avni EF, Dacher JN, Stallenberg B, Collier F, Hall M, Schulman CC. Renal duplications: the impact of perinatal ultrasound on diagnosis and management. *Eur Urol* 1991; **20**: 43–48.

6. Hartman GW, Hodson CJ. The duplex kidney and related abnormalities. *Clin Radiol* 1969; **20**: 387.

7. Whitaker J, Danks DM. A study of the inheritance of duplication of the kidneys and ureters. *J Urol* 1966; **95**: 176.

8. Glassberg KI, Braren V, Duckett JW et al. Suggested terminology for duplex systems, ectopic ureters and ureteroceles. *J Urol* 1984; **132**: 1153–1154.

9. Atwell JD, Cook PL, Howell CJ, Hyde I, Parker BC. Familial incidence of bifid and double ureters. *ADC* 1974; **49**: 390–393.

10. Meyer R. Zur anatomie und entwicklungsgeschickte der ureterverdoppelung. *Virchows Arch Path Anat Physiol Klin Med* 1907; **187**: 408–434.

11. Weigert C. Ueber einige bildungsfehler der ureteren. *Virchows Arch Path Anat Physiol Klin Med* 1877; **70**: 490–501.

12. Mackie GG, Stephens FD. Duplex kidneys: a correlation of renal dysplasia with the position of the ureteric orifice. *J Urol* 1975; **14**: 274–280.

13. Montfort G, Guys JM, Coquet M, Rith K, Louis C, Bocciardi A. Surgical management of duplex ureteroceles. *J Pediatr Surg* 1992; **27**: 634–638.

14. Gauthier F, Montupet P, Renouard C et al. Management of uropathies diagnosed prenatally. Discussion based on a series of 53 cases. [French]. *Chir Pediatr* 1987; **28**: 215–219.

15. Jee LD, Rickwood AMK, Williams MPL, Anderson PAM. Experience with duplex system anomalies detected by prenatal ultrasonography. *J Urol* 1993; **149**: 808–810.

16. Mandell J, Blyth BR, Peters CA, Retik AB, Estroff JA, Benacerraf BR. Structural genitourinary defects detected *in utero*. *Radiology* 1991; **178**: 193–196.

17. Woodard JR. The impact of fetal diagnosis on the management of obstructive uropathy. *Postgrad Med J* 1990; **66** (suppl 1): s37–43.

18. Winters WD, Lebowitz RL. Importance of prenatal detection of hydronephrosis of the upper pole. *Am J Roentgenol* 1990; **155**: 125–129.

19. Brown T, Mandell J, Lebowitz RL. Neonatal hydronephrosis in the era of sonography. *Am J Radiol* 1987; **148**: 959–963.

20. Ekter AS, Dhillon HK, Duffy PG, Ransley PG. *Prophylactic Incision of Ureteroceles in Prenatally Diagnosed Duplex Kidneys.* Birmingham: British Association of Urological Surgeons, 1994.

21. Elder JS, Duckett JW. Perinatal urology. In: Gillenwater JL, Grayhack JT, Howards SS, Duckett JW (eds) *Adult and Paediatric Urology*, vol 2. St Louis: Mosby Year Book, 1991, pp 1711–1810.

22. Snyder HM. Anomalies of the ureter. In: Gillenwater JY, Grayhack JT, Howards SS, Duckett JW (eds) *Adult and Paediatric Urology*, vol 2, 2nd edn. St Louis: Mosby Year Book, 1991, pp 1831–1862.

23. Mandell J, Colodny AH, Lebowitz R, Bauer SB, Retik AB. Ureteroceles in infants and children. *J Urol* 1980; **123**: 921.

24. Kaplan WE, Nasrallah P, King LR. Reflux in complete duplication in children. *J Urol* 1978; **120**: 220.

25. Husmann DA, Allen TD. Resolution of vesicoureteral reflux in completely duplicated systems: fact or fiction? *J Urol* 1991; **145**: 1022–1023.

26. Caldamone AA, Snyder HM, Duckett JW. Ureteroceles in children: followup of management with upper tract approach. *J Urol* 1984; **131**: 1130–1132.

27. Share JC, Lebowitz RL. The unsuspected double collecting system on imaging studies and at cystoscopy. *Am J Roentgenol* 1990; **155**: 561–564.

28. Aaronson IA, Cremin BJ. Duplex upper urinary tract, ectopic ureter, ureterocele. In: *Clinical Paediatric Radiology*, 1st edn. Edinburgh: Churchill Livingstone, 1984; pp 149–172.

29. Bisset GS, Strife JL. The duplex collecting system in girls with urinary tract infection: prevalence and significance. *Am J Radiol* 1987; **148**: 497–500.

30. Fehrenbacker LG, Kelalis PP, Stickler GB. Vesicoureteric reflux and ureteral duplication in children. *J Urol* 1972; **107**: 862–864.

31. Lee PH, Diamond DA, Duffy PG, Ransley PG. Duplex reflux: a study of 105 children. *J Urol* 1991; **146**: 657–659.

32. Peppas DS, Skoog SJ, Canning DA, Belman AB. Nonsurgical management of primary vesicoureteral reflux in complete ureteral duplication: is it justified? *J Urol* 1991; **146**: 1594–1595.

33. Ahmed S, Bocaut HA. Vesicoureteral reflux in complete ureteral duplication: surgical options. *J Urol* 1988; **140**: 1092–1094.

34. Kister W, Schärli AF, Winiker H. Ureteral reimplantation *en bloc* for refluxing duplicated ureters. *Pediatr Surg Int* 1994; **9**: 373–376.

35. Committee IRS. Medical versus surgical treatment of primary vesicoureteric reflux: a prospective international reflux study in children. *J Urol* 1981; **125**: 277–283.

36. Ben-Ami T, Gayer G, Hertz M, Lotan D, Boichis A. The natural history of reflux in the lower pole of duplicated collecting systems: a controlled study. *Pediatr Radiol* 1989; **19**: 308.

37. Weinstein AJ, Bauer SB, Retik AB, Mandell J, Colodny AH. The surgical management of megaureters in duplex systems: the efficacy of ureteral tapering and common sheath reimplantation. *J Urol* 1988; **139**: 328–331.

38. Persad R, Kamineni S, Mouriquand PDE. Recurrent symptoms of urinary tract infection in eight patients with refluxing ureteric stumps. *Br J Urol* 1994; **74**: 720–722.

39. Belman AB, Filmer RB, King LR. Surgical management of duplication of the collecting system. *J Urol* 1974; **112**: 220.

40. Hendren WH, Mitchell ME. Surgical correction of ureteroceles. *J Urol* 1979; **121**: 590–597.

41. Dewan PA, O'Donnell B. Polytef injection of refluxing duplex ureters. *Eur Urol* 1991; **19**: 35–38.

42. Caione P, Zaccara A, Capozza N, Gennaro MD. How prenatal ultrasound can affect treatment of ureteroceles in neonates and children. *Eur Urol* 1989; **16**: 195–199.

43. Cohen SJ. Ureteroceles. *Postgrad Med J* 1990; **66** (suppl 1): S47–S53.

44. Rickwood AMK, Reiner I, Jones M, Pournaras C. Current management of duplex system ureteroceles: experience with 41 patients. *Br J Urol* 1992; **70**: 196–200.

45. Scherz HC, Kaplan GW, Packer MG, Brock WA. Ectopic ureteroceles: surgical management with preservation of continence – a review of 60 cases. *J Urol* 1989; **142**: 538–541.

46. Thomas DFM, Whitaker RH. Reflux and duplex systems. In: Whitaker RH (ed) *Current Perspectives in Paediatric Urology*. London: Springer-Verlag, 1989; pp 1–16.

47. Kroovland RL, Perlmutter AD. A one stage approach to ectopic ureterocele. *J Urol* 1979; **122**: 367–369.

48. King LR, Koslowski JM, Schacht MJ. Ureteroceles in children. *JAMA* 1983; **249**: 1461–1465.

49. Decter RM, Roth DR, Gonzales ET. Individualised treatment of ureteroceles. *J Urol* 1989; **142**: 535–537.

50. Sen S, Ahmed S. Management of double system ureteroceles. *Aust NZ J Surg* 1987; **57**: 655–660.

51. Tank ES. Experience with endoscopic incision and open unroofing of ureteroceles. *J Urol* 1986; **136**: 241–242.

52. Dénes FT, Lopes RN, Arap S, Silva FAQ, Góes GMD. Prolapsed ureterocele. *Eur Urol* 1985; **11**: 106–109.

53. Cobb LM, Desai PG, Price SE. Surgical management of infantile (ectopic) ureteroceles: report of a modified approach. *J Pediatr Surg* 1982; **16**: 745–748.

54. Leong J, Mikhael B, Schillinger JF. Refluxing ureteroceles. *J Urol* 1980; **124**: 136–139.

55. Lam AH, Sachinwalla TN. Imaging of ureteral duplication with a non functioning component. *Australas Radiol* 1990; **34**: 64–67.

56. Montfort G, Morrison-Lacombe G, Coquet M. Endoscopic treatment of ureteroceles revisited. *J Urol* 1985; **133**: 1031–1033.

57. Uehling DT, Bruskewitz RC. Initiation of vesico-ureteral reflux after heminephrectomy for ureterocele. *Urology* 1989; **33**: 302–304.
58. Rich MA, Keating MA, III HMS, Duckett JW. Low transurethral incision of single system intravesical ureteroceles in children. *J Urol* 1990; **144**: 120–121.
59. Blyth B, Passerini-Glazel G, Camuffo C, III HMS, Duckett JW. Endoscopic incision of ureterocele: intravesical versus ectopic. *J Urol* 1993; **149**: 556–560.
60. Centron J, Melin Y, Valayer J. Simplified treatment of ectopic ureterocele in 35 children. *Eur Urol* 1981; **7**: 321,
61. Huisman TK, Kaplan GW, Brock WA, Packer MG. Ipsilateral ureteroureterostomy and pyeloureterostomy: a review of 15 years of experience with 25 patients. *J Urol* 1987; **138**: 1207–1210.
62. Williams DI, Woodard JR. Problems in the management of ectopic ureteroceles. *J Urol* 1964; **92**: 635.
63. Johnston JH, Johnson LM. Experiences with ectopic ureteroceles. *Br J Urol* 1969; **41**: 61.
64. Thompson IM, Amar AD. Clinical importance of ureteral duplication and ectopia. *JAMA* 1958; **168**: 881–886.
65. Gill B. Ureteric ectopy in children. *Br J Urol* 1980; **52**: 257–263.
66. Mandell J, Bauer SB, Colodny AH, Lebowitz RL, Retik AB. Ureteral ectopia in infants and children. *J Urol* 1981; **126**: 219–222.
67. Ellerker AG. The extravesical ectopic ureter. *Br J Surg* 1958; **45**: 344–353.
68. Johnston JH, Davenport TJ. The single ectopic ureter. *Br J Urol* 1969; **41**: 428–433.
69. Ahmed S, Barker A. Single system ectopic ureters: a review of 12 cases. *JPS* 1992; **27**: 491–496.
70. Scott JES. The single ectopic ureter and the dysplastic kidney. *Br J Urol* 1981; **53**: 300–305.
71. Gotoh T, Morita H, Tokunaka S, Koyanagi T, Tsuji I. Single ectopic ureter. *J Urol* 1983; **129**: 271–274.
72. Brannan W, Henry HH. Ureteral ectopia: report of 39 cases. *J Urol* 1973; **109**: 192–195.
73. Ahmed S, Morris LL, Byard RW. Ectopic ureter with complete ureteric duplication in the female child. *JPS* 1992; **27**: 1455–1460.
74. Mogg RA. Some observations on the ectopic ureter and ureterocele. *J Urol* 1967; **97**: 1003–1012.
75. Das S, Amar AD. Extravesical ureteral ectopia in male patients. *J Urol* 1981; **125**: 842–846.
76. Williams DI, Royle M. Ectopic ureter in the male child. *Br J Urol* 1969; **41**: 421–427.
77. Finan BF, Mollitt DL, Golladay ES, Redman JF. Giant ectopic ureter presenting as abdominal mass in an infant. *Urology* 1987; **30**: 246–247.
78. Cobb LM, Panagiotou E, Bowan A, Price SE. Ectopic ureter with seminal vesicle insertion in an infant with tracheo-oesophageal fistula and possible adult polycystic kidney disease. *J Urol* 1983; **129**: 1036–1039.
79. Kesavan P, Ramakrishnan MS, Fowler R. Ectopia in unduplicated ureters in children. *Br J Urol* 1977; **49**: 481–493.
80. Nussbaum AR, Dorst JP, Jeffs RD, Gearhart JP, Sanders RC. Ectopic ureter and ureterocele: their varied sonographic manifestations. *Radiology* 1986; **159**: 227–235.
81. Wyly JB, Lebowitz RL. Refluxing urethral ectopic ureters: recognition by the cyclic voiding cystourethrogram. *Am J Roentgenol* 1984; **142**: 1263–1267.
82. Amar AD. Improved methods in the diagnosis of ureteral duplication and ectopia. *Can Med Assoc J* 1966; **95**: 813–817.
83. Erlich RM, Koyle MA, Shanberg AM. A technique for ureteral stump ablation. *J Urol* 1988; 1240–1241.
84. Smith FL, Ritchie EL, Maizels M et al. Surgery for duplex kidneys with ectopic ureters: ipsilateral ureteroureterostomy versus polar nephrectomy. *J Urol* 1989; **142**: 532–534.
85. Marshall S. Reimplantation of the dilated ectopic ureter of the duplex system as a separate unit. *J Urol* 1986; **135**: 574–575.
86. Williams DI, Lightwood RG. Bilateral single ectopic ureters. *Br J Urol* 1972; **44**: 267–273.
87. Blundon KE, Lane JW. Diagnostic difficulties in ureteral ectopia. *J Urol* 1960; **84**: 463–469.
88. Dange AS, Sen S, Zachariah N, Chaco J, Mammen KE. Single system ureteral ectopia. *Pediatr Surg Int* 1994; **9**: 377–380.
89. Das S, Amar AD. Ureteropelvic junction obstruction with associated renal anomalies. *J Urol* 1984; **131**: 872–874.
90. Ossandon F, Androulakis P, Ransley PG. Surgical problems in pelviureteral junction obstruction of the lower moiety in incomplete duplex systems. *J Urol* 1981; **125**: 872–875.
91. Androulakis PA, Ossandon F, Ransley PG. Intrinsic pathology of the lower moiety ureter in the duplex kidney with ectopic ureterocele. *J Urol* 1981; **125**: 873–874.
92. Kaplan N, Elkin M. Bifid renal pelves and ureters. Radiographic and cinefluorographic observations. *Br J Urol* 1968; **40**: 235–244.
93. O'Reilly PH, Lawson RS, Sheilds RA, Testa HJ, Edwards EC, Carroll RN. A radioisotope method of assessing uretero-ureteric reflux. *Br J Urol* 1978; **50**: 164–168.
94. Tressider GC., Blandy JP, Murray RS. Pyelo-pelvic and uretero-ureteric reflux. *Br J Urol* 1970; **42**: 728–735.
95. Amar AD. Treatment of reflux in bifid ureters by conversion to complete duplication. *J Urol* 1972; **108**: 77.
96. Bauer SB, Perlmutter AD, Retik AB. Anomalies of the upper urinary tract. In: Walsh PC, Retik AB, Stamey TA Jr EDV (eds) *Campbell's Urology*, vol 2, 6th edn. Philadelphia: WB Saunders, 1992; pp 1357–1442.

97. Albers DD, Geyer JR, Barnes SD. Blind ending branch of bifid ureters: report of three cases. *J Urol* 1968; **99**: 160.

98. Albers DD, Geyer JR, Barnes SD. Clinical significance of blind ending branch of bifid ureter: report of 3 additional cases. *J Urol* 1971; **105**: 634.

99. Konturri M, Kaski P. Blind ending bifid ureter with ureteroureteral reflux. *Scand J Nephrol Urol* 1972; **6**: 91.

100. Beasley SW, Kelly JH. Inverted Y duplication of the ureter in association with ureterocele and bladder diverticulum. *J Urol* 1986; **136**: 899–900.

101. Ecke M, Klatte D. Inverted Y ureteral duplication with a uterine ectopy as a cause of enuresis. *Urol Int* 1989; **44**: 116–118.

102. Britt DB, Borden TA, Woodhead DM. Inverted Y ureteral duplication with a blind ending branch. *J Urol* 1972; **108**: 387.

103. Perkins PJ, Kroovland RL, Evans AT. Ureteral triplication. *Radiology* 1973; **108**: 533–538.

104. Dunetz GN, Bauer SB. Complete duplication of the bladder and urethra. *Urology* 1985; **25**: 179–182.

105. Kossow JH, Morales PA. Duplication of bladder and urethra and associated anomalies. *Urology* 1973; **1**: 71.

106. Woodhouse CRJ, Williams DI. Duplications of the lower urinary tract in children. *Br J Urol* 1979; **51**: 481–487.

107. Bauer SB, Perlmutter AD, Retik AB. Anomalies of the upper urinary tract. In: Walsh PC, Retik AB, Stamey TA, Jr EDV (eds) *Campbell's Urology*, vol 2, 6th edn. Philadelphia: WB Saunders, 1992; pp 1357–1442.

108. Campbell MF. Anomalies of the kidney. In: Campbell MF, Harrison JH (eds) *Urology*. Philadelphia: WB Saunders, 1970; pp 1447–1452.

109. Abeshouse B, Bhisitkul I. Crossed renal ectopia with and without fusion. *Urol Int* 1959; **9**: 63–91.

110. Dretler S, Olsson C, Pfister R. The anatomic, radiologic and clinical characteristics of the pelvic kidney: an analysis of 86 cases. *J Urol* 1971; **105**: 623–627.

111. Hill J, Bunts R. Thoracic kidney: case reports. *J Urol* 1960; **84**: 460–462.

112. Malek R, Kelalis P, Burke E. Ectopic kidney in children and frequency of association with other malformations. *Mayo Clin Proc* 1971; **46**: 461–467.

113. Hendren W, Donahoe P. Renal fusions and ectopia. In: Welch K, Randolph J, Ravitch M, O'Neill J, Rowe M (eds) *Pediatric Surgery*, vol 2. Chicago: Year Book Medical, 1986; pp 1134–1145.

114. Jeanty P, Romero R, Kepple D, Stoney D, Coggins T, Fleisher A. Prenatal diagnoses in unilateral empty renal fossa. *J Ultrasound Med* 1990; **9**: 651–654.

115. Hill L, Grzybek P, Mills A, Hogge W. Antenatal diagnosis of fetal pelvic kidneys. *Obstet Gynecol* 1994; **83**: 333–336.

116. Gleason P, Kelalis P, Husmann D, Kramer S. Hydronephrosis in renal ectopia: incidence, etiology and significance. *J Urol* 1994; **151**: 1660–1661.

117. Boatman D, Culp Jr D, Culp D, Flocks R. Crossed renal ectopia. *J Urol* 1972; **108**: 30–31.

118. Hertz M, Rubenstein Z, Shahin N, Melzer M. Crossed renal ectopia: clinical and radiological findings in 22 cases. *Clin Radiol* 1977; **28**: 339–344.

119. Kelalis P, Malek R, Segura J. Observations on renal ectopia and fusion in children. *J Urol* 1973; **110**: 588–592.

120. Kyrayiannis B, Stenos J, Deliveliotis A. Ectopic kidneys with and without fusion. *Br J Urol* 1979; **51**: 173–174.

121. McDonald J, McClellan D. Crossed renal ectopia. *Am J Surg* 1957; **93**: 995–1002.

122. Caine M. Crossed renal ectopia without fusion. *Br J Urol* 1956; **28**: 257–258.

123. Glenn JF. Analysis of 51 patients with horseshoe kidney. *New Engl J Med* 1959; **261**: 684–687.

124. Dees J. Clinical importance of congenital anomalies of the upper urinary tract. *J Urol* 1941; **46**: 659.

125. Whitehouse G. Some urographic aspects of the horseshoe kidney anomaly – a review of 59 cases. *Clin Radiol* 1975; **25**: 107–114.

126. Segura J, Kelalis P, Burke E. Horseshoe kidney in children. *J Urol* 1972; **108**: 333–336.

127. Pitts W, Muecke E. Horseshoe kidneys: a 40 year experience. *J Urol* 1975; **113**: 743–746.

128. Kölln C, Boatman D, Schmidt J, Flocks R. Horseshoe kidney: a review of 105 patients. *J Urol* 1972; **107**: 203–204.

129. Wilson C, Azmy A. Horseshoe kidney in children. *Br J Urol* 1986; **58**: 361–363.

130. Bronshtein M, Yoffe N, Brandes J, Blumenfeld Z. First and early second trimester diagnosis of fetal urinary tract anomalies using transvaginal sonography. *Prenat Diagn* 1990; **10**: 653–666.

131. Zondek LH, Zondek T. Horseshoe kidney and associated congenital malformations. *Urol Int* 1964; **18**: 347.

132. Boatman D, Kölln C, Flocks R. Congenital anomalies associated with horseshoe kidney. *J Urol* 1972; **107**: 205–207.

133. Whitaker R, Hunt G. Incidence and distribution of renal anomalies in patients with neural tube defects. *Eur Urol* 1987; **13**: 322–323.

134. Lippe B, Geffner M, Deitrich R, Boechat M, Kangarloo H. Renal malformations in patients with Turner syndrome: imaging in 141 patients. *Pediatrics* 1988; **82**: 852–856.

135. Boullier J, Chehval M, Purcell M. Removal of a multicystic half of a horseshoe kidney: significance of preoperative evaluation in identifying abnormal surgical anatomy. *J Pediatr Surg* 1992; **27**: 1244–1246.

136. Van-Every M. *In utero* detection of horseshoe kidney with unilateral multicystic dysplasia. *Urology* 1992; **40**: 435–437.

137. Mesrobian H, Kelalis P, Hrabovsky E, Othersen H, DeLorimer A, Nesmith B. Wilms tumour in horseshoe kidneys: a report from the National Wilms tumour study. *J Urol* 1985; **133**: 1002–1004.

138. Mollard P, Braun P. Primary ureterocalycostomy for severe hydronephrosis in children. *J Pediatr Surg* 1980; **15**: 87–91.

139. Potter E. Bilateral renal agenesis. *J Pediatr* 1946; **29**: 68–76.

140. Potter E. Bilateral absence of ureters and kidneys. A report of 50 cases. *Obstet Gynecol* 1965; **94**: 3–12.

141. Kierse M, Meerman R. Antenatal diagnosis of Potter syndrome. 1978; **52**(1(S)): 64s–67s.

142. Romero R, Cullen M, Grannum P et al. Antenatal diagnosis of renal anomalies with ultrasound. III. Bilateral renal agenesis. *Am J Obstet Gynecol* 1985; **151**: 38–43.

143. McGohan J, Myracle M. Adrenal hypertrophy: possible pitfall in the sonographic diagnosis of renal agenesis. *J Ultrasound Med* 1986; **5**: 265–268.

144. Bronshtein M, Amit A, Achiron R, Noy I, Blumenfeld Z. The early prenatal sonographic diagnosis of renal agenesis: techniques and possible pitfalls. *Prenat Diag* 1994; **14**: 291–297.

145. Mihara M, Ito Y, Fukushima K, Yamashita F, Tsunosue M. Ultrasonic screening for renal abnormalities in three-year-old children. *Acta Paediatr* 1992; **81**: 326–328.

146. Sheih C, Hung C, Wei C, Lin C. Cystic dilatations within the pelvis in patients with ipsilateral renal agenesis or dysplasia. *J Urol* 1990; **144**: 324–327.

147. Hitchcock R, Burge D. Renal agenesis: an acquired condition? *J Pediatr Surg* 1994; **29**: 454–455.

148. Mesrobian H, Rushton H, Bulas D. Unilateral renal agenesis may result from *in utero* regression of multicystic dysplasia. *J Urol* 1993; **150**: 793–794.

149. Harsthorne N, Shepard T, Barr M. Compensatory renal growth in fetuses with unilateral renal agenesis. *Teratology* 1991; **441**: 7–10.

150. Nicolaides K, Cheng H, Abbas A, Snijders R, Gosden C. Fetal renal defects: associated malformations and chromosomal defects. *Fetal Diagn Ther* 1992; **7**: 1–11.

151. Emanuel B, Nachman R, Aronson N, Weiss H. Congenital solitary kidney. *Am J Dis Child* 1974; **127**: 17–19.

152. Trigaux J, Van-Beers B, Delchambre F. Male genital tract malformations associated with ipsilateral renal agenesis: sonographic findings. *J Clin Ultrasound* 1991; **19**: 3–10.

153. Acien P, Ruiz J, Hernandez J, Susarte F, del-Moral M. Renal agenesis in association with malformation of the female genital tract. *Am J Obstet Gynecol* 1991; **165**: 1368–1370.

154. Atiyeh B, Hussman D, Baum M. Contralateral renal anomalies in patients with renal agenesis and noncystic renal dysplasia. *Pediatrics* 1993; **91**: 812–815.

155. Argueso L, Ritchey M, Boyle E, Milliner D, Bergstralh E, Kramer S. Prognosis of patients with unilateral renal agenesis. *Pediatr Nephrol* 1992; **6**: 412–416.

156. N'Guessan G, Stephens F. Supernumerary kidney. *J Urol* 1983; **130**: 649–653.

157. Meyer R. Zur anatomie und entwicklungsgeschickte der ureterverdoppelung. *Virchows Arch Path Anat Physiol Klin Med* 1907; **187**: 408–434.

158. Weigert C. Ueber einige bildungsfehler der ureteren. *Virchows Arch Path Anat Physiol Klin Med* 1877; **70**: 490–501.

17

Cystic renal disease in childhood

D.F.M. Thomas and M.M. Fitzpatrick

Introduction

The bewildering nomenclature historically used in the classification of cystic renal disorders of childhood has not enhanced our understanding of these important and relatively common forms of congenital renal pathology. Terms such as multicystic, polycystic, aplasia and Potter's type I, II and III, shed little light on the underlying defect of embryogenesis, clinical significance or pattern of inheritance.

Clinically the most common source of confusion stems from failure to distinguish accurately between multicystic dysplastic kidney (MDK), a structural embryological defect which in its usual unilateral form carries a good prognosis, and polycystic renal disease (polycystic kidneys), a genetically determined, more diffuse disorder of the renal parenchyma associated with important extrarenal manifestations.

Figure 17.1 summarizes the important distinguishing features of the different forms of paediatric cystic renal disease.

Incidence of cystic renal disease in childhood

The true incidence of cystic renal disease in the paediatric population is difficult to gauge. Autopsy data, derived from a selected paediatric population, inevitably yield a higher incidence of serious renal pathology. In addition to those children whose deaths have been caused directly by renal pathology, paediatric autopsies frequently reveal non-lethal uropathies in children with multiple congenital anomalies. Conversely, the true incidence of certain 'silent' asymptomatic forms of unilateral cystic pathology, e.g. multicystic dysplastic kidney, simple cysts, etc. is only now becoming apparent as the use of ultrasound becomes more routine.

Reviewing a series of 6521 consecutive autopsies in infants and children, Mir and associates [1] at the Children's Hospital University of Helsinki found evidence of renal cysts in 136 cases (2%). Of these 136 infants and children, 103 died in the first month of life. Coexisting extrarenal anomalies were identified in 102 of the 136 cases and the well-recognized association between oesophageal atresia and renal abnormalities was noted in 29 (21%) of their cases.

Polycystic renal disease

Polycystic kidney disease in children is an inherited disorder with diffuse cystic involvement of both kidneys, without dysplasia [2]. There are two major forms presenting in childhood, autosomal recessive polycystic kidney disease (ARPKD) and autosomal dominant polycystic kidney disease (ADPKD). Considerable overlap exists both in clinical presentation and radiographic features.

		AETIOLOGY	ASSOCIATED ABNORMALITIES
MULTICYSTIC DYSPLASTIC KIDNEY	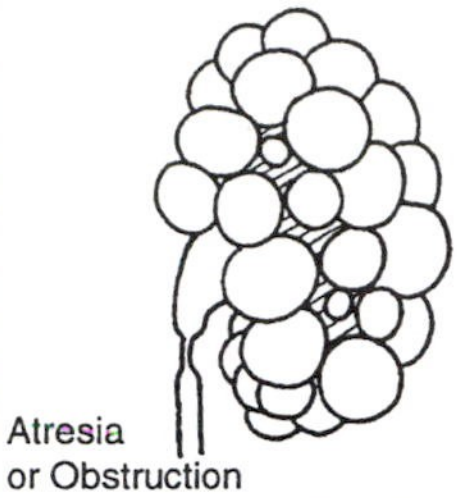 Atresia or Obstruction	Inheritance poorly studied. Probably sporadic	***Urological*** Contralateral PUJ obstruction, Vesico Ureteric reflux, ***Non urological*** eg Oesophageal Atresia
AUTOSOMAL DOMINANT POLYCYSTIC DISEASE	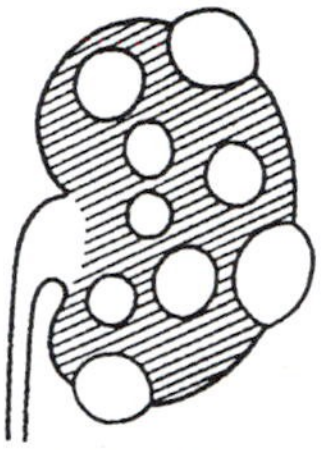	Inherited Autosomal Dominant	Cerebral Vessel Aneurysms or Hepatic Cysts
AUTOSOMAL RECESSIVE POLYCYSTIC DISEASE	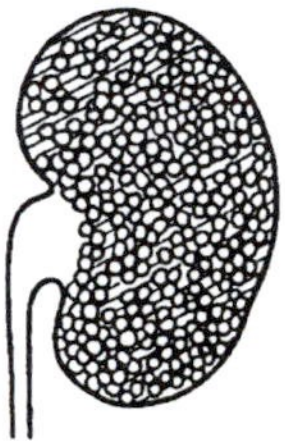	Inherited Autosomal Recessive	Congenital Hepatic Fibrosis
MULTILOCULAR CYST	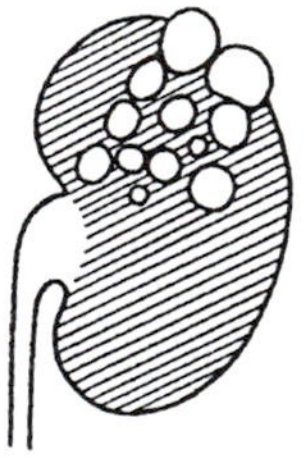	Sporadic Anomaly or Neoplastic	
SIMPLE CYST	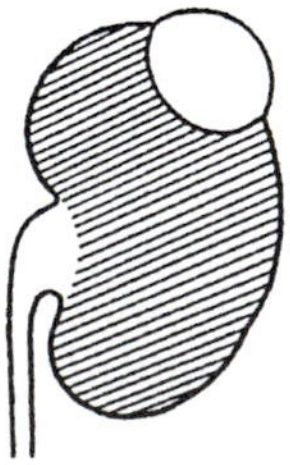	Acquired (rare in infancy)	

Figure 17.1 Cystic renal pathology of childhood, characteristics, aetiology and associated abnormalities.

Autosomal recessive polycystic kidney disease

This disorder involves cystic dilatation of renal collecting ducts and some biliary dysgenesis and periportal fibrosis. The exact incidence is unknown. However, current estimates based on published data put the incidence of ARPKD between 1 in 10 000 and 1 in 40 000 [3].

Antenatal diagnosis

The diagnosis is suggested by antenatal ultrasound findings of enlarged kidneys, oligohydramnios, and absence of urine in the bladder. It has been noted that sonographic features (Figure 17.2) may be present in the second trimester but usually are not apparent until after 30 weeks [4]. Increased maternal α-fetoprotein has been reported but this is a non-specific finding.

Pathology

In the newborn the kidneys are large but normal in shape. Microscopically the cysts are usually less than 2 mm in size and have been shown to be dilated collecting ducts [5–7]. As

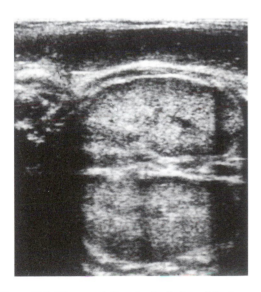

Figure 17.2 Ultrasound. Longitudinal view of fetal abdomen showing diffusely enlarged fetal kidneys. Characteristic prenatal ultrasound features of autosomal, recessive polycystic kidney disease.

the child grows, larger renal cysts develop, and fibrosis and hyperplasia become more prominent, producing a pattern more like that seen in the autosomal dominant polycystic kidney disease. A degree of biliary dysgenesis and hepatic fibrosis is always present and with time, hepatomegaly and portal hypertension become evident in most children.

Clinical presentation and course

Most patients present in infancy [3,8–10]. Some present at birth with huge flank masses that can complicate delivery. Severely affected infants may have pulmonary hypoplasia and features of Potter's syndrome. Respiratory distress is often an early complication, and infants with true pulmonary hypoplasia often die soon after birth with pulmonary failure. Death from renal failure is uncommon in the newborn period. Infants who survive the neonatal period usually have a decreased glomerular filtration rate, but their renal function may improve with renal maturation.

Almost all affected children have a concentrating defect and a degree of polyuria and polydypsia [3,8–10]. Hypertension is common and can be a presenting feature [3,11]. It is important that hypertension is treated aggressively as this may lead to progression of renal insufficiency.

An older child may present with the complications of hepatic fibrosis and portal hypertension, including hepatosplenomegaly, bleeding oesophageal varices, portal thrombosis and hypersplenism [12,13]. A serious complication in children with significant hepatic involvement is bacterial ascending cholangitis [9].

Radiological features (Table 17.1)

The intravenous pyelogram in infancy generally shows large delayed nephrograms [14]. Computed tomography (CT) with enhancement shows linear or radial opacification in enlarged kidneys [9]. The ultrasound findings are generally those of large kidneys with an increased echogenicity obscuring the corticomedullary junction [15]. The liver in affected infants is usually normal in size but dilated intrahepatic biliary ducts or poor visualization of the peripheral portal veins due to fibrous

Table 17.1 Radiological distinction between autosomal recessive polycystic kidney disease (ARPKD) and autosomal dominant polycystic kidney disease (ADPKD)

	ARPKD	*ADPKD*
Ultrasound	Bilateral, enlarged, diffusely echogenic kidneys, occasional macrocysts (<2 cm)	Enlarged kidneys with macrocysts (>2 cm) of varying sizes, may be unilateral
	Hepatic periportal fibrosis; intrahepatic biliary dilatation	Extrarenal cysts (liver, pancreas, ovary, spleen)
IVP	Enlarged kidneys with poor function, delayed mottled nephrogram	Enlarged kidneys with caliceal splaying around macrocysts

tissue may be demonstrated [16]. In older children the IVP findings are less specific and tend to resemble those seen in ADPKD.

Clinical management

With improvements in neonatal intensive care, the survival of affected neonates has improved and it may now be difficult to predict which newborns requiring ventilation have pulmonary hypoplasia incompatible with survival [2]. It is important that those infants without significant renal impairment are closely followed, since most will have a concentrating defect and may therefore be at risk during periods of dehydration associated with intercurrent infections. Hypertension, if present, must be treated aggressively and if urinary tract infection occurs, appropriate imaging should be undertaken. Electrolyte and acid–base balance should be carefully monitored and treated appropriately.

The treatment of chronic renal failure in children with ARPKD is as with other children in chronic renal failure, and this has improved over the last decade with aggressive management of renal bone disease, use of erythropoietin and an emphasis on nutritional support. Dialysis and/or transplantation are indicated when these children reach end-stage renal failure. Renal transplantation offers definitive replacement therapy, and at the time of transplantation, nephrectomies may be indicated to control hypertension, or to allow for graft placement if the native kidneys are massively enlarged. In children with predominant hepatic involvement, monitoring for the potential complications of portal hypertension is very important.

Prognosis

This is difficult to assess, but survival of all but the most severely affected newborns who have significant pulmonary hypoplasia seems now possible. In a recent series actuarial survival rates calculated from birth revealed 86% alive at 3 months, 79% at 1 year, 51% at 10 years and 46% at 15 years [10].

Autosomal dominant polycystic kidney disease

This disorder is characterized by the presence of renal cysts at any point along the nephron and by a characteristic pattern of extrarenal manifestations of the gastrointestinal and cardiovascular system [5,17]. This is the most common inherited human kidney disease; its prevalence ranges from 1 in 200 to 1 in 1000 [17]. The gene responsible has been localized to the short arm of chromosome 16, closely linked to the α-haemoglobin gene [17,18]. This allows for presymptomatic, even antenatal diagnosis in informative families; however, diagnosing ADPKD years before the onset of symptoms has potential major problems and ethical implications.

Antenatal diagnosis

Antenatal ultrasound findings of enlarged kidneys with or without cysts and absent urine in the bladder have been reported in families with known ADPKD, but these findings are not often evident until the third trimester [19,20].

Presentation and clinical course

A wide spectrum of presentation is encountered in paediatric practice, ranging from severe neonatal manifestations, which are very rare and indistinguishable from ARPKD, to the incidental discovery of cysts on renal ultrasound scanning in asymptomatic children [2,8,11]. Again hypertension can affect infants and indeed is common even in those with normal renal function. Older children may present with hypertension, abdominal pain, palpable abdominal masses, haematuria, urinary tract infections, abdominal or inguinal hernias and, very rarely, renal failure.

Extrarenal manifestations are rare in childhood, but when present can help to differentiate ADPKD from ARPKD. These may include hepatic, pancreatic or ovarian cysts [21,22]. There are reports in the literature of cerebral vessel aneurysms in children with ADPKD [23] and of endocardial fibroelastosis [24].

Management

Asymptomatic children in ADPKD families who are at risk, should be followed annually for the development of haematuria, hypertension or palpable abdominal masses. The development of hypertension, renal failure and end-stage renal failure need to be treated appropriately. The risk of hypertension is correlated with renal cyst number and size and poorly controlled hypertension is a major factor in premature renal functional deterioration [25,26]. Urinary tract infections need to be promptly and appropriately treated, occasionally cyst drainage may be necessary to control infection, and in extreme cases nephrectomy may be indicated.

Prognosis

Neonatal ADPKD may have a poor prognosis but this remains uncertain [2,27]. Presentation of ADPKD in the older child, however, has a good prognosis – over 80% of children diagnosed by ultrasound in one large series maintained normal renal function throughout childhood [27].

Multicystic dysplastic kidney

Before the advent of routine prenatal ultrasound, the multicystic dysplastic kidney (MDK) was regarded as something of a urological curiosity, a rare anomaly generally presenting as an abdominal mass in the neonatal period. Nephrectomy was undertaken as a matter of routine. It is becoming apparent, however, that the MDK is a far more common anomaly than was previously suspected. In most instances, however, the lesion is small, unilateral and difficult, if not impossible, to detect clinically during routine neonatal examination in affected infants who are otherwise healthy and outwardly normal. The heightened interest in this renal anomaly in recent years stems from the controversies surrounding the 'prophylactic' surgical removal of these asymptomatic lesions. In turn, the indications for nephrectomy centre on the perceived risk of late complications and the natural history of MDKs left *in situ*.

Incidence

Our data [28] and those reported by Rickwood et al. from Liverpool [29] place the incidence of unilateral MDK at around 1 in 4000 live births. The incidence of bilateral MDK is approximately 1 in 20 000 pregnancies [28, 30,31].

Pathogenesis and inheritance

Macroscopically the MDK consists of an irregular, characteristically 'knobbly' mass of tense, discrete cysts of varying size with small intervening islands of dysplastic parenchymal tissue (Figure 17.3). MDKs are usually associated with atresia of the proximal ureter at the pelviureteric junction, but MDKs are also occasionally found in conjunction with distal ureteric obstruction.

The underlying aetiological mechanism appears to be an obstructive insult dating from the earliest stages of gestation. In turn this probably results from a ureteric bud abnormality resulting in failure to establish patency of the collecting system and disordered induction of metanephric mesenchyme.

Although MDK has generally been regarded as a sporadic anomaly, the occurrence of

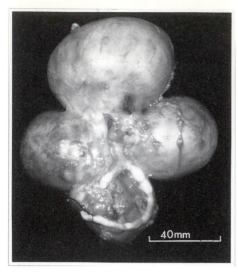

Figure 17.3 Nephrectomy specimen. Multicystic dysplastic kidney – note 'beaded' atretic proximal ureter. (Courtesy of P. G. Ransley.)

unilateral MDKs in siblings has been encountered by ourselves [32] and others [33]. The family study of renal dysplasia undertaken by Al Saadi et al. [34] identified affected siblings in only 1 out of 21 families studied. However, this was a post-mortem study and the definition of renal dysplasia was extended to include other forms of renal pathology apart from multicystic renal dysplasia. Krull et al. [35] retrospectively studied 48 children with multicystic renal dysplasia, of whom fewer than half had been diagnosed prenatally. While no incidence of familial occurrence of multicystic renal dysplasia was identified, various other forms of renal diseases were found in eight of the families studied. MDK is one of the anomalies encompassed by hereditary renal adysplasia (HRA), an autosomal dominant condition with incomplete penetrance and variable expression, of which bilateral or unilateral renal agenesis are the most important components [36]. Roodhooft et al. [37] found silent urological abnormalities in 9% of the parents of cases of bilateral renal agenesis. The documented association with renal agenesis, vesicoureteric reflux (conditions with a known genetic basis), and pelviureteric junction (PUJ) obstruction (in which a familial inheritance is sometimes implicated) indicates that genetic factors may play a more important role in the aetiology of MDK than was previously recognized. Systematic family and genetic studies

aimed at defining the importance of these genetic factors could be of value in counselling and might ultimately shed new light on the genetic regulation of embryological development of the urinary tract.

Presentation

Prenatal ultrasound

Nowadays the majority of cases are identified as an incidental finding on routine prenatal ultrasound (Figure 17.4). Although the prenatal ultrasound appearances are usually characteristic, the differential diagnosis between multicystic dysplastic kidney and severe hydronephrosis (PUJ obstruction) can still pose an occasional diagnostic challenge – even for the experienced radiologist. Bilateral MDKs generally represent a straightforward prenatal diagnosis: the fetal abdomen is occupied by echolucent cysts, the bladder is empty and oligohydramnios is invariably present (Figure 17.5). In our experience most MDKs are evident on second-trimester ultrasound, but Kelleher et al. [38] reported that only 33% of their prenatally detected cases were identified on ultrasound before 20 weeks' gestation.

Postnatal presentation

Abdominal mass

Prior to the advent of prenatal ultrasound, MDKs most commonly presented as an abdominal mass in the neonatal period. Abdominal masses are not common in new-

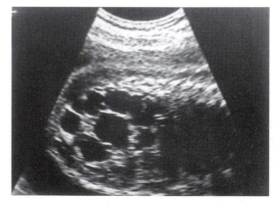

Figure 17.4 Characteristic prenatal ultrasound appearances of multicystic dysplastic kidney.

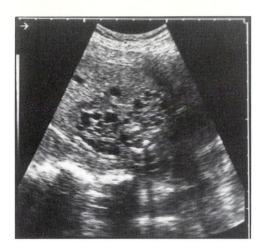

Figure 17.5 Prenatal ultrasound appearances of bilateral multicystic dysplastic kidneys, i.e. fetal abdomen occupied by renal cysts, oligohydramnios.

born infants, but when they do occur more than half are renal in origin. Griscom [39], reviewing a series of 117 neonatal abdominal masses, reported that 63 (54%) arose within the kidney. MDK was the most commonly encountered abdominal mass, i.e. 25 cases (21%), with hydronephrosis (PUJ obstruction) accounting for 20 cases (17%). Other neonatal renal masses include polycystic kidneys, renal neoplasms and renal vein thrombosis. Most renal neonatal abdominal masses, e.g. hydronephrosis, intestinal duplication, cysts, ovarian cysts, etc., have a smooth surface on palpation, whereas the surface of a MDK is characteristically irregular and 'knobbly'.

Respiratory distress
Bilateral multicystic renal dysplasia is a lethal anomaly, not only because of the total absence of functioning renal tissue but also because the associated oligohydramnios gives rise to pulmonary hypoplasia. On the rare occasions when bilateral MDKs have not been detected prenatally or when the offer of termination has been declined, the inevitable outcome for any liveborn infant is early neonatal death from pulmonary insufficiency.

Urinary infection
In the past MDKs occasionally came to light during the investigation of urinary infections. In these rare instances, however, the urinary infection is usually associated with a coexisting urological anomaly, notably vesicoureteric reflux (VUR), rather than the MDK itself (a combination of ureteric atresia and the non-communicating nature of the cysts prevents the access of ascending bacterial infection into the lesion itself.)

Renal failure
A unilateral MDK poses no threat to overall renal function unless the contralateral kidney is also congenitally abnormal or has sustained postnatal damage, e.g. as the result of reflux nephropathy. In practice, it is exceedingly rare for MDK to present with renal failure in childhood, but when this does occur it is generally the outcome of PUJ obstruction in the contralateral kidney.

Diagnosis

Postnatal ultrasound

In addition to documenting the ultrasound appearances of MDK in the affected kidney, the initial postnatal ultrasound study is aimed at looking for evidence of dilatation indicating contralateral PUJ obstruction or VUR. The diagnostic ultrasound characteristics of multicystic dysplastic kidney have been defined by Stuck et al. [40] as:

1. Presence of interfaces between the cysts.
2. Non-medial location of the largest cyst.
3. Absence of identifiable renal sinus.
4. Multiplicity of non-communicating overall round cysts.
5. Absence of parenchymal tissue.

Isotope imaging, e.g. ^{99m}Tc-DMSA, ^{99m}Tc-MAG3

The results of isotope imaging rarely influence clinical management in the first few weeks of life and functional studies are best deferred until 4–6 weeks of age when findings can be interpreted more reliably than in the early neonatal period. Most centres favour static imaging with ^{99m}Tc-DMSA but in the presence of dilatation in the contralateral kidney a dynamic study, e.g. ^{99m}Tc-MAG3 has the additional benefit of generating drainage curve data. Typically MDK has no demonstrable isotope uptake, i.e. zero function, whereas most hydronephrotic kidneys retain some differential function – although this may amount to little more than a few per cent.

The combination of ultrasound and isotope imaging should enable the diagnosis of MDK to be made with sufficient certainty to avoid the need for nephrectomy on purely diagnostic grounds alone. Intermediate forms of the anomaly have been described in which some of the features of MDK are combined with some of those of PUJ obstruction [41]. On the rare occasions when low levels of residual isotope uptake are detected, nephrectomy is preferred.

Voiding cystourethrogram

VUR is the anomaly most commonly observed in association with MDK, with a reported incidence of 28–43% [38,42–44] (Table 17.2). In this situation VUR affecting the contralateral upper tract is generally low grade and self limiting. Whether a voiding cystourethrogram

(VCU) should be performed routinely in all infants with a MDK is arguable. The investigation is invasive and often distressing to the infants and their parents. For this reason, we prefer to reserve voiding cystography for those children with evidence of ureteric or contralateral pelvicaliceal dilatation on ultrasound.

Other investigations

Intravenous urography (IVU) and other investigations such as percutaneous cyst puncture add little to the information derived from the modalities described above and as such serve no useful role in the routine investigative protocol.

Management

Management of the child with a prenatally detected MDK can be subdivided into the

Table 17.2 Frequency of coexistent urinary tract anomalies associated with multicystic dysplastic kidney

Contralateral pathology	Frequency	Population studied
Bilateral MDKs	5 out of 27 cases (19%)	Fetal population Kleiner 1986 [31]
	2 out of 12 cases (17%)	Fetal population Gordon et al. 1988 [28]
Vesicoureteric reflux*	23 out of 64 cases (36%)	Unilateral MDK Kelleher et al. 1993 [38]
	8 out of 29 cases (28%)	Unilateral MDK Flack and Bellinger 1993 [42]
	28 out of 65 cases (43%)	MDK Registry Data Wacksman and Phipps 1993 [43]
	9 out of 49 cases (18%)	Atiyah et al. 1992 [44]
	68 out of a total of 207 cases (33%)	
Contralateral PUJ	2 out of 23 cases (9%)	Unilateral MDK Gordon et al. 1988 [28]
	2 out of 29 cases (7%)	Unilateral MDK Flack and Bellinger 1993 [42]
	2 out of 19 cases (11%)	Unilateral MDK Kleiner 1986 [15]
	6 out of 49 cases (12%)	Atiyah et al. 1992 [44]
	12 out of a total of 120 cases (10%)	

* Predominantly low-grade contralateral reflux.

specific management of the MDK itself and the urological management of any coexisting anomalies.

Coexisting urological problems

Vesicoureteric reflux

Where VUR has been identified it is best managed conservatively in the first instance, i.e. with antibiotic prophylaxis and urine surveillance. Parents and general practitioners of children who have not been routinely investigated by voiding cystography should be aware that the existence of VUR has not been positively excluded.

Ureteric reimplantation for contralateral VUR is rarely required and in our experience proved necessary in only 2 out of more than 70 children with prenatally detected MDKs.

Contralateral PUJ obstruction

This is potentially the most serious coexisting anomaly; it occurs in up to 10% of cases [28,41] (Table 17.2). The decision to proceed to pyeloplasty, however, should be guided by a combination of ultrasound, isotope renography and, arguably, an IVU. A measured assessment of the indications for surgical intervention is preferable to a hasty, ill-considered decision to proceed to neonatal pyeloplasty.

Management of the multicystic dysplastic kidney

Clinical presentation – abdominal mass

Few paediatric urologists would argue with the surgical removal of a MDK presenting as a large obvious abdominal mass in the neonatal period. In this clinical situation, however, it is only rarely necessary to proceed to nephrectomy as a matter of urgency. In most instances, nephrectomy can be deferred and performed on a semielective basis at a few weeks of age once the diagnostic work-up has been completed. Nephrectomy can be accomplished through a relatively small flank or lumbotomy incision if the cysts are aspirated prior to removal of the kidney.

Prenatally or incidentally detected multicystic dysplastic kidney

In the absence of symptoms or a discernible mass, the 'prophylactic' surgical removal of a MDK is more difficult to justify. Without

evidence of the maternal ultrasound scan, the majority of the asymptomatic lesions would have remained unrecognized. The role of surgery in the management of prenatally detected MDKs remains controversial. The arguments can be summarized as follows:

1. *An intuitive argument – dysplastic tissue serving no useful purpose is best removed.* One must recognize, however, that the overwhelming majority of prenatally detected MDKs are incidental findings in asymptomatic infants. Sounder, more scientifically based arguments are needed before submitting large numbers of children to general anaesthesia and surgery.

2. *Hypertension* – an undoubted association exists – although the magnitude of the hypertension risk is likely to be extremely low in relation to the true frequency of the anomaly. An English language literature search [28] spanning the two decades from 1968 to 1988 unearthed only three case reports of hypertension which resolved following removal of the MDK. Isolated case reports have subsequently appeared in the literature [45]. If MDKs were giving rise to hypertension on a significant scale one would expect this to be reflected in the published literature on hypertension in childhood and early adult life. This is not the case. Taylor et al. [46] reporting a series of 42 children with 'surgical' renal hypertension did not encounter a single MDK. Similarly, Hendren et al. [47] did not report a single MDK amongst their series of 22 children with hypertension of renal aetiology. A possible link between MDKs and hypertension in adult life might be more difficult to identify but, broadly speaking, the available evidence [28] does not indicate that MDKs present with hypertension in adult life.

3. *Malignancy.* A literature review undertaken by Noe et al. [48] uncovered seven documented cases of renal tumours arising in a multicystic dysplastic kidney. Of these four were Wilm's tumours (in children ranging in age from 10 months to 4 years). Oddone et al. [49] have also reported a Wilm's tumour arising in the upper pole of a MDK in a 9-month-old infant, and Cuckow et al. [50] have reported a probable Wilm's tumour in a 2-year-old child. None of the reported

malignancies have resulted in death. In relation to the true frequency of MDK the number of documented malignancies represents a very low order of risk. On the basis of published data, Noe et al. [48] have calculated that at least 20 000 MDKs would have to be removed in order to prevent one death from Wilm's tumour. Kelleher et al. [38] recommended that MDKs greater than 6 cm in length at 1 year of age should be removed, although this is an empirical recommendation since there is no evidence linking size or the persistence of cystic elements to the risk of late complications.

Natural history

The tendency for multicystic dysplastic kidneys to involute spontaneously is now well documented. The process of involution is not confined to postnatal life. Mesrobian et al. [51] have reported three fetuses with unequivocal ultrasound evidence of unilateral multicystic dysplasia *in utero*, in whom no detectable renal tissue could be demonstrated on ultrasound or isotope renography in postnatal life. Of the 64 MDKs reported in Kelleher's series [38], 35% disappeared during the course of pre- and postnatal ultrasound follow-up. Other authors have also documented the phenomenon of involution of MDKs on serial postnatal ultrasound. These findings indicate that involution of a MDK probably accounts for a proportion (possibly a sizeable proportion) of cases of apparent unilateral renal agenesis encountered in adult life.

Practical considerations

Management of prenatally detected MDKs varies from centre to centre. Our policy is currently as follows:

1. Large, clinically evident multicystic dysplastic kidneys – are removed surgically at around 4 weeks of age.
2. Asymptomatic prenatally detected MDKs (the majority) are managed conservatively, i.e. left *in situ*. Ultrasound and blood pressure follow-up is maintained until around 5 years of age and blood pressure follow-up alone maintained thereafter.

3. Children with prenatally detected MDKs are not submitted to voiding cystography in the absence of ureteric dilatation or urinary infection. This invasive investigation is performed, however, if postnatal ultrasound reveals evidence of ureteric dilatation or if urinary tract infection is documented.

Multilocular renal cysts

Multilocular renal cyst, a rare renal lesion of uncertain aetiology, has also been termed cystic nephroma, benign multilocular cystic nephroma, etc. The pathogenesis is unclear, indeed doubt remains whether it should be regarded as a developmental anomaly or a benign form of cystic neoplasia. The occurrence is sporadic and there is no evidence to point to any familial tendency. Histologically multilocular cyst can be distinguished from other forms of renal pathology by the criteria defined by Powell et al. [52], i.e.:

1. The lesion is solitary, multilocular and usually unilateral.
2. The cysts do not communicate with the renal pelvis.
3. The loculi are non-communicating and have an epithelial lining.
4. The main cyst and loculi do not contain renal elements.
5. Any residual tissue surrounding the multilocular cyst is histologically normal.

Children account for approximately half the cases (in one review [53] of 38 children, the mean age was 17 months). After infancy there is an unexplained hiatus in the age distribution until early adult life. Paediatric cases generally present with a mass, haematuria or pain – or occasionally as an incidental finding. Multilocular renal cysts can be readily distinguished from other forms of cystic disease by a combination of ultrasound and CT imaging (Figure 17.6). Although partial nephrectomy or 'shelling out' appear attractive surgical options [54] (and conservation of the kidney has been described), this may be technically difficult if not impossible to accomplish. In practice, nephrectomy is the most realistic form of treatment.

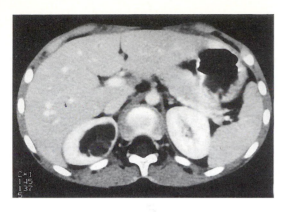

Figure 17.6 Multilocular renal cyst. CT cut demonstrating normal left kidney, septate multilocular space occupying cystic lesion in right kidney.

Solitary renal cysts

Simple, i.e. solitary, renal cysts, are a common finding in adults of middle age and onwards, but they are exceedingly rare in infants and small children. This observation supports the view that adult simple cysts are acquired rather than congenital in aetiology. Simple cysts are defined by the following pathological criteria:

1. The cyst is unilocular.
2. The cyst does not communicate with the collecting system.
3. A single layer of epithelium lines the cyst wall.
4. There is no evidence of upper tract or infundibular obstruction.
5. Apart from the solitary cyst the renal parenchyma is otherwise normal.

The diagnosis of a simple renal cyst in the paediatric age group should be viewed with caution. Other pathology that can occasionally give rise to confusion includes dilatation of the upper pole moiety of a duplex kidney, multilocular renal cyst (see above) and central necrosis within a renal tumour. Where doubt remains, additional imaging with CT or MRI may be required to complement the ultrasound findings. Once alternative pathology has been excluded, management of simple cysts is determined largely by the presence or absence of symptoms. Symptomatic simple cysts are best treated by de-roofing or partial nephrectomy, since cyst aspiration is likely to result in recurrence. Asymptomatic simple cysts, discovered as incidental ultrasound findings, can be managed conservatively with ultrasound follow-up.

References

1. Mir S, Rapola J, Koskimies. Renal cysts in pediatric autopsy material. *Nephron* 1983; **33**: 189–195.
2. McDonald RA, Avner ED. Inherited polycystic kidney disease in children. *Semin Nephrol* 1991; **11**: 632–642.
3. Cole BR. Autosomal recessive polycystic kidney disease. In: Gardner KD, Bernstein J (eds) *The Cystic Kidney*. Dordrecht, Netherlands: Kluwer, 1990; pp 327–350.
4. Zerres K, Hansmann M, Mallmann R, Gembruch U. Autosomal recessive polycystic kidney disease: problems of prenatal diagnosis. *Prenat Diagn* 1988; **8**: 215–229.
5. Dalgaard OZ. Bilateral polycystic disease of the kidneys: a follow-up of two hundred and eighty-four patients and their families (Suppl). *Acta Med Scand* 1957; **328**: 1–255.
6. Faraggiana T, Bernstein J, Strauss L, Churg J. Use of lectins in the study of histogenesis of renal cysts. *Lab Invest* 1985; **53**: 575–579.
7. Verani R, Walker P, Silva FG. Renal cystic disease of infancy: results of histochemical studies. *Pediatr Nephrol* 1989; **3**: 37–42.
8. Gagnadoux M-F, Habib R, Levy M. Cystic renal diseases in children. *Adv Nephrol* 1989; **18**: 33–58.
9. Kääriäinen H, Koskimies O, Norio R. Dominant and recessive polycystic kidney disease in children: evaluation of clinical features and laboratory data. *Pediatr Nephrol* 1988; **2**: 296–302.
10. Kaplan BS, Fay J, Shah V, Dillon MJ, Barratt TM. Autosomal recessive polycystic kidney disease. *Pediatr Nephrol* 1989; **3**: 43–49.
11. Cole BR, Conley SB, Stapleton FB. Polycystic kidney disease in the first year of life. *J Pediatr* 1987; **111**: 693–699.
12. Lieberman E, Salinas-Madrigal L, Gwinn JL et al. Infantile polycystic disease of the kidneys and liver: clinical, pathological radiological correlations and comparison with congenital hepatic fibrosis. *Medicine* 1971; **50**: 277–318.
13. Blyth H, Ockenden BG. Polycystic disease of kidneys and liver presenting in childhood. *J Med Genet* 1971; **8**: 257–284.
14. Chilton SJ, Cremin BJ. The spectrum of polycystic disease in children. *Pediatr Radiol* 1981; **11**: 9–15.
15. Boal DK, Teele RL. Sonography of infantile polycystic kidney disease. *Am J Radiol* 1980; **135**: 575–580.
16. Premkumar A, Berdon WE, Levy H, Amodio J, Abramson SJ, Newhouse JH. The emergence of

hepatic fibrosis and portal hypertension in infants and children with autosomal recessive polycystic kidney disease: initial and follow-up sonographic and radiographic findings. *Pediatr Radiol* 1988; **18**: 123–129.

17. Gabow PA. Autosomal dominant polycystic kidney disease. In: Gardner KD, Bernstein J (eds) *The Cystic Kidney*. Dordrecht, Netherlands: Kluwer, 1990; pp 295–326.

18. Reeders ST, Hildebrand CE. Report of the committee on the genetic constitution of chromosome 16. *Cytogenet Cell Genet* 1989; **51**: 299–318.

19. Pretorius DH, Lee ME, Manco-Johnson ML, Weingast GR, Sedman AB, Gabow PA. Diagnosis of autosomal dominant polycystic kidney disease *in utero* and in the young infant. *J Ultrasound Med* 1987; **6**: 249–255.

20. Main D, Mennuti MT, Cornfield D, Coleman B. Prenatal diagnosis of adult polycystic kidney disease. *Lancet* 1983; **ii**: 337–338.

21. Everson GT. Hepatic cysts in autosomal dominant kidney disease. *Mayo Clin Proc* 1990; **65**: 1020–1025.

22. Milutinovic J, Schabel SI, Ainsworth SK. Autosomal dominant polycystic kidney disease with liver and pancreatic involvement in early childhood. *Am J Kidney Dis* 1989; **13**: 340–344.

23. Proesmans W, Van Damme B, Casaer P, Marchal G. Autosomal dominant polycystic kidney disease in the neonatal period: association with a cerebral arteriovenous malformation. *Pediatrics* 1982; **70**: 971–975.

24. de Chadarevian J-P, Kaplan BS. Endocardial fibroelastosis, myocardial scarring and polycystic kidneys. *Int J Pediatr Nephrol* 1981; **2**: 273–275.

25. Gabow PA, Chapman AB, Johnson AM et al. Renal structure and hypertension in autosomal dominant polycystic kidney disease. *Kidney Int* 1990; **38**: 1177–1180.

26. Gabow PA, Johnson AM, Kaehny WD et al. Factors affecting the progression of renal disease in autosomal dominant polycystic kidney disease. *Kidney Int* 1992; **41**: 1311–1319.

27. Sedman A, Bell P, Manco-Johnson M, Schrier R et al. Autosomal dominant polycystic kidney disease in childhood: a longitudinal study. *Kidney Int* 1987; **31**: 1000–1005.

28. Gordon AC, Thomas DFM. Multicystic dysplastic kidney: is nephrectomy still appropriate? *J Urol* 1988; **140**: 1231–1234.

29. Rickwood AMK, Anderson PAM, Williams MPL. Multicystic renal dysplasia detected by prenatal ultrasonography. Natural history and results of conservative management. *Br J Urol* 1992; **69**: 538–540.

30. Brand IR, Kaminopetros K, Cave M, Irving HC, Lilford RJ. Specificity of antenatal ultrasound in the Yorkshire Region: a prospective study of 2261 ultrasound detected anomalies. *Br J Obstet Gynecol* 1994; **101**: 392–397.

31. Kleiner B, Filly RA, Mack L, Callen PW. Multicystic dysplastic kidney: observations of contralateral disease in the fetal population. *Radiology* 1986; **161**: 27–29.

32. Thomas DFM. MDKs in Siblings. Data presented to the Society of Pediatric Urological Surgeons, Philadelphia, 1995.

33. Murugasu B. Familial renal adysplasia. *Am J Kidney Dis* 1991; **18**: 490–494.

34. Al Saadi AA, Yoshimoto M, Bree R et al. A family study of renal dysplasia. *Am J Genet* 1984; **19**: 669–677.

35. Krull F, Hoyer P, Habenicht R et al. Die multizystische Nierendysplasie. *Monatsschr Kinderheilk* 1990; **138**: 202–205 [German].

36. McPherson E, Carey J. Kramer A et al. Dominantly inherited renal adysplasia. *Am J Med Genet* 1987; **26**: 836–850.

37. Roodhooft AM, Birnholz J, Holmes L. Familial nature of congenital absence and severe dysgenesis of both kidneys. *N Engl J Med* 1984; **310**: 1341–1345.

38. Kelleher JP, Dillon HK, Duffy PG, Ransley PG. The Antenatally Diagnosed Multicystic Dysplastic Kidney: now you see it, now you don't. Data presented to the Annual Meeting of the British Association of Urological Surgeons, Harrogate 1993; abstract no. 128.

39. Griscom NT. The roentgenology of neonatal abdominal masses. *Am J Roentgenol* 1965; **93**: 447–463.

40. Stuck KJ, Koff SA, Silver TM. Ultrasonic features of multicystic dysplastic kidney: expanded diagnostic criteria. *Radiology* 1982; **143**: 217–221.

41. Carey PO, Howards SS. Multicystic dysplastic kidneys and diagnostic confusion on renal scan. *J Urol* 1988; **139**: 83–84.

42. Flack CE, Bellinger MF. The multicystic dysplastic kidney and contralateral vesicoureteral reflux: protection of the solitary kidney. *J Urol* 1993; **150**: 1873–1874.

43. Wacksman J, Phipps L. Report of the Multicystic Kidney Registry: preliminary findings. *J Urol* 1993; **150**: 1870–1872.

44. Atiyah B, Husmann D, Baum M. Contralateral renal abnormalities in multicystic-dysplastic kidney disease. *J Pediatr* 1992; **121**: 65–67.

45. Susskind MR, King LR. Hypertension and the multicystic kidney (abstract 12), Eighty-second Annual Meeting American Urological Association, *J Urol* 1987; **139** (suppl): 106A.

46. Taylor RG, Azmy AF, Young DG. Long-term follow-up of surgical renal hypertension. *J Pediatr Surg* 1987; **22**: 228–230.

47. Hendren WH, Kim SH, Herrin JT, Crawford JD. Surgically correctable hypertension of renal origin in childhood. *Am J Surg* 1982; **143**: 432–441.

48. Noe HN, Marshall JH, Edward O. Nodular renal blastema in the multicystic kidney. *J Urol* 1989; **142**: 486–488.

49. Oddone M, Marino C, Sergi C et al. Wilm's tumour arising in a multicystic kidney. *Pediatr Radiol* 1994; **24**: 236–238.

50. Cuckow PM, Arthur R, Cullinane C, Najmaldin A. Tumours Arising from Multicystic Dysplastic Kidneys. Poster presented to ESPU Meeting, Toledo, Spain, April 1995.

51. Mesrobian H-GJ, Rushton HG, Bulas D. Unilateral renal agenesis may result from *in utero* regression of multicystic renal dysplasia. *J Urol* 1993; **150**: 793–794.

52. Powell T, Shackman R, Johnson HD. Multilocular cysts of the kidney. *Br J Urol* 1951; **23**: 142–152.

53. Akhtar M, Qadeer A. Multilocular cyst of kidney with embryonic tissue. *Urology* 1980; **16**: 90–94.

54. Thomas DFM, Androulakakis PA, Ransley PG. Conservation of the kidney following an unusual presentation of multilocular cyst in a 7 year old child. *J Urol* 1982; **128**: 363–365.

18

Congenital disorders of the bladder

A.M.K. Rickwood

Neuropathic bladder

Aetiology

Myelomeningocele (Figure 18.1) remains by far the commonest cause of congenital neuropathic bladder (Table 18.1), despite a declining birth incidence of this condition plus selective treatment of such infants as they are born. Most other causes also have an obvious spinal anomaly, although one of the more prevalent, sacral agenesis, is often overlooked at birth and during infancy, especially when occurring as an isolated lesion rather than in association with some other anomaly (imperforate anus, etc.).

Table 18.1 Neuropathic bladder dating from the newborn period: Department of Urology, Royal Liverpool Childrens Hospital, 1984–90

	No.	%
Congenital		
Myelomeningocele	420	86
Sacral agenesis	28	6
Lumbosacral lipoma	24	5
Other spinal lesions	8	1.6
Occult	2	0.4
Acquired		
Cord ischaemia	2	0.4
Tumour	3	0.5
Dermal sinus	2	0.4
(Intradural abscess)		
Total	489	

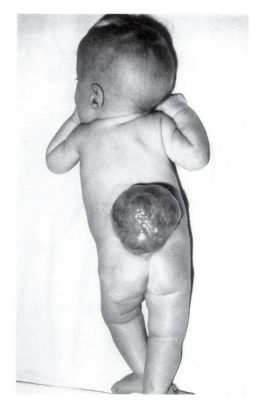

Figure 18.1 Myelomeningocele. Although declining in incidence and frequently detected prenatally, meningomyelocele remains the commonest cause of the congenital neuropathic bladder.

Acquired neuropathic bladder in the new-born period is exceptional. Cord infarction occasionally occurs in small, premature, infants already compromised by conditions leading to hypotension and hypoxaemia. Intraspinal extension of congenital neuroblastoma is a rare cause of neuropathic bladder. Congenital dermal sinuses, typically sited at the lumbosacral junction, can be complicated by extradural or intradural abscess formation, usually by *Staphylococcus aureus* or *Escherichia coli*, and prompt drainage can reverse any bladder involvement.

Pathophysiology

The detrusor is innervated parasympathetically via the second, third and fourth sacral seg-ments and these same levels also somatically innervate the striated musculature of the pelvic floor, including the external urethral sphincter. Ascending sensory fibres from the bladder run adjacent to the spinothalamic tracts and descending motor fibres to the pyramidal tracts. In the neurologically intact individual bladder reflexes, including coordination of detrusor and sphincter, are mediated at brain-stem level rather than sacrally.

Although the pathophysiology of neuropathic bladder was originally determined in cord-injured patients, the same mechanisms apply to those with congenital abnormalities of the cord [1] and depend principally upon whether the lesion affects the cord sacrally, with destruction of the innervation of the bladder and sphincters (areflexic bladder), or

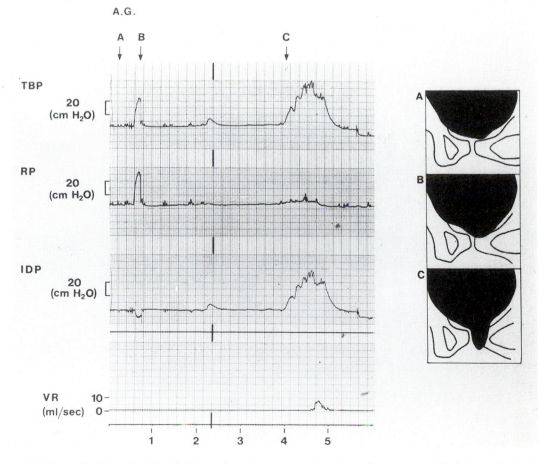

Figure 18.2 Hyperreflexic bladder. The bladder neck is closed at rest (a) and remains competent (b) during a rise in intra-abdominal pressure (b). Voiding is by a hyperreflexic detrusor contraction with opening of the bladder neck and initially complete detrusor-sphincter dyssynergia (c). TBP = total bladder pressure (cmH$_2$O); RP = rectal pressure; IDP = intrinsic (detrusor) pressure; FR = flow rate (ml/s).

whether suprasacrally to leave the innervation of these structures intact but isolated from higher centres (hyperreflexic bladder). With the latter type, bladder filling induces sacrally mediated reflex detrusor voiding contractions (Figure 18.2). The same sensory input also triggers a mass pelvic reflex so that there is simultaneous contraction both of the detrusor and of the external urethral sphincter (detrusor-sphincter dyssynergia). Although the external sphincter ultimately relaxes, this is often only partially so that voiding is obstructed. Detrusor-sphincter dyssynergia leads to high-pressure detrusor contractions which tend to fade away before the bladder is empty (non-sustained contractions). Because the innervation of the pelvic floor is intact, the sphincteric mechanism is competent: voiding occurs only by detrusor contractions and the bladder is inexpressible. With sacral cord lesions (areflexic bladder) there are no detrusor con-

tractions and voiding occurs by overflow or by raising intra-abdominal pressure (e.g. by suprapubic compression). Although the sphincteric mechanism is also paralysed, for reasons unknown the proximal urethra exerts a level of static obstruction varying from one patient to another. Where this is low, both residual urine volume and functional bladder capacity are small; where high, good functional bladder capacity is at the expense of a large residual urine volume.

In practice many congenital neuropathic bladders exhibit an intermediate pattern, with a combination of detrusor hyperreflexia and sphincteric incompetence so that voiding is both by detrusor contractions and by raising intra-abdominal pressure (Figure 18.3). Sixty per cent of myelomeningocele patients have such dysfunction, while among the remainder 25% have supra-sacral (hyperreflexic) and 15% sacral (areflexic) bladders. Intermediate

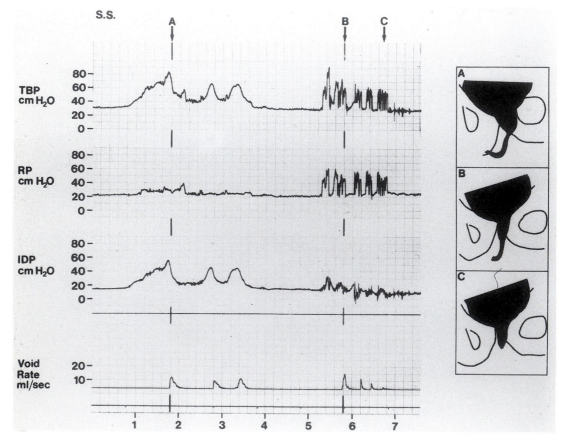

Figure 18.3 Intermediate bladder. Voiding occurs both by hyperreflexic detrusor contractions (a) and by abdominal straining (b), ultimately with static sphincteric obstruction (c).

bladders also predominate with all other congenital cord lesions, pure diastematomyelia excepted.

In the normal bladder baseline intravesical pressure rises only minimally within the physiological range of capacity. With all forms of neuropathic bladder, and especially in the intermediate type, baseline detrusor pressure often rises appreciably as the bladder fills (detrusor non-compliance). Where there is an element of sphincteric incompetence, detrusor non-compliance serves to further reduce functional bladder capacity. More importantly, when the sphincter mechanism is competent or where there is a high level of static sphincteric obstruction, detrusor non-compliance may lead to elevated levels of intravesical pressure causing secondary ureterovesical obstruction or, on occasion, secondary vesicoureteric reflux. It seems that this tends to occur when intravesical pressures persistently exceed 20–25 cmH$_2$O.

Although qualitative changes in function of the congenital neuropathic bladder are comparatively unusual during childhood and adult life, this is not so during infancy. A 'safe' bladder neonatally does not always remain so during infancy.

Factors serving to limit the ability of the neuropathic bladder to store and void urine are summarized in Table 18.2.

Neuropathic bladder and the upper renal tracts

Various primary anomalies of the upper renal tracts (renal agenesis, horseshoe kidney, crossed fused ectopia, etc.) are more common in myelomeningocele patients than in the population at large, but they rarely influence management.

Table 18.2 Factors affecting the ability of the neuropathic bladder to store and void urine

Storage failure	*Voiding failure*
Detrusor hyperreflexia	Detrusor-sphincter dyssynergia
Detrusor non-compliance	Static sphincteric obstruction
Sphincteric incompetence	Non-sustained detrusor contractions
Combinations	Combinations

Secondary complications (ureterovesical obstruction, vesicoureteric reflux) are notoriously prevalent in patients with congenital neuropathic bladder and particularly among those with myelomeningocele. Although severe changes at birth are rare (and renal failure neonatally virtually unknown), some element of upper tract obstruction is present in 7–15% of neonates with myelomeningocele, while a further 8–20% have vesicoureteric reflux [2]. Deterioration thereafter during infancy is common: in one series the combined incidence of obstruction and reflux neonatally – 20% – had increased to 49% at 2 years of age [2]. Several factors are identifiable as causing these complications:

1. *Bladder outflow obstruction* (detrusor-sphincter dyssynergia, static sphincteric obstruction) is almost always associated with residual urine and while upper renal tract complications are unusual in the absence of residual urine, and never occur when the bladder is permanently empty due to gross sphincteric incompetence, the converse does not always hold in that the upper renal tracts may remain normal in the presence of persistent, appreciable, residual urine (Figure 18.4). Thus it seems that outflow obstruction alone does not lead to renal complications.
2. *Detrusor non-compliance*, when combined with outflow obstruction, leads to permanently elevated intravesical pressure and this conjunction is probably the commonest cause of obstructive uropathy in patients with neuropathic bladder.
3. *Detrusor hyperreflexia*, causing episodic rises in intravesical pressure, has also been established as a factor in secondary upper urinary tract obstruction.
4. *Vesicoureteric reflux* is of evident importance when associated with urinary tract infection and can lead to permanent renal scarring. Experimentally, high-pressure sterile reflux, as can occur with neuropathic bladder, also leads to scarring. Whether this is so of humans is unknown, although it is recognized that a combination of urinary infection and high-pressure reflux is often rapidly and severely damaging to the kidney.
5. *Urinary tract infection* occurs in 5–25% of myelomeningocele patients during early

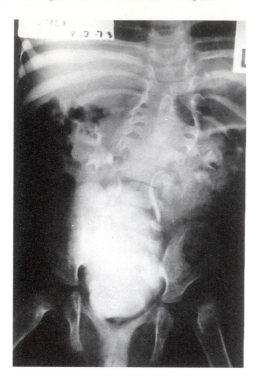

Figure 18.4 IVU in a female infant with neuropathic bladder. The upper renal tracts remain normal despite a huge residual urine.

infancy [3], and while clearly potentially dangerous in those with vesicoureteric reflux, is of arguable importance otherwise. Although urinary infection is usually (though not always [2]) associated with secondary obstructive uropathy, it is now generally believed that such infection is the result rather than the cause of this complication.

Assessment of the neonate with neuropathic bladder

Clinical

Most conditions likely to be associated with neuropathic bladder are easily recognizable at birth. Certain forms of spina bifida occulta, without overlying cutaneous abnormalities, and sacral agenesis, form an exception to this rule and the bladder disorder may only come to light as a result of urinary retention, urinary infection or, rarely, symptoms resulting from an element of renal failure. Sacral agenesis in particular should always be excluded, by palpation, in any neonate or infant presenting with urinary infection or retention.

Some 7% of myelomeningocele patients escape bladder involvement (though never those with thoracolumbar lesions). This occurs only when there is a combination of an incomplete cord lesion, with both sensory and motor sparing, and positive conus reflexes (anocutaneous, glans-bulbar). Motor sparing is difficult to ascertain neonatally but conus reflexes are readily demonstrable as also sensory sparing by general arousal to peri-anal pinprick. Thus, no matter how slight the neurological deficit otherwise, neuropathic bladder is certain in the presence of a sensory complete cord lesion or negative conus reflexes. Conversely, where there are both sensory sparing and positive reflexes, bladder function may ultimately prove to be normal. Positive conus reflexes are associated with suprasacral (hyperreflexic) bladder dysfunction and negative reflexes with sacral (areflexic) or intermediate dysfunction. In the former circumstance the infant is usually observed to pass a spontaneous (though often interrupted) urinary stream, while in the latter there is either continuous dribbling or a urinary stream occurring only when the infant cries or strains. Expressibility of the bladder implies a degree of sphincteric incompetence, although it should be noted that suprapubic pressure may provoke a hyperreflexic detrusor contraction so simulating 'expressibility'. Inability to express the bladder indicates either sphincteric competence or that the bladder is permanently empty due to gross sphincteric incompetence.

Imaging studies

Ultrasonography is the best means of detecting hydronephrosis, residual urine and thickening of the bladder wall (often the first sign of developing detrusor non-compliance). Routine cystography is worthwhile because of the high incidence of vesicoureteric reflux and which is not always associated with hydronephrosis; the examination is best performed with simultaneous urodynamic assessment where this facility is available. ^{99m}Tc-DMSA scintigraphy is advisable in those with vesicoureteric reflux, although not before 1 month of age, nor, if permanent renal damage is to be assessed, within 1 month of any symptomatic urinary infection.

Urodynamic assessment

A full description of urodynamic equipment, technique and interpretation is provided by Mundy et al. [4] Urodynamic assessment in neonates is best combined with simultaneous video-radiological studies, using contrast medium for filling, and is ideally performed by the clinician also responsible for the patient's future management.

Such studies show that it is possible to identify the 'unsafe' bladder neonatally [5], that is one where a combination of outflow obstruction plus detrusor non-compliance and/or detrusor hyperreflexia is apt to lead to persistently elevated intravesical pressure. Follow-up of such cases has established that in the absence of treatment secondary renal complications are significantly more common than in those with 'safe' bladders. Nonetheless, 'safe' bladders can change for the worse during infancy, so that no case should be regarded as being entirely free of risk.

Management

General

Hitherto neonatal management of the infants with neuropathic bladder has been mainly expectant with active measures reserved for the minority having established upper renal tract complications at birth or developing these at an early stage. Regular bladder expression, by suprapubic pressure, has long been practised: there is no substantive evidence that this does any harm, even when there is vesicoureteric reflux, nor, either, that it does any good.

The general unsatisfactory results of such conservative management [2] suggest that a more active policy could be advantageous. In one small prospective trial, half those cases identified as having an 'unsafe' bladder urodynamically were managed from birth by intermittent catheterization and at 2 years of age they had significantly fewer renal complications than the remainder managed expectantly [6]; preliminary reports of other trials show a similar trend.

Surveillance

Ultrasonography represents the best means of regular surveillance and while the frequency with which it is performed should reflect the perceived risk of complications, this should rarely exceed 4-month intervals during the first year of life. Increasing residual urine or thickening of the bladder wall often precede development of hydronephrosis. The value of 'routine' urine specimens is doubtful, but specimens are desirable with any clinically suspected urinary infection and, if confirmatory, should prompt reassessment of the upper renal tracts and, sometimes, bladder function also.

Management of established complications

Acute urinary retention occasionally follows neonatal closure of myelomeningocele, possibly in a manner analogous to the spinal shock following cord trauma. This phenomenon is usually transient and is manageable by a period of intermittent catheterization.

Management of obstructive upper renal tract complications depends upon their severity. Modest degrees can be expected to respond to (continued) intermittent catheterization but seldom to more severe dilation. Here a period of indwelling urethral catherization represents a useful temporizing measure but one which should rarely extend beyond one month's duration. Endoscopic sphincterotomy (in boys) or vigorous internal urethrotomy (in girls) are effective remedies but risk damaging the sphincteric mechanism as a whole so making for future difficulties in managing urinary incontinence. Cutaneous vesicostomy represents the most satisfactory medium-term solution [7] (Figure 18.5); closure of the vesicostomy is usually deferred until 3–4 years of age when some more definitive treatment can be established. The once-popular supravesical urinary diversions (usually cutaneous ureterostomies) are now very rarely indicated.

Antibiotic prophylaxis is advisable in cases with vesicoureteric reflux. As with obstruction, lesser degrees of vesicoureteric reflux are manageable by intermittent catheterization, where active treatment is considered necessary at all, but major degrees of reflux seldom respond satisfactorily. Operative correction of such reflux is rarely advisable neonatally or during early infancy and is best managed by cutaneous vesicostomy.

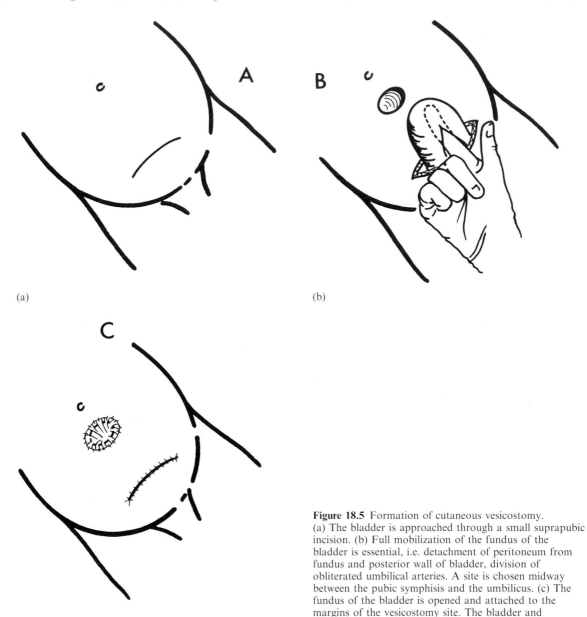

Figure 18.5 Formation of cutaneous vesicostomy. (a) The bladder is approached through a small suprapubic incision. (b) Full mobilization of the fundus of the bladder is essential, i.e. detachment of peritoneum from fundus and posterior wall of bladder, division of obliterated umbilical arteries. A site is chosen midway between the pubic symphisis and the umbilicus. (c) The fundus of the bladder is opened and attached to the margins of the vesicostomy site. The bladder and overlying incision are then closed.

Long-term progress and management

With current forms of treatment secondary upper renal tract complications, once an appreciable cause of morbidity and mortality [8], are now largely avoidable. Parents are naturally concerned as to later management of urinary incontinence. To an extent this is determined by the patient's other disabilities and for the severely handicapped there remains a role for indwelling urinary catheters for girls, penile urinals for boys and, occasionally, for permanent urinary diversion in children of both sexes. For the less disabled there is usually the prospect of some form of appliance-free urinary continence. Patients with positive conus reflexes, and a competent sphincteric mechanism, do well on a regimen of intermittent catheterization (though often only in conjunction with permanent anticholinergic medication), as also do those with negative conus reflexes and a large residual urine. A combination of negative conus reflexes and a small residual urine volume usually implies a degree of sphincteric incompetence requiring surgical correction to give adequate functional bladder capacity. This may take the form of bladder neck suspension or repair in girls, with voiding by intermittent catheterization, or the artificial urinary sphincter in boys, usually with voiding by abdominal straining. These procedures may need to be combined with augmentation cystoplasty, using bowel segments, where there is also appreciable detrusor non-compliance or hyperreflexia. The results of such major surgery can never be guaranteed, and while good in the short and medium term, their long-term outcome remains to be established.

The exstrophic anomalies

General

These comprise a spectrum of lesions arising in the hind end of the fetus with the commonest, classical vesical exstrophy, occupying a central position as regards severity. The embryogenic aberration common to all is failure of the primitive streak mesoderm to invade the allantoic extension of the cloacal (infraumbilical) membrane, so that ectoderm and endoderm remain abnormally in contact in the developing lower abdominal wall. The absence of the intervening mesoderm represents an unstable state leading to disintegration of the infraumbilical membrane, so that the pelvic viscera become laid open upon the abdominal surface, although the abdominal musculature, derived from the thoracic somite mesoderm, is normal on each side of this midline defect. The abnormally extensive cloacal membrane acts as a wedge holding apart the developing structures to cause pelvic diastasis, and, cranially, a wide linea alba or, more severely, an exomphalos. The same effect may lead to double phallus or, in the female, partial or complete duplication of the genital tract from failure of fusion of the genital tubercles or of the mullerian ducts.

The type of lesion occurring depends upon the extent of the allantoic expansion of the cloacal membrane and upon the stage in development at which this dehisces. Classical vesical exstrophy with epispadias results from breakdown of an extensive membrane after completion of the urorectal septum at about the 16-mm stage, so that the primitive urogenital sinus is exteriorized. A less extensive infraumbilical membrane, limited to the pubic area, leads to epispadias, without exstrophy, while if only the superior portion of the membrane remains uninvaded by mesoderm its dehiscence leads to superior vesical fissure. The most plausible explanation of the most severe lesion, vesico-intestinal fissure, as its alternative denomination, cloacal exstrophy, implies, is that it represents the same basic anomaly but that dehiscence of the cloacal membrane, and its infraumbilical extension, occur earlier, at the 5-mm stage. Exstrophy occurring at this time leads to exteriorization of a central bowel field between the two bladder fields. The exstrophic bowel involves the ileocaecal region and it is believed that the blind-ending colon distal to this represents postanal or tail gut rather than hind gut proper [9].

All the exstrophic anomalies are rare and have a 2–3 : 1 male to female preponderance. The incidence of classical vesical exstrophy is estimated, in various communities, to lie between 1 in 10 000 and 1 in 50 000 live births. There is an impression that in recent years, and for no evident reason, classical exstrophy has become rarer, while cloacal exstrophy has increased somewhat. In principle the more severe anomalies are detectable by ultrasonography prenatally but this is unusual and in the event they may be mistaken for exomphalos or gastroschisis. The genetic basis of the exstrophic anomalies is uncertain. Examples of vesical exstrophy have occasionally been recorded in siblings, including some of different sexes, and in monovular twins. The risk of recurrence in an individual family is estimated between 1 in 100 and 1 in 300, while the chance of a mother with exstrophy or epispadias giving birth to offspring with either complaint has been calculated at 700 times the norm [10].

Vesical exstrophy with epispadias
Anatomy

The entire lower urinary tract is laid open. The size of the exstrophied bladder varies from one of almost normal surface area (Figure 18.6) to

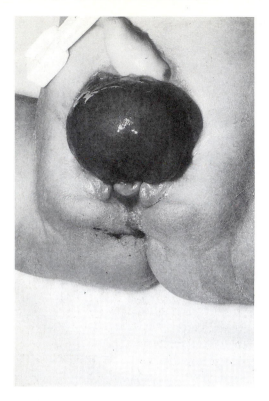

Figure 18.6 Vesical exstrophy in a female neonate: in this case the bladder is of almost normal dimensions.

one where little more than the trigone is represented. At birth the mucosa is smooth and the detrusor supple but with exposure the mucosa rapidly becomes hyperaemic and friable, with subsequent development of cystitis cystica and squamous metaplasia, while the detrusor becomes oedematous and rigid and may ultimately become replaced by fibrous tissue. The innervation of the detrusor is seemingly normal neonatally but again tends to deteriorate in time. The anus is always anteriorly placed and directed forwards and sometimes a degree of sphincteric laxity allows rectal prolapse to occur. In a few females there is more extreme anal displacement so that the orifice, which is somewhat stenotic, lies at the distal extremity of the urethral strip with the vaginal orifice immediately above it. The umbilical structures are downwardly displaced with the cord vessels emerging immediately above the apex of the bladder.

In males there is complete epispadias with the urethra represented by a strip of mucosa on the dorsum of the short, upturned, penis. The scrotum is broad and shallow and inguinal herniae are common, while testicular maldescent exists in some cases. As a rule the less the pubic diastasis the better developed the penis and scrotum, although often at the expense of a relatively small bladder. In females the epispadiac urethra is usually short and occasionally no urethral mucosa is discernible. The clitoris is bifid and the labia widely separated so that the vaginal orifice is clearly visible.

Primary anomalies of the upper renal tracts are exceptional and congenital abnormalities of other systems are unusual. The secondary changes occurring in the exposed bladder occasionally cause obstructive hydroureteronephrosis.

Management

The immediate concern is to protect the bladder from undue exposure; Gelonet is often used, although 'Clingfilm' seems to serve rather better. Except where the bladder is unusually small, or where some other anomaly presents a more pressing problem, it is desirable to close the lesion within the neonatal period. This ensures that the bladder is protected and also does much for parents' morale. In males closure is restricted to the bladder and prostatic urethra while in females the whole of such urethra as exists is reconstructed. No attempt is made at this stage to construct a competent sphincteric mechanism, indeed it is advantageous that the bladder remains permanently almost empty since vesicoureteric reflux usually exists following its closure.

The cosmetic result – and probably the ultimate functional result also – is materially improved if the pelvic ring can be approximated anteriorly. Due to the influence of maternal relaxins this can reputedly be effected within the first 48 hours of life without need for pelvic osteotomy. The author has not found this to be satisfactory and prefers to defer bladder closure until 1–4 weeks of age and to combine this with formal pelvic osteotomies. The most satisfactory closure of the pelvic ring is obtainable using anterior, Salter, osteotomies. The visceral repair follows immediately. The bladder is circumcised from the surrounding skin, with ligation of the umbilical vessels superiorly, and the bladder walls on each side are freed extraperitoneally so that their trimmed edges can be brought together and sutured in the midline without tension. In girls the entire urethral strip is mobilized on each side and tubularized by anterior midline sutures; in boys this process is confined to the prostatic urethra. No attempt is made to construct a 'bladder neck' as such, although it is customary to divide the pubo-urethral ligaments from the pubic bones on each side and to imbricate these anteriorly over the proximal urethra. With the bladder and urethral repair completed, the pubic rami are approximated anteriorly and fixed together with a stout monofilament suture. This manoeuvre brings together the edges of the rectus abdominis on each side, which are then sutured together vertically in the midline and similarly the fat and skin overlying them (Figure 18.7). Bladder drainage is secured for 3–6 weeks postoperatively via a suprapubic catheter and the pelvic repair is maintained for a similar period by Bryant's traction, a hip spica or even a firm crepe bandage. A minor degree of breakdown of the distal urethral repair is common and of little consequence. Occasionally the entire repair disintegrates so that the exstrophic state is reconstituted. This does not preclude a further repair, by the same method, provided the bladder remains supple and invertible.

An outline of longer-term management follows. As mentioned, vesicoureteric reflux is the norm following bladder closure and for that reason some advise antibiotic prophylaxis. In boys the epispadias is repaired at 2–3 years of age and it is often advantageous to obtain penile enlargement by prior administration of testosterone. Achieving urinary continence is more problematical and is usually deferred until 7–10 years of age. Good results have been reported from a few centres by bladder neck repair alone [11], but most other units have failed to replicate such success [12]. The problem lies in the relatively small size of the bladder in most cases, which causes a rapid rise in pressure as the organ fills so that either the bladder neck repair disintegrates or, when remaining sound, leads to poor bladder emptying and secondary upper urinary tract obstruction due to raised intravesical pressure. This problem can be overcome by augmentation cystoplasty using bowel segments [13]. In girls the sphincteric mechanism is reconstituted by tubularization of the trigone, with the ureters reimplanted at a higher level in the bladder, and with voiding by intermittent self-catheterization. The results, in the medium term at least, are excellent. Boys are more difficult to manage since few (if any) will self-catheterize urethrally. One option is to combine augmentation cystoplasty with placement of an artificial urinary sphincter at the bladder outlet. Voiding, by abdominal straining tends to be incomplete, so that it is wise to construct also a continent abdominal stoma, usually using the appendix which can be catheterized two or three times a day to ensure periodic complete bladder emptying. An alternative, again using augmentation cystoplasty and a continent abdominal stoma, is to close off the bladder outlet completely so that voiding is entirely by catheterization of the stoma.

Sexual intercourse usually presents no problems for affected females and, except for the minority with a bicornuate uterus, most are fertile. There is sometimes a long-term problem with genital prolapse. Adult males are capable of sexual intercourse provided upward chordee has been corrected with the epispadias repair

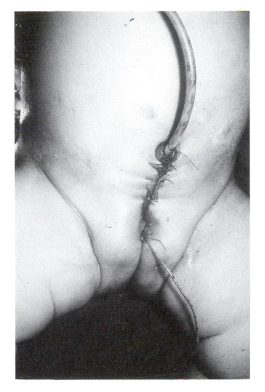

Figure 18.7 Completion of operative reconstruction of bladder exstrophy in a female infant: iliac osteotomy has enabled the pelvic ring and abdominal wall to be approximated in the midline anteriorly.

but because any ejaculation is retrograde few are likely to father children. Lastly it remains to be mentioned that there is an appreciable toll of upper renal tract complications (reflux nephropathy, secondary obstruction) which even today is not entirely avoidable.

As mentioned, primary reconstruction is not feasible when the bladder is small nor is it advisable if secondary changes have rendered the bladder rigid and uninvertible. In such cases closure can usually be effected at a later age, 2–3 years, if combined with augmentation cystoplasty.

Thus functional reconstruction is potentially possible in almost all cases. However much misery and disenchantment on the part of parents and child result if an over-sanguine view of this process is given at the outset. It should always be emphasized that the surgery involved is major and complex, with no guarantee of a successful short- or long-term outcome, and that at the end of the day permanent urinary diversion may prove to be the only satisfactory solution to the various problems.

Cloacal exstrophy

General

In contrast to classical vesical exstrophy, infants with cloacal exstrophy are often born prematurely and a majority have other associated anomalies, both of the upper urinary tracts (renal agenesis, multicystic dysplasia, etc.) and of other systems, including the heart, diaphragm, extremities, intestines, thoracic cage and spine (myelomeningocele or sacral agenesis) [14]. On occasion these materially influence management, including whether to treat at all.

Anatomy

Although details vary, the basic pattern is one of two hemi-bladders, each with a ureteric orifice, separated by a central zone of intestine with upper and lower orifices (Figure 18.8). The upper orifice, which usually prolapses, represents the ileocaecal region and leads to the terminal ileum, while the lower leads to a short colon ending blindly in front of the sacrum. A third, appendicular, orifice is sometimes apparent and occasionally the appendix is duplicated. Superiorly there is a broad exomphalos containing ileum and sometimes a portion of the liver.

In males the phalli are almost always duplicated, rudimentary and epispadiac. The testes usually lie intra-abdominally or may be unilaterally or bilaterally absent. In females the uterus is virtually always bicornuate with com-

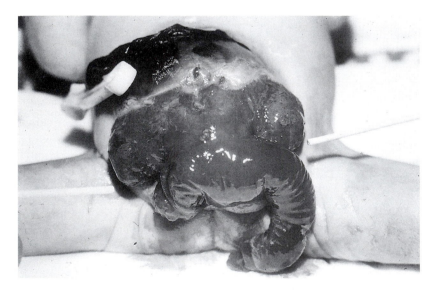

Figure 18.8 Cloacal exstrophy in a male neonate. Ileum is prolapsed through the upper orifice of the central bowel field and there is a broad exomphalos superiorly.

plete vaginal duplication. In some individuals there are no evident external or internal genitalia.

Management

For those with other major anomalies no active treatment may be appropriate. Although survival has occasionally occurred in the absence of surgical reconstruction, death usually rapidly supervenes due to profuse fluid losses through the relatively short intestinal tract.

Where active treatment is undertaken, urgent consideration of gender is necessary in male patients. Only exceptionally can a satisfactory penis be constructed and in this circumstance apart, reassignment to the female gender is usually advisable. The infant's birth should not be registered until this decision has been taken. Primary reconstruction is usually in two stages, the first, neonatally, involving the gastrointestinal tract. Where at all possible, the colon, even though short, should be incorporated into the faecal stream else there is apt to be failure to thrive due to malabsorption from intestinal hurry [15]. Probably the ideal reconstruction is to leave the central bowel field *in situ*, to act, in effect, as an 'auto-augmentation' of the bladder. To this end, the terminal ileum and colon are detached from the bowel field and anastomosed end to end while the blind-ending colon distally is brought out as a terminal, definitive colostomy. Bilateral orchidectomy is performed if male to female gender reassignment has been elected. The second stage follows at 1–3 months of age and involves bladder reconstruction, incorporating the central bowel field where this remains in place, along lines described for classical vesical exstrophy. Where there is gender reassignment as much of the urethra as exists is tubularized and transposed ventrally between the separated corpora. If necessary, a distal 'urethra' can be completed using a tubed inverted 'U' perineal skin flap based posteriorly. The two corpora are reduced, if unduly prominent, and then brought together in the midline anterior to the urethra, along with their glans, to form a 'clitoris'. In true females with vaginal duplication a single midline organ is constructed as far cranially as possible. This is effected by division of their medial walls and approximation of the viscera with anterior and posterior suture lines. A good pelvic osteotomy is essential for this extensive reconstruction and enables the omphalocele to be repaired at this second stage.

In longer-term management, the colostomy is best regarded as permanent since successful functional anal reconstruction is very rarely feasible with present techniques and never if there is also myelomeningocele or sacral agenesis. Bladder management follows the lines described for classical exstrophy. If the central bowel field has been left as an 'auto-augmentation', the bladder usually has good, low-pressure capacity and it is necessary only to construct a competent sphincteric mechanism by tubularization of the trigone along with reimplantation of the ureters at a higher level in the bladder. Voiding is by self-catheterization. Vaginal reconstruction, in cases having undergone gender reassignment, is deferred to later childhood or adolescence and may be effected using bowel, where sufficient is available, or, more often, by myocutaneous flaps based upon the gracilis muscles. In true females, fertility is impossible if there is uterine duplication.

Other exstrophic anomalies

Epispadias

With males the defect varies from one where no more than the glans penis is involved (Figure 18.9) to one where the entire urethra up to the bladder neck is laid open dorsally (Figure 18.10). In the latter circumstance the sphincteric mechanism is almost always involved and parents should be warned that this will require surgical reconstruction when the child is older but that this is by no means always successful. The penile deformity is usually corrected at 18 months of age. In the very rare female variety the entire urethra is always involved, as also the sphincteric mechanism, both requiring surgical attention, ideally in a single stage at around 3 years of age.

Superior vesical fissure

As a rule this unusual lesion amounts to little more than a superior vesicocutaneous fistula

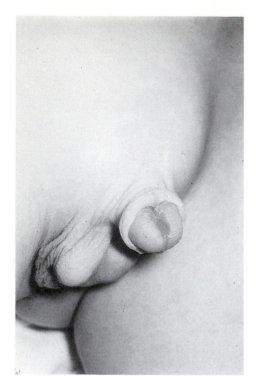

Figure 18.9 Glandular epispadias in a male infant.

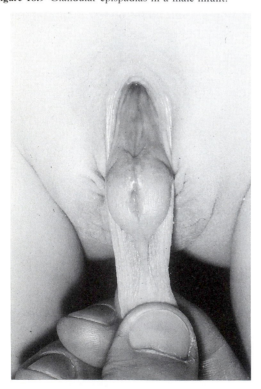

Figure 18.10 Complete epispadias in a male patient.

and its closure, neonatally, presents no problems. Bladder and sphincter function are usually entirely normal.

Covered exstrophy

In this lesion the bladder and urethra are normally formed. There is pubic diastasis with separation of the recti in the lower abdominal wall and the skin over this central defect is rugose and in immediate contact with the underlying bladder. Cosmetic reconstruction is feasible without the need for pelvicosteotomy. Occasionally the sphincteric mechanism is incompetent.

References

1. Rickwood AMK, Thomas DG, Philp NH, Spicer RD. Assessment of congenital neuropathic bladder by combined urodynamic and radiological studies. *Br J Urol* 1982; **54**: 502–511.
2. Light K, van Blerk PJP. Causes of renal deterioration in patients with myelomeningoceles. *Br J Urol* 1977; **49**: 257–260.
3. Chapman WH, Shurtleff DB, Eckert DW, Ansell JS. A prospective study of the urinary tract from birth in patients with myelomeningocele. *J Urol* 1969; **102**: 363–366.
4. Mundy AR, Stephenson TD, Wein AJ. *Urodynamics, Principles, Practice, Applications.* London: Churchill Livingstone, 1984.
5. Bauer SB, Hallett M, Khashbin S et al. Predictive value of urodynamic evaluation of newborns with myelodysplasia. JAMA 1984; **252**: 650–652.
6. Geroniotis E, Koff SA, Enrile B. Prophylactic use of clean intermittent self-catheterisation in the treatment of infants and young children with myelomeningocele and neurogenic bladder dysfunction. *J Urol* 1988; **139**: 85–86.
7. Snyder HC, Kalichman MA, Charney E, Duckett JW. Vesicostomy for neurogenic bladder with spina bifida: follow up. *J Urol* 1983; **130**: 924–926.
8. Eckstein HB, Cooper DGW, Howard AR. Causes of death in children with myelomeningocele or hydrocephalus. *Arch Dis Child* 1967; **42**: 163–167.
9. Johnston TB. Extroversion of the bladder complicated by intestinal openings in the region of the extroverted area. *J Anat* 1913; **48**: 89–93.
10. Shapiro E, Lepor H, Jeffs RD. The inheritance of classical bladder exstrophy. *J Urol* 1984; **132**: 308–310.
11. Lepor H, Jeffs RD. Primary bladder closure and bladder neck reconstruction in males with bladder exstrophy. *J Urol* 1983; **130**: 1142–1145.

12. Johnston JH, Kogan SJ. The exstrophic anomalies and their surgical correction. *Curr Prob Surg* 1974; **2**: 1–24.

13. Diamond DA, Ransley PG. Bladder neck reconstruction with omentum, silicone and augmentation cystoplasty – a preliminary report. *J Urol* 1985; **136**: 252–255.

14. Soper RT, Kilger K. Vesicointestinal fissure. *J Urol* 1984; **92**: 490–501.

15. Howell C, Caldamone A, Snyder HC, Zeigler M, Duckett JW. Optimal management of cloacal exstrophy. *J Pediatr Surg* 1983; **18**: 365–369.

19

Prenatal diagnosis and management of genital abnormalities

E. Shapiro and B.R. Elejalde

Introduction

This chapter will review the prenatal diagnosis and management of genital abnormalities. Over the past two decades, there has been significant advances in antenatal diagnosis and intervention for urological disease. Initially, prenatal ultrasound was used for detecting fetal number, position and size. This imaging modality has evolved through advancements in imaging technology and observer experience to allow late first-trimester diagnosis of gender, skeletal and urinary tract abnormalities [1].

In addition to prenatal ultrasound, amniocentesis and chorionic villus sampling are important diagnostic tools for antenatal diagnosis. Amniocentesis can be performed as early as 9 weeks [2] and chorionic villus sampling can be utilized prior to 12 weeks. These examinations enable early diagnosis of chromosomal or genetic abnormalities in high-risk patients [3]. Percutaneous umbilical venous sampling utilizing ultrasound guidance permits direct sampling of the fetal vascular system and provides a means for delivering fetal therapy [4]. More recently, polymerase chain reaction techniques have been used to evaluate fetal cell DNA abnormalities in maternal serum samples [5]. Advances in molecular biological techniques will continue to provide additional screening capabilities in the future.

Malformations of the genitalia occur as single malformations, as developmental field defects or as components of congenital and inherited syndromes. These malformations can occur in a family who has a previously affected member or, more commonly, in a family who does not have any history of the defect or any recognizable risk. Prenatal diagnosis of genital abnormalities is offered to families who have a known risk (i.e. an affected family member). In these cases, the most important component of the genetic prenatal diagnosis of genital malformations is a complete family history and physical examination of the affected family members. In the case of a single isolated malformation, prenatal diagnosis is dependent upon imaging techniques or the identification of a cytogenetic, biochemical, immunological or molecular marker for the malformation.

Embryology

In order to use advanced prenatal technologies for the diagnosis and management of genital abnormalities, a brief review of the embryological timing of the events involved with sexual differentiation and the development of the external genitalia will be presented [6,7].

The chromosomal sex directs the development of the paired bipotential gonads into either a testis or an ovary after the sixth week of gestation. The testis develops in the presence of a Y chromosome. Although factors on the X, Y and autosomal chromosomes are all important in testicular development, the most important factor, testicular determining factor, is located on the Y chromosome. In the absence of this factor, testicular differentiation does not occur and an ovary will develop at 11–12 weeks [8]. Prior to 8 weeks, the male and female genitalia appear morphologically identical [9]. By the eighth week, the testis elaborates testosterone from the Leydig cells which stimulates the wolffian duct to differentiate into the vas deferens, seminal vesicle, and epididymis [10]. The testis also elaborates mullerian-inhibiting substance from the sertoli cells, which causes mullerian duct regression [11,12]. Both of these developmental events occur locally by diffusion to ipsilateral target tissues. Virilization of the male external genitalia proceeds under the influence of dihydrotestosterone which results from conversion of testosterone by the enzyme 5-α reductase [10]. By week 12, testosterone levels are maximal and the external genitalia have differentiated. Between 14 and 15 weeks, the genital tubercle elongates, the urogenital folds close over the urogenital groove forming the urethra and the genital swellings enlarge to form the scrotum [13].

Testicular descent into the scrotum occurs after 26 weeks' gestational age. Testicular descent occurs in 62% of male fetuses by 28–30 weeks and in 93% after 32 weeks' gestational age [14]. If the gonad does not differentiate into a testis, female genitalia develop in the absence of mullerian-inhibiting substance. By the ninth week, the wolffian ducts regress in the female and the mullerian ductal structures differentiate into the fallopian tube, uterus and upper two-thirds of the vagina [15]. The lower one-third of the vagina is derived from the urogenital sinus [16]. By 24 weeks, the urogenital sinus vagina and mullerian vagina form a contiguous lumen [17].

The external genitalia of the female also differentiate in the absence of hormonal influences. At 8 weeks, the genital tubercle develops into the glans of the clitoris and the urogenital sinus forms the vestibule [18]. The urethral folds and genital swellings form the labia minora and labia majora, respectively [19,20]. Feminization of the external genitalia is complete by 28 weeks' gestation.

Prenatal fetal sex determination

During pregnancy, there is often curiosity about the fetal sex. Fetal sex can be determined by cytogenetic and molecular analysis. Prenatal ultrasound is an important adjunct in the determination of fetal sex. These methods are complementary in the diagnosis of malformations of the genitalia and of syndromes that have abnormal genitalia as one of their manifestations.

While the fetal sex can be examined in each fetus that undergoes an ultrasonographic examination, there are specific indications for determining fetal gender which include:

1. Patients with a history of X-linked disorders (i.e. haemophilia, aqueductal stenosis or Duchenne's muscular dystrophy), when there are no precise cytogenetic, molecular or biochemical methods for the diagnosis of the affected individuals. This indication is changing as molecular technology becomes available for many X-linked diseases.
2. Assignment of dizygocity in twin gestation.
3. Exclusion of maternal cell contamination during amniocentesis when a mixed population of cells is present on karyotype.
4. The need to confirm fetal sex to diagnose other structural abnormalities (i.e. posterior urethral valves).
5. Familial syndromes in which genital abnormalities are common (i.e. Opitz syndrome) [21].

Stocker [22] and Schorzman [23] were the first to report the sonographic determination of fetal sex. Other authors have reported their experience [2,14,24–27]. When the fetus' legs are apart, allowing visualization of the genital area, the male and female genitalia can be accurately distinguished as early as 14 weeks (B.R. Elejalde, unpublished data, 1992). The genitalia become easier to distinguish as the fetus grows and the genitalia enlarge and become more differentiated.

Birnholz [14] visualized the external genitalia with 99% accuracy in 69% of 855 fetuses between 15 weeks' gestation and term. Definitive visualization of the external genitalia was achieved in greater than 90% of cases after the fifth month. The external genitalia were visualized in detail by ultrasound in only one-third of the cases between the fourth and fifth month, two-thirds of cases between the fifth and sixth month, and in more than 90% of cases after that time. Reece et al. [26] subsequently reported visualization of the fetal external genitalia in 83.5% between weeks 15 and 20 using the longitudinal and coronal

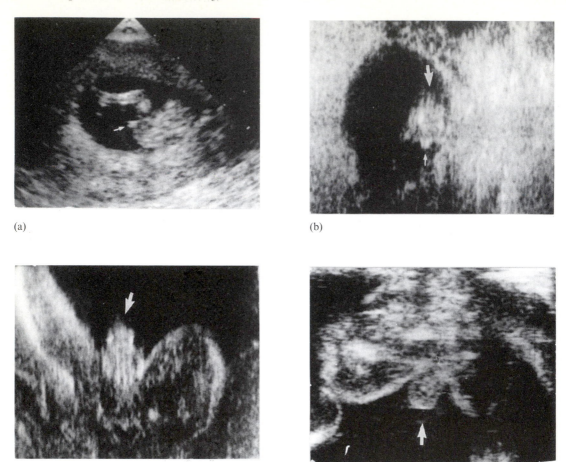

(a)

(b)

(c)

(d)

views of the fetal pelvis. Accuracy was reported to be 100% in males and 90% in females.

Elejalde [2] reported that at 14 weeks, the genitalia were seen in 19% of the cases with an error rate of 3.8%. As proficiency has improved, the genitalia can currently be seen in 81% of cases at 14 weeks. By the twentieth week of gestation, the genitalia are seen in 98% of the cases and no errors have been detected (B.R. Elejalde, 1992, unpublished data).

Prenatal ultrasound examination of the male genitalia can visualize the phallus as early as 10–11 weeks' gestation (Figures 19.1(a)–(h)), but the ultrasonographic assignment of sex is not possible at this stage. The genitalia are visualized in an oblique transverse plane and in the coronal plane. The sagittal views of the genitalia are difficult to perform and not very informative. As the pregnancy progresses, the phallus becomes larger in males and the scrotum can be seen. The female genitalia can also be examined prenatally using ultrasound (Figure 19.2(a)–(f)). In females, the labia majora and minora are visible by 15 weeks' gestation. By the twentieth week of gestation, the genitalia of both male and female can be seen in detail. The pulsations of the dorsal penile artery can be observed occasionally [2]. The urethra can be visualized when the fetus urinates (Figure 19.1(e)) and the labia majora and minora and the clitoris are easily discernible.

Birnholz [14] also compared his sonographic observations of testicular descent to Scorer's findings. No descent of the testis was seen in fetuses weighing less than 800 g. Forty per cent of fetuses weighing 900–1000 g and 80% of fetuses weighing 2000 g demonstrated testicular

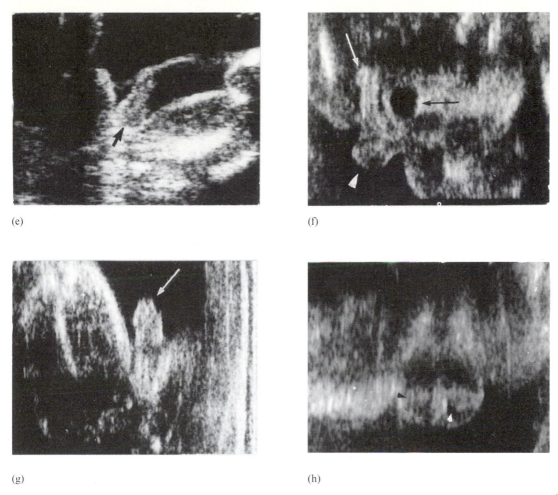

(e)

(f)

(g)

(h)

Figure 19.1 Prenatal ultrasound examination of male genitalia. (a) Midline view of male genitalia at 11 weeks' gestation. The arrow shows a prominent penis; the scrotum is not visible. (b) Coronal view of the lower half of the fetal body. The scrotum (small arrow) and the fetal spine (large arrow) are seen. (c) Transverse view of the penis (arrow) and scrotum at 21 weeks' gestation. Note the walls of the urethra in the middle of the penile shaft. (d) Transverse view of the scrotum at 22 weeks' gestation. (e) Erect penis (arrow) during urination at 22 weeks. (f) Penis (white arrow), scrotum (white arrowhead) and bladder (black arrow) at 22 weeks' gestation. (g) Penis at 30 weeks with well-defined glans and prepuce. (h) Coronal view of the scrotum at 32 weeks. The testes (black arrowhead) are descended and there are small bilateral hydroceles (white arrowhead).

descent. In no case was descent seen before 26 weeks. Therefore, this morphological feature is not useful in providing early sonographic information on the determination of fetal sex nor can it be used to estimate fetal maturity, since the timing of testicular descent is variable after 26 weeks.

Prenatal ultrasound of the scrotal contents have shown that hydroceles are a common finding [28,29]. The scrotum begins to show a collection of fluid as a faint band and accumulates progressively until the testicles descend

(Figure 19.1(h)). The ultrasound appearance of a hydrocele is a sonolucent area surrounding the testis. It may be difficult to determine if the hydrocele is communicating or non-communicating, unless there is a change in the size of the sonolucent structure on serial examinations [30].

Fetal sex cannot be determined in approximately 10% of fetuses after 24 weeks, due to the fetal position or maternal obesity [14]. Visualization of the penis can be confused with the umbilical cord or fetal fingers [30].

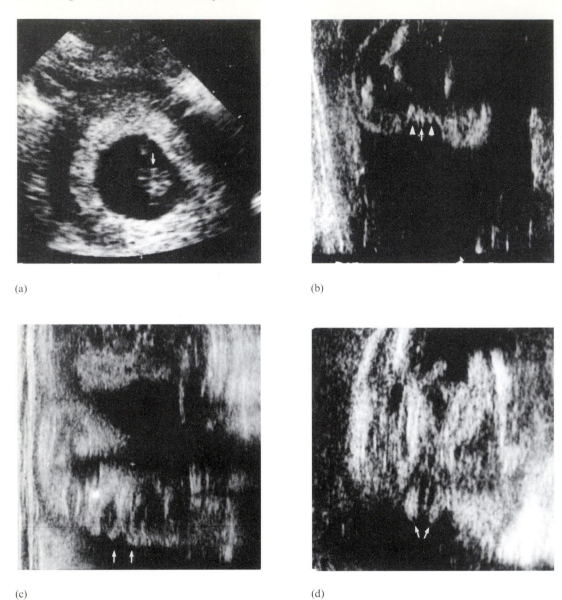

(a)

(b)

(c)

(d)

Although the technical capabilities of ultrasound have improved over the years enabling us to determine fetal gender prenatally, chromosomal confirmation is imperative before concluding that significant genetic or medical conditions exist [30]. When the ultrasound findings and the cytogenetically determined sex are discordant, it is necessary to repeat the ultrasonographic examination. When female genitalia are seen on ultrasound and the karyotype is 46, XY, these cases may represent testi- cular feminization or pure gonadal dysgenesis, for example. When the ultrasound findings suggest male genitalia and the karyotype is 46, XX, these cases may represent congenital adrenal hyperplasia or other intersex conditions. One should never assume that the cytogenetic sex is more accurate than the ultrasonographic examination. They are complementary and their combined interpretation allows for the accurate diagnosis of these types of conditions.

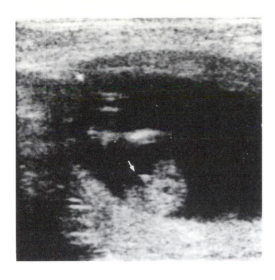

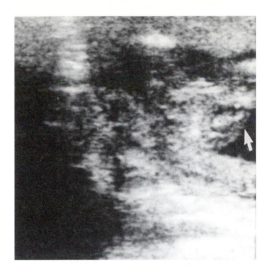

(e)   (f)

Figure 19.2 Prenatal ultrasound examination of the female genitalia. (a) Female genitalia at 10 weeks' gestation; note the prominent clitoris (arrow). (b) Coronal plane at 15 weeks showing the labia majora (arrowheads) and labia minora (arrow). (c) Transverse view of the labia majora (arrows) and interlabial space (between arrows) at 36 weeks. (d) Transverse view of the labia majora (arrows) and minora protruding over the perineum. (e) Transverse view of prominent 'phallus' at 13 weeks (arrow). (f) Same fetus as seen in (e) at 15 weeks. Clitoris is less prominent and a 46,XX karyotype was confirmed.

Uterovaginal anomalies

Prenatal ultrasound has also been used to visualize obstructed uterovaginal anomalies [30]. The anomalies are seen in two forms [31]. One form of hydrometrocolpos is due to isolated vaginal obstruction secondary to imperforate hymen, a transverse vaginal septum or segmental vaginal atresia. A second type of hydrometrocolpos occurs in association with a persistent urogenital sinus and cloacal anomalies. Uterovaginal anomalies are uncommon and are seen in 1 in 16 000 live births [32]. The cystic dilatation of the vagina and uterus results from accumulation of mucous secretions from the cervical mucous glands stimulated by maternal oestrogen [30,33]. A persistent urogenital sinus can be associated with intersex conditions or can be the result of arrested normal embryological development of the vagina [34,35]. Examination of the external genitalia can be misleading, since clitoral hypertrophy and ambiguous genitalia are often seen in intersex disorders. Although imperforate hymen is rarely seen in association with other malformations, hydrometrocolpos due to vaginal atresia, persistent urogenital sinus or

cloacal anomalies are commonly seen in association with other congenital malformations of the urinary and gastrointestinal tract and skeletal systems [30]. Hydrometrocolpos may also be one of the ultrasonographically recognizable signs of several genetic syndromes including the following autosomal dominant syndromes: camptobrachydactyly, hand–foot–uterus syndrome, Hay–Wells syndrome (ankyloblepharon, ectodermal defects, cleft lip and palate) and Ulnar–Mammary (Pallister) syndrome. The following autosomal recessive disorders may be associated with hydrometrocolpos: Johanson–Blizzard syndrome and Kaufman–McKusick (hydrometrocolpos, polydactyly, congenital heart disease). Hydrometrocolpos is associated with other anomalies, including: imperforate anus, renal agenesis, vaginal and uterine duplications, oesophageal atresia and lumbosacral anomalies [36–38], and in some cases, rectovaginal fistula, anal atresia, and vaginal and uterine duplications can occur.

Hydrometrocolpos due to uterovaginal anomalies has been detected sonographically as early as 26 weeks' gestation [31]. The sonographic findings include a large spherical or ovoid cystic pelvic abdominal mass with an almost imperceivable thin wall. This thin attenuated fluid-filled structure represents the vagina (hydrocolpos). The uterus can be differentiated by its thick muscular wall which has minimal distensibility. The ·fluid-filled mass most frequently contains a fluid-debris level. It is anechoic when there is a mixture of urine and uterovaginal secretions and/or meconium in the fetus with a cloacal anomaly [39]. Also, cloacal anomalies can have duplex genital tract malformations.

A solid-like echogenic mass can be seen with hydrometrocolpos secondary to imperforate hymen, transverse vaginal septum or vaginal atresia [39–41]. Imperforate hymen may lead to a bulging mass that can extend to the perineum and be visualized between the labia [41]. The bladder is not often seen in these fetuses due to extrinsic compression by the fluid-filled mass. Hydronephrosis and hydroureter may also result from extrinsic compression of the urinary tract. Hydro(metro)colpos should be in the differential diagnosis of a fetus with a cystic midline mass or a multicystic mass with internal echoes or a fluid-debris level arising from the pelvis. Ovarian duplication, meconium cysts and rectovaginal fistula with imperforate anus can also present with a similar sonographic appearance.

Ovarian cysts

Ovarian cysts can be detected by prenatal ultrasound [30]. These fluid-filled ovarian tumours are rare and most commonly occur unilaterally. Unilocular cysts are more common than septated cysts. Cysts can range in size from those that are very small to structures which fill the abdomen. Benign cysts are of germinal origin such as single cysts, thecalutein cysts and corpus luteum cysts. Granulosa cell tumours, benign cystic teratomas and mesonephromas are extremely rare in the newborn [42,43]. Ovarian cysts are not usually found in association with other congenital anomalies. Cases have been reported in which ovarian cysts have been found in association with congenital hypertrophic pyloric stenosis, hydrocephalus, absence of the corpus callosum and congenital hypothyroidism [44,45].

The prenatal ultrasound characteristics of an ovarian cyst are a fluid-filled intra-abdominal mass in a female fetus. Internal echoes may be seen. The urinary and gastrointestinal tract must be examined and appear separate from this mass [45–50]. Polyhydramnios has been seen in approximately 10% of patients with ovarian cysts, possibly due to extrinsic compression of the intestinal tract leading to small bowel obstruction [51].

Antenatal diagnosis of larger ovarian cysts can impact on the mode of delivery as well as management of the neonate [30]. Serial ultrasound examinations should be performed to monitor the gross appearance of the cysts. In order to avoid dystocia or intrapartum rupture which can lead to fetal death, an elective caesarean section or an attempt to drain the cyst under ultrasound guidance has been recommended [43]. Torsion and bleeding of a pedunculated ovarian cyst can occur and should be suspected if a hypoechoeic mass is subsequently noted to be hyperechoeic [50]. Newborns with ovarian cysts should be evaluated for hypothyroidism, although these two abnormalities rarely occur together [51]. Prenatal differential diagnosis of these masses include urachal and mesenteric cysts, enteric duplications, duodenal atresia and dilated bowel. Enteric duplications are usually tubular in shape. Duodenal atresia is associated with the 'double bubble' appearance as well as polyhydramnios.

Postnatally, large cysts should be surgically excised, even though the incidence of malignancy is extremely low [42,43], and the ovary should be preserved. Large cysts can be associated with ascites [52], torsion [53], rupture [54], haemorrhage [55], infection [56] and bowel obstruction [57].

Urethral abnormalities

Urethral abnormalities are not commonly diagnosed on prenatal ultrasound since dilatations of the urethra are associated with rare conditions. Posterior urethral valves occur in 1 in 5000 to 8000 male births. This congenital obstructive uropathy is associated with marked dilatation of the bladder and upper urinary tract. The posterior urethra is dilated and on occasion can be visualized ('key hole' sign) antenatally, further confirming this diagnosis [1]. The prune belly syndrome is extremely rare and occurs in 1 in 29 000–40 000 births. This syndrome is associated with the classical triad of findings, including lax abdominal wall musculature, dilatation of the urinary tract and bilateral undescended testes. An associated genital abnormality in males with prune belly syndrome is absence of the corporal bodies and fusiform megalourethra. The penis may have other associated abnormalities, including penile torsion, dorsal chordee, ventral chordee and hypospadias. The dilated megalourethra can be seen on an antenatal sonogram and will aid in confirming the diagnosis of prune belly syndrome in a patient with a distended bladder and dilated upper urinary tract [27].

In addition to the prenatal sonographic diagnosis of genital abnormalities, prenatal diagnosis and treatment of genital abnormalities due to congenital adrenal hyperplasia has been reported [48,50,55]. Congenital adrenal hyperplasia due to the 21-hydroxylase deficiency is the most common cause of ambiguous genitalia in the newborn and one of the most common autosomal recessive conditions. Congenital adrenal hyperplasia is transmitted as an autosomal recessive inborn error of adrenal steroid metabolism. It is the only intersex condition that, if unrecognized, threatens the survival of the infant. It has an incidence of 1 in 12 000 newborn with ethnic variability. In Caucasians, the incidence is 1 in 12 800, in Japanese 1 in 15 000, in the Yupik Eskimo 1 in 680 and in Italians 1 in 5500 to 1 in 10 000. Males and females are equally affected. The severe classic disorder results in excess adrenal secretion of androgens, causing virilization of the external genitalia of affected female fetuses during the critical period of sexual differentiation which occurs between 9 and 13 weeks' gestation [6,58].

Mornet [59] estimated that gene conversions account for 74% of the cases of 21-hydroxylase deficiency. Complete deletion of the gene produces 20% of the classic salt-wasting form of the condition. There are at least six allelic forms of the condition. Traditionally, the prenatal diagnosis of congenital adrenal hyperplasia in a fetus at risk can be performed during the first trimester by HLA typing or by DNA analysis of genes within the HLA complex, using probes for 21-hydroxylase genes, C4 genes, HLA genes, or a combination of these genes in chorionic villus cells [60–62]. The identification of the genes that produce this condition, as well as the specific mutations, allows for precise diagnosis of the condition using amniotic fluid or chorionic villus samples obtained any time after 9 weeks' gestation [63–65]. Chorionic villus material is obtained by either placing a small flexible polyethylene catheter through the cervix or transabdominally placing a needle inside the chorium frondosum, under ultrasound guidance and aspirating a small amount (approximately 25 mg) of chorionic villi. This tissue is processed for cytogenetic and biochemical testing [66,67]. Sex chromosomal analysis is available within a few days of the procedure and genotyping is available in about 2–3 weeks. Molecular techniques using DNA restriction fragment length polymorphisms detected by DNA probes for the genes in the HLA complex may be an additional means of diagnosing 21-hydroxylase deficiency. These procedures may be performed on biopsy specimens from chorionic villi or amniotic fluid cells [68].

Theoretically, suppression of the fetal pituitary adrenal axis with glucocorticoid during gestational weeks 9–17 should prevent the development of ambiguous genitalia in female fetuses at risk [69]. In families with one affected sibling, prenatal diagnosis of 21-hydroxylase deficiency has been most important, since there is a 25% risk of a subsequent affected sibling. Shapiro [70] reported the use of dexamethasone suppression at 8 weeks' gestation in a 34-year-old female whose son had congenital adrenal hyperplasia due to severe salt-losing 21-hydroxylase deficiency. The chorionic villi biopsy revealed a 46,XX chromosomal pattern. Cultured cells from the biopsy confirmed the fetus to be of identical HLA haplotype to the previous affected sibling. Dexamethasone 0.25 mg orally four times a day was initiated and the drug was well tolerated. Serial fetal ultrasound evaluations revealed no fetal malformations [70]. The prenatal sonographic appearance of the labia and clitoris did not appear abnormal throughout the third trimester (Figure 19.3). At 41 weeks' gestation, the patient delivered a female neonate with minimal prominence of the clitoris, mildly rugated labia and a single perineal

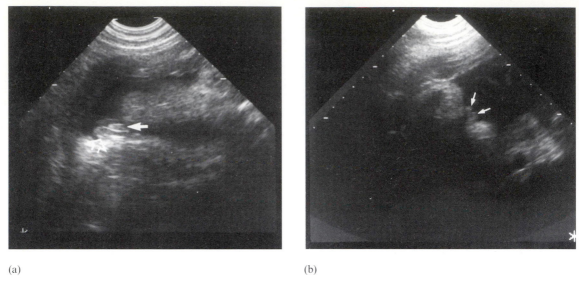

(a)   (b)

Figure 19.3 (a) Sonographic appearance of labia (open arrow) and clitoris (closed arrow) during the third trimester of pregnancy. (b) Sonographic appearance of labia (arrows) as viewed from below at level of buttocks.

opening with minimal posterior labial fusion (Figure 19.4). A genitogram was performed through the single perineal opening and revealed a short urogenital sinus, from which arose a long urethra and normal appearing bladder. A normal vagina entered low and a cervical impression was seen at the apex (Figure 19.5). Postnatal tapering of maternal steroids was performed with no long-term sequelae. Side-effects have been reported and include hyperglycaemia, excessive weight gain, chronic epigastric pain and increased facial hair growth [71].

Additional cases of first-trimester prenatal fetal adrenal suppression with dexamethasone have been reported [72]. To date, the overall experience with this treatment regimen suggests that fetal adrenal suppression in high-risk pregnancies appears to be an important adjunct in the antenatal management of congenital adrenal hyperplasia due to 21-hydroxylase deficiency.

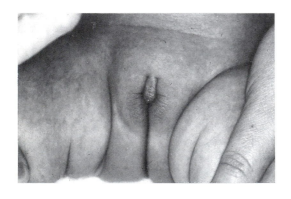
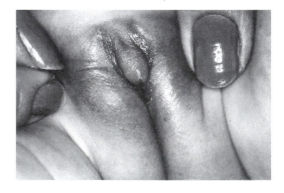

(a)   (b)

Figure 19.4 (a) External genitalia of female newborn treated *in utero* with maternal administration of dexamethasone from week 4 of pregnancy. Minimal virilization is noted. (b) Prominence of clitoris and posterior labial fusion present.

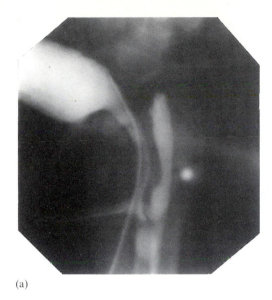

(a)

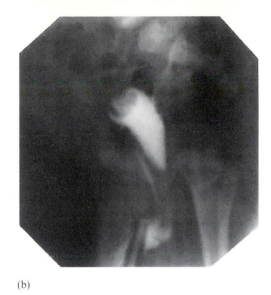

(b)

Figure 19.5 Genitogram through single perineal opening demonstrates short urogenital sinus. (a) Elongated urethra and normal bladder are seen. (b) Post-void film shows normal vagina entering low and cervical impression is demonstrated at its apex.

References

1. Mandell J, Peters CA, Retik AB. Prenatal and post-natal diagnosis and management of congenital abnormalities. In: Walsh PC, Retik AB, Stamey TA, Vaughan Jr ED (eds) *Campbell's Urology*. Philadelphia: WB Saunders, 1992; pp 1563–1589.
2. Elejalde BR, De Elejalde MM, Heitman T. Visualization of the fetal genitalia by ultrasonography: a review of the literature and analysis of its accuracy and ethical implications. *J Ultrasound Med* 1985; **4**: 633–639.
3. Doran TA. Chorionic villus sampling as the primary diagnostic tool in prenatal diagnosis. Should it replace genetic amniocentesis? *J Reprod Med* 1990; **35**: 935.
4. Seeds JW, Bowe WA. Ultrasound guided fetal intravascular transfusion in severe rhesus immunization. *Am J Obstet Gynecol* 1986; **154**: 1105.
5. Bianchi D, Flint A, Pizzimenti M et al. Isolation of fetal DNA from nucleated erythrocytes in maternal blood. *Proc Nat Acad Sci* 1990; **87**: 3279.
6. George FW, Wilson JD. Embryology of the genital tract. In: Walsh PC, Retik AB, Stamey TA, Vaughan Jr ED (eds) *Campbell's Urology*. Philadelphia: WB Saunders, 1992; pp 1496–1508.
7. Maizels M. Normal development of the urinary tract. In: Walsh PC, Retik AB, Stamey TA, Vaughan Jr ED (eds) *Campbell's Urology*. Philadelphia: WB Saunders, 1992; pp 1301–1343.
8. Wilson JD, Goldstein JL. Classification of hereditary disorders of sexual development. In: Bergsma D (ed) Genetic Forms of Hypogonadism. Birth Defects XI: 1–16.
9. Gillman J. The development of the gonads in man, with a consideration of the role of fetal endocrines and the histogenesis of ovarian tumors. *Carnegie Contrib Embryol* **210**: 32, 83.
10. Siiteri PK, Wilson JD. Testosterone formation and metabolism during male sexual differentiation in the human embryo. *J Clin Endocrinol Metab* 1974; **38**: 113.
11. Donahoe PK, Ito Y, Hendren WH III. A graded organ culture assay for detecting of mullerian inhibiting substance. *J Surg Res* 1977; **23**: 141.
12. Josso N. Antimullerian hormone: new perspectives for a sexist molecule. *Endocrine Rev* 1986; **7**: 421.
13. Spaulding MH. The development of the external genitalia in the human embryo. *Carnegie Contrib Embryol* 1921; **13**: (61), 67.
14. Birnholz JC. Determination of fetal sex. *New Eng J Med* 1983; **309**: 942–944.
15. FitzGerald JJT (ed). Abdominal and pelvic organs. In: *Human Embryology*. New York: Harper & Row, 1978, p 106.
16. Toaff ME. Origin of the epithelium of atretic hemivaginas. *Am J Obstet Gynecol* 1984; **149**: 237 (letter).
17. Waterman RE. Human embryo and fetus. In: Hafez ESE, Kenemans P (eds) *Atlas of Human Reproduction*. Hingham, MA: Kluwer Boston.
18. Hamilton WJ, Mossman HW (eds). The urogenital system. In: *Human Embryology Prenatal Development of Form and Function*. New York: Macmillan Press, 1976; p 377.

19. Bellinger MF, Duckett JW. Accessory phallic urethra in the female patient. *J Urol* 1982; **127**: 1159.

20. Stephens FD. *Congenital Malformations of the Urinary Tract.* New York: Praeger.

21. Jones KL (ed). *Smith's Recognizable Patterns of Human Malformations*, 3rd edn. Philadelphia: WB Saunders, pp 707–763.

22. Stocker J, Evans L. Fetal sex determination by ultrasound. *Obstet Gynecol* 1977; **50**: 462.

23. Schorzman LL. Sex determination *in utero. Med Ultrasound* 1977; **1**: 25.

24. Dunne MG, Cunat JS. Sonographic determination of fetal gender before 25 weeks gestation. *Am J Radiol* 1983; **140**: 741–743.

25. Natsuyama E. Sonographic determination of fetal sex from twelve weeks of gestation. *Am J Obstet Gynecol* 1984; **149**: 748–757.

26. Reece EA, Winn HN, Wan M et al. Can ultrasonography replace amniocentesis in fetal gender determination during the early second trimester? *Am J Obstet Gynecol* 1987; **156**: 579–581.

27. Benacerraf BR, Saltzman DH, Mandell J. Sonographic diagnosis of abnormal fetal genitalia. *J Ultrasound Med* 1989; **8**: 613–617.

28. Conrad AR, Rao SAS. Ultrasound diagnosis of fetal hydrocele. *Radiology* 1978; **127**: 232.

29. Miller EI, Thomas RH. Fetal hydrecele detected *in utero* by ultrasound. *Br J Radiol* 1979; **52**: 624–625.

30. Romero R, Pilu G, Jeanty P et al. (eds). The genital tract. In: *Prenatal Diagnosis of Congenital Anomalies.* East Norwalk, CN: Appleton & Lange.

31. Nussbaum Blask AR, Sanders RC, Gearhart JP. Obstructed uterovaginal anomalies: demonstration with sonography. Part I. neonates and infants. *Pediatr Radiol* 1991; **179**: 79–83.

32. Westerhout FC, Hodgman JE, Anderson GV et al. Congenital hydrocolpos. *Am J Obstet Gynecol* 1964; **89**: 957.

33. Mahoney PJ, Chamberlain JW. Hydrometrocolpos in infancy: congenital atresia of the vagina with abnormally abundant cervical secretions. *J Pediatr* 1940; **17**: 772.

34. Williams DI, Bloomberg S. Urogenital sinus in the female child. *J Pediatr Surg* 1976; **11**: 51–56.

35. Hahn-Pedersen J, Kvist N, Nielsen OH. Hydrometrocolpos: current views of pathogenesis and management. *J Urol* 1984; **132**: 537–540.

36. Lide TN, Coker WG. Congenital hydrometrocolpos. Review of the literature and report of a case with uterus duplex and incompletely septate vagina. *Am J Obstet Gynecol* 1952; **64**: 1275.

37. Graivier L. Hydrocolpos. *J Pediatr Surg* 1969; **4**: 563.

38. Reed MH, Griscom NT. Hydrometrocolpos in infancy. *Am J Radiol* 1973; **118**: 1.

39. Hill SJ, Hirsch JH. Sonographic detection of fetal hydrometrocolpos. *J Ultrasound Med* 1985; **4**: 323–325.

40. Wilson DA, Stacy TM, Smith EI. Ultrasound diagnosis of hydrocolpos and hydrometrocolpos. *Radiology* 1978; **128**: 451–454.

41. Davis GH, Wapner RJ, Kurtz AB et al. Antenatal diagnosis of hydrometrocolpos by ultrasound examination. *J Ultrasound Med* 1984; **3**: 371–374.

42. Carlson DH, Griscom NT. Ovarian cysts in the newborn. *Am J Radiol* 1972; **116**: 664–672.

43. Jouppila P, Kirkinen P, Tuononen S. Ultrasonic detection of bilateral ovarian cysts in the fetus. *Eur J Obstet Gynecol Reprod Biol* 1982; **131**: 87.

44. Evers JL, Rolland R. Primary hypothyroidism and ovarian activity: evidence of an overlap in the synthesis of pituitary glycoproteins. Case report. *Br J Obstet Gynecol* 1981; **88**: 195–202.

45. Sandler MA, Smith SJ, Pope SG et al. Prenatal diagnosis of septated ovarian cysts. *J Clin Ultrasound* 1985; **13**: 55.

46. Valenti C, Kassner EG, Yermakov V et al. Antenatal diagnosis of a fetal ovarian cyst. *Am J Obstet Gynecol* 1975; **123**: 216–219.

47. Crade M, Gillooly L, Taylor KJM. *In utero* demonstration of an ovarian cyst mass by ultrasound. *J Clin Ultrasound* 1980; **8**: 251–252.

48. Mitsutake K, Abe I, Masumoto R et al. Prenatal diagnosis of fetal abdominal masses by real-time ultrasound. *Kurume Med J* 1981; **28**: 329–334.

49. Tabsh KMA. Antenatal sonographic appearance of a fetal ovarian cyst. *J Ultrasound Med* 1982; **1**: 329–331.

50. Preziosi P, Fariello G, Maiorana A et al. Antenatal sonographic diagnosis of complicated ovarian cysts. *J Clin Ultrasound* 1986; **14**: 196.

51. Jafri SZH, Bree RL, Silver JM et al. Fetal ovarian cysts: sonographic detection and association with hypothyroidism. *Radiology* 1984; **150**: 809–812.

52. Ahmed S. Neonatal and childhood ovarian cysts. *J Pediatr Surg* 1971; **6**: 702.

53. Karrer FW, Swenson SA. Twisted ovarian cyst in a newborn infant: report of a case. *Arch Surg* 1961; **83**: 921.

54. Tietz KG, Davis JB. Ruptured ovarian cyst in a newborn infant. *J Pediatr* 1957; **51**: 564.

55. Monson R, Rodgers BM, Nelson RM et al. Ruptured ovarian cyst in a newborn infant. *J Pediatr* 1978; **93**: 324.

56. Marshall JR. Ovarian enlargements in the first year of life: review of 45 cases. *Ann Surg* 1965; **16**: 372.

57. Dieter RA Jr, Kindrachuk W, Muller RP. Neonatal intestinal obstruction due to torsion of an ovarian cyst. *J Fam Pract* 1977; **10**: 533.

58. Griffin JE, Wilson JD. Disorders of sexual differentiation. In: Walsh PC, Retik AB, Stamey TA, Vaughan Jr ED (eds) *Campbell's Urology.* Philadelphia: WB Saunders, 1992; pp 1509–1542.

59. Mornet E, Boue J, Raux-Demay M et al. First trimester prenatal diagnosis of 21-hydroxylase deficiency by linkage analysis to HLA-DNA probes and by 17-

hydroxyprogesterone determination. *Hum Genet* 1986; **73**: 358–364.

60. Mornet E, Crete P, Kuttenn F et al. Distribution of deletions and seven point mutations on CYP21B genes in three clinical forms of steroid 21-hydroxylase deficiency. *Am J Hum Genet* 1991; **48**: 79–88.

61. Pollack MS, Carroll MC, Black S et al. Congenital 21-hydroxylase deficiency as a new mutation: detection during prenatal diagnosis by HLA typing and DNA analysis. *Hum Immunol* 1986; **17**: 183 (abstract).

62. Killeen AA, Seelig S, Ulstrom RA et al. Diagnosis of classical steroid 21-hydroxylase deficiency using an HLA-B locus-specific DNA-probe. *Am J Med Genet* 1988; **29**: 703–712.

63. Couillin P, Boue J, Nicholas H et al. Prenatal diagnosis of congenital adrenal hyperplasia (21-OH deficiency type) by HLA typing. *Prenat Diagn* 1981; **1**: 25–33.

64. Pang S, Pollack MS, Loo M et al. Pitfalls of prenatal diagnosis of 21-hydroxylase deficiency congenital adrenal hyperplasia. *J Clin Endocrinol Metab* 1985; **61**: 89–97.

65. Hughes IA, Dyas J, Riad-Fahmy D et al. Prenatal diagnosis of congenital adrenal hyperplasia: reliability of amniotic fluid steroid analysis. *J Med Genet* 1987; **24**: 344–347.

66. Brambati B, Oldrini A, Ferrazzi E et al. Chorionic villi sampling: general methodological and clinical approach. In: Fraccaro M, Simoni G, Brambati B (eds) *First Trimester Fetal Diagnosis*. New York: Springer-Verlag, pp 7–18.

67. Callaway C, Falcon C, Grant G et al. HLA typing with cultured amniotic and chorionic villus cells for early prenatal diagnosis or parentage testing without one parent's availability. *Hum Immunol* 1986; **16**: 200–204.

68. White PC, New MI, Dupont B. Structure of human steroid 21-hydroxylase genes. *Proc N Acad Sci* 1986; **83**: 5111.

69. David M, Forest MG. Prenatal treatment of congenital adrenal hyperplasia resulting for 21-hydroxylase deficiency. *J Pediatr* 1984; **105**: 799–803.

70. Shapiro E, Santiago JV, Crane JP. Prenatal fetal adrenal suppression following *in utero* diagnosis of congenital adrenal hyperplasia. *J Urol* 1989; **142**: 663–666.

71. Dorr HG, Sippell WC, Bidlingmaier F et al. Experience with intrauterine therapy of congenital adrenal hyperplasia (CAH) due to 21-hydroxylase deficiency. In: Endocrine Society Program and Abstracts, 70th Annual Meeting, New Orleans, June 8–11, 1988, Bethesda, MD: Endocrine Society, p 21.

72. Pang S, Pollack MS, Marshall RN et al. Prenatal treatment of congenital adrenal hyperplasia due to 21-hydroxylase deficiency. *Med Intellig* 1990; **322**: 111–115.

20

Postnatal investigation and management of genital and intersex anomalies

R.H. Whitaker and D.M. Williams

Introduction

In order to explain the various abnormalities of development that lead to intersex disorders, with or without ambiguous genitalia, it is necessary to understand normal development (Figure 20.1). There are important physiological and embryological events that lead to normal gonads, internal and external sexual organs and function [1].

An important concept is that the development of the male fetus is an active, rapid process whilst female differentiation is passive and slower.

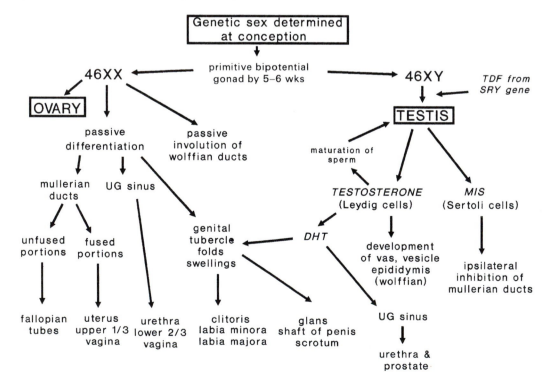

Figure 20.1 Map of normal development.

Male development

The first important factor known to influence the developing gonad of the 46XY zygote is *testis determining factor* (TDF), the production of which at 6–7 weeks is controlled by the SRY gene on the distal portion of the short arm of the Y chromosome [2]. First Sertoli cells appear in the primitive testis which, together with the germ cells that migrated from the yolk sac, become enclosed as testicular cords. Soon Leydig cells differentiate outside the cords and finally the testis becomes a rounded organ.

Mullerian inhibiting substance (MIS) is produced from 7 weeks onwards by the Sertoli cells under the influence of a gene on the tip of the short arm of chromosome 19 [3]. It diffuses locally to the ipsilateral mullerian (paramesonephric) duct to cause involution at 9–11 weeks [4]. In the male, all that remains of this duct thereafter is the appendix testis and prostatic utricle.

Testosterone production by the Leydig cells is maximum at 16 weeks. Its production is stimulated initially by placental human chorionic gonadotrophin (HCG) and later by fetal pituitary gonadotrophins. It diffuses into the wolffian ducts to cause their differentiation into vasa, seminal vesicles and epididymes between 8 and 12 weeks. It also diffuses into the androgen-sensitive cells of the developing genitalia, where it may be converted by the enzyme 5-α reductase to a potent metabolite, dihydrotestosterone (DHT). Testosterone and DHT exert their effect by combining with intracellular androgen receptor and these complexes enter the nucleus to bind with chromosomal DNA target sites to influence gene expression (Figure 20.2).

The testosterone–receptor complex regulates the feedback loop of gonadotrophin production from the hypothalamus/pituitary axis, stimulates spermatogenesis and has a continuing effect on the virilization of the wolffian duct derivatives, whilst the DHT–receptor complex causes virilization of the external genitalia and urogenital sinus, and causes maturation at male puberty.

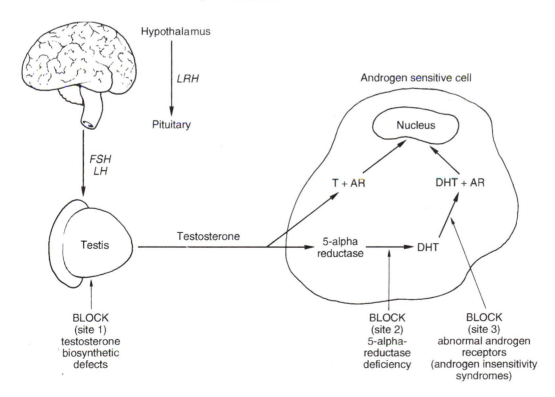

Figure 20.2 Normal pathway of androgen production in the androgen-sensitive cell with the three main sites of block. AR = androgen receptor; T = testosterone.

Female development

In the absence of TDF, the 46XX gonad develops into an ovary between 12 and 25 weeks; follicles develop maximally by the end of this time under the influence of fetal pituitary follicular stimulating hormone (FSH). In the absence of testosterone the wolffian ducts involute. Similarly, without the inhibition of MIS, there is passive female differentiation of the mullerian ducts, urogenital sinus and primitive external genitalia (Figure 20.1).

The cloaca splits into the urogenital sinus (UGS) anteriorly and the rectum posteriorly. The UGS becomes part of the bladder, urethra and lower two-thirds of the vagina.

Abnormal sexual development

Several defects can lead to abnormal sexual development:

- Chromosomal anomalies and gonadal dysgenesis.
- Virilization of female fetus (female pseudohermaphroditism).
- Inadequate virilization of male fetus (male pseudohermaphroditism).

The commoner conditions are summarized in Table 20.1. Not all are associated with ambiguous genitalia; thus patients may present in childhood, at puberty or later with lumps in the groins, gynaecomastia or infertility. However, for diagnostic purposes it is convenient to describe all such conditions together.

Chromosomal anomalies and gonadal dysgenesis

A variety of chromosomal problems can arise during either meiosis or mitosis. These include non-dysjunction, deletion, translocation, rearrangement and breakage. The results are summarized as *missing/mosaic*, *additions* or *apparently normal chromosomes*.

Missing/mosaic

- 45XO   Turner's syndrome
- 45XO/46XY   Mixed gonadal dysgenesis
- 46XX/46XY   True hermaphrodite
                      (31%) [5,6]

Turner's syndrome (45XO, mosaics or variant)

In the absence of a Y chromosome these patients are female with unambiguous genitalia and streak gonads (Table 20.1).

Mixed gonadal dysgenesis (mostly mosaic 45XO/46XY)

These patients may have abnormal or ambiguous genitalia with a spectrum of abnormality (Table 20.1). The gonads may be asymmetrical, often with a palpable testis in the groin or scrotum on one side which has Sertoli and Leydig cells only. Opposite there may be a streak gonad and, due to ipsilateral lack of MIS [4], ipsilateral persistence of mullerian structures (fallopian tube and bi- or unicornuate uterus).

Rearing as male is possible if there is a good phallus which responds well to stimulation with testosterone but the majority with ambiguous genitalia are reared as females. This is often wise as the mosaic pattern is associated with short stature, infertility and the need to remove the gonads because of the malignancy risk [7].

For female rearing a gonadectomy with genitoplasty is needed, whilst for male rearing dysgenetic tissue is removed and the hypospadias repaired.

True hermaphrodite (46XX/46XY)
See below.

Additions

- 47XXY–49XXXXXY   Klinefelter's, etc.
- (various combinations)
- 47XXX

Klinefelter's syndrome (47XXY–49XXXXXY or mosaic 46XX/47XXY)
These patients have a Y chromosome and hence testes (Table 20.1).

Apparent normal

- 46XX   Male (translocation of fragments of Y chromosome onto X chromosome)
- 46XY   Female (loss of SRY gene from Y chromosome)
- 46XX   True hermaphrodite (57–80%) [5,6]

Table 20.1 Synopsis of three groups of patients with abnormalities of sexual development

	Karyotype	Gonad	Genitalia	Clinical notes
Chromosomal anomalies and gonadal dysgenesis				
Turner's syndrome	45XO or variant	Streaks or ovaries	Female	Short stature, sexual infantilism, primary amenorrhoea, inconstant physical features (webbing of neck and increase in carrying angle)
Mixed gonadal dysgenesis	45XO/46XY	Streak ±UDT	Male, female or ambiguous	Short stature, mixed internal organs, phallus short and hypospadiac, late virilization, infertility, gynaecomastia and gonadal tumour risk
Klinefelter's syndrome	47XXY or variant	Testes and seminal tubule dysgenesis	Male	Tall (long legs), small firm testes, aspermic, gynaecomastia in 50%, mental and emotional difficulties common
46XX male	46XX	Testes	Male or ambiguous	Often hypospadias and UDT, short stature, infertility, rare
True hermaphroditism	46XX, 46XY 46XX/46XY	Ovary and testis or ovotestis	Ambiguous or male	Variable internal and external organs, bifid scrotum, hypospadias, surgery according to sex of rearing
Pure gonadal dysgenesis	46XX	Streak	Female	Tall, sexual infantilism, amenorrhoea, no clitoral hypertrophy, no gonadal tumour risk
Pure gonadal dysgenesis	46XY	Streak	Female	Variable clitoral hypertrophy, failure of sexual development, primary amenorrhoea, gonadal tumour risk
Female virilization (female pseudohermaphroditism)				
Virilizing congenital adrenal hyperplasia (e.g. 21-hydroxylase deficiency)	46XX	Ovaries	Ambiguous	Virilized, salt loss in 75% of 21OH deficiency, uterus and upper vagina present, clitoral hypertrophy, raised plasma 17OH progesterone, autosomal recessive, 1 : 13 000 Caucasian births
Transplacental androgens	46XX	Ovaries	Ambiguous	Virilized, exogenous androgen or from virilizing tumour in mother. Now rare
Male undervirilization (male pseudohermaphroditism)				
Testosterone biosynthetic defects (e.g. 17β-hydroxy-steroid dehydrogenase deficiency)	46XY	Testes (UDT)	Ambiguous	Male internal organs, severe hypospadias, variable virilization at puberty, variable breast development
DHT biosynthetic defects (5α-reductase deficiency)	46XY	Testes	Ambiguous	Virilize at puberty but penis remains small. Failure to convert testosterone to DHT within cell. Autosomal recessive
Complete androgen insensitivity syndrome	46XY	Testes (UDT)	Female	Female external organs, short vagina, no uterus, breast development at puberty, gonadal tumour risk. End organ response failure
Partial androgen insensitivity syndrome	46XY	Testes	Ambiguous	Small hypospadiac phallus, variable labioscrotal fusion, ± UDT, virilization and gynaecomastia at puberty. Partial end organ response failure
Hernia uteri inguinale (persistent mullerian duct syndrome)	46XY	Testes	Male	Normal phallus, uterus and tube may be in inguinal hernia, ± UDT, poor sperm and hormone production, gonadal tumour risk

- 46XY   True hermaphrodite (13%) [5,6]
- 46XX   Streak gonads – pure gonadal dysgenesis
- 46XY   Streak gonads – pure gonadal dysgenesis

46XX males

This is a rare condition in which affected patients are phenotypically male usually with no genital ambiguity. Wolffian duct structures are normal and mullerian derivatives are suppressed, indicating normal early production of MIS and testosterone. At puberty there is often gynaecomastia and hyalinization of the testes which become small and firm. In most cases the DNA from the short arm of the Y chromosome, containing the recently recognized SRY gene, is transposed to the distal end of the short arm of an X chromosome [2].

Hypospadias and undescended testes need operative treatment.

True hermaphroditism (46XX, 46XY or 46XX/ 46XY)

By definition such patients have both ovarian and testicular tissue either separately or as ovotestes (Table 20.1). The external genitalia are usually ambiguous. The internal organs are variable but usually asymmetrical according to the influence of the ipsilateral gonad. In the presence of an ovotestis a fallopian tube is present in 50%, a vas in 25% and ambiguous structures in 25% [5]. A uterus is usually present but may be hypoplastic or unicornuate.

A decision on the most appropriate sex of rearing is based mainly on the adequacy of the phallus, hence female rearing is usual. The surgical choices are genitoplasty or hypospadias repair. In the presence of a Y chromosome all dysgenetic tissue must be removed due to the malignancy risk [7].

Some of these patients with 46XX chromosomes have menses and occasional pregnancies have been reported [8].

Pure gonadal dysgenesis (46XX or 46XY)

There are two forms of pure gonadal dysgenesis, 46XX and 46XY, in which there are bilateral inactive streak gonads (Table 20.1).

As such patients have normal female appearance they are seldom recognized in the neonatal period. They have hypoplastic mullerian internal organs and no wolffian structures.

A Y chromosome gives an increased gonadal tumour risk [7].

Virilization of female (female pseudohermaphroditism – 46XX)

The most common form of 46XX virilization is congenital adrenal hyperplasia (CAH) in which the basic anomaly is a block in steroid biosynthesis which results in an accumulation of metabolic precursors acting as substrates for increased androgen production [9]. An alternative source of excess androgen is exogenous intake or, rarely, an androgen secreting tumour in the mother (Table 20.1).

Congenital adrenal hyperplasia (46XX)

CAH accounts for approximately 70% of children with ambiguous genitalia [8]. It affects both sexes, leading to ambiguous genitalia in females, with or without salt loss (Table 20.1). Boys usually present as neonates with salt loss (vomiting, shock, hyponatraemia, hyperkalaemia).

The adrenal gland normally produces three classes of steroid hormone – glucocorticoids, mineralocorticoids and sex hormones; these are produced by a series of enzymatic steps from cholesterol (Figure 20.3). Deficiency of any of these enzymes results in a lack of end products usually including cortisol. The normal feedback loop is triggered by cortisol to the pituitary to control ACTH output. Without this control mechanism there is excessive ACTH secretion which causes the adrenal glands to hypertrophy.

21-Hydroxylase deficiency accounts for more than 95% of cases of CAH. This enzyme is encoded by two genes on the short arm of chromosome 6, one of which has become inactive due to a series of deleterious mutations [10]. In its absence there is excess accumulation of the steroid precursor, 17-hydroxyprogesterone, which is diagnostic of this condition (Figure 20.5). This precursor is metabolized to androstenedione, a weak androgen, and finally to testosterone (Figure 20.3).

Approximately 75% of cases also have a block in the 21-hydroxylase-mediated step in aldosterone biosynthesis, which results in increased urinary sodium excretion and potassium retention.

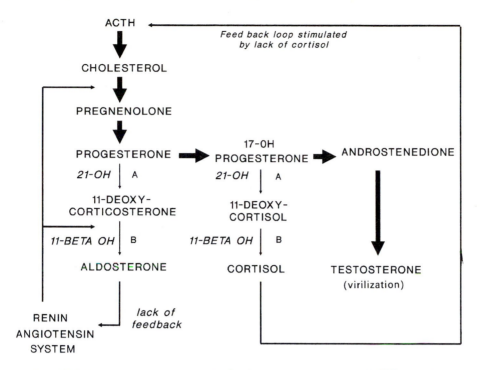

Figure 20.3 Steroid hormone biosynthesis showing the consequences of (A) 21-hydroxylase (21-OH) and (B) 11-β hydroxylase (11-β OH) deficiencies.

Clinical features

In females the excess androgen production leads to a spectrum of virilization varying from mild clitoromegaly to an apparent 'male' appearance with a terminal urethral meatus but an empty scrotum (Table 20.1). The internal genitalia are invariably normal female. The excess ACTH causes some hyperpigmentation in either sex.

11β-Hydroxylase deficiency is a rarer cause of CAH. There is mild elevation of 17-hydroxy-progesterone but as the enzyme block is further down the pathway there is greater elevation of 11-deoxycortisol and 11-deoxy-corticosterone (Figure 20.3). The latter has mineralocorticoid activity so, in addition to the consequences of excess androgen, affected infants become hypertensive in time.

Treatment of CAH

Urgent diagnosis and treatment is needed to correct cortisol and aldosterone deficiency with hydrocortisone and fludrocortisone, respectively. Thereafter the aim is to provide the minimum dosages necessary to inhibit the excess ACTH and renin/angiotensin stimulation and hence allow normal growth and maturation and fluid and electrolyte balance [9].

Affected girls may need extensive genitoplasty as soon as the child is medically stable. The results of surgery are excellent. Details are discussed later.

With adequate medical and surgical management there is the prospect of normal sexual function and fertility.

Transplacental androgens (46XX)

This is now a rare form of female virilization (Table 20.1).

Inadequate virilization of males (male pseudohermaphroditism – 46XY)

Most of the anomalies (Table 20.1) are due either to inadequate production of testosterone and/or DHT or to a deficiency in the peripheral effects of these hormones. Occasionally, in a 46XY fetus, there is failure of production of

MIS which leads to an ipsilateral persistence of mullerian duct derivatives. In this condition of hernia uteri inguinale (persistent mullerian duct syndrome) (Table 20.1) there are testes, but the child presents with a hernia or for an orchidopexy at which time a fallopian tube and uterus are found [8,11].

Figure 20.2 shows the three main sites for defects. Patients present as males with varying degrees of lack of virilization or as infertile 'females' (Table 20.1).

The three groups are as follows:

Decreased production of testosterone

There are several testosterone biosynthetic defects due to enzyme deficiencies in the androgen production pathway, such as deficiency of 17β hydroxysteroid dehydrogenase or 3β steroid dehydrogenase. MIS is produced normally so that no mullerian structures remain. Patients with these defects usually present with ambiguous genitalia (Table 20.1) and the diagnosis is confirmed by measurement of plasma and urinary androgen precursors as well as testosterone levels before and after HCG stimulation (Figure 20.6) [12].

Decisions concerning sex of rearing are discussed below and these determine the choice of appropriate surgery.

Abnormal testosterone metabolism

In 5α reductase deficiency there is a failure to convert testosterone to DHT. Without DHT there is minimal virilization of the fetus but at puberty a surge of androgen production causes marked virilization. In the Dominican Republic, where this condition is not uncommon, it was accepted readily that affected children were raised as girls and that at puberty they adopted the male role [13]. Diagnostic tests include measurement of the testosterone/DHT ratio in plasma and the ratio of 5α to 5β androgen metabolites in urine after stimulation with HCG [14] (Figure 20.6).

Surgery is chosen according to the sex of rearing.

Defective end organ response (androgen insensitivity)

Resistance to the action of androgens, the so-called androgen insensitivity syndrome, is associated with abnormal sexual development. Approximately two-thirds of cases are familial, showing an X-linked pattern of inheritance. The gene is located on the long arm of the X chromosome, Xq11–12, and has now been extensively studied [15].

Two phenotypic forms are recognized (Table 20.1). In *complete androgen insensitivity syndrome (CAIS)* (previously testicular feminization syndrome) there is total resistance of the tissues to the effects of androgens and the child has normal appearing female external genitalia (Figure 20.6). The condition may present in infancy or childhood with labial swellings or herniae which are found to contain testes. More commonly, it presents in adolescence with primary amenorrhoea. There is absence of internal female genitalia on ultrasound and/or laparoscopy and testicular histology shows Leydig cells and tubules but no spermatogenesis. Plasma testosterone concentrations are within the age-appropriate range, or sometimes higher as a result of increased stimulation by LH. A number of mutations of the androgen receptor gene have been identified in patients with CAIS [16].

In *partial androgen insensitivity syndrome (PAIS)* the genital ambiguity is variable (Table 20.1). Familial hypospadias may represent a variant of PAIS [17].

The diagnosis of PAIS depends first on demonstrating a normal testosterone and DHT response to HCG stimulation (Figure 20.6). Measurement of androgen precursors in plasma and their metabolites in urine after HCG stimulation should exclude testosterone biosynthetic defects. Pelvic ultrasound generally shows absence of female internal genitalia, although vaginal remnants may persist. Testicular histology shows immaturity with prominent Leydig cells. In some patients with PAIS a mutation has been found in the androgen receptor gene [16]. However, in many cases no mutation can be identified and it must be assumed that partial androgen insensitivity is the result of defects on other, as yet unrecognized, genes which have a role in sexual development.

Patients with CAIS are reared as female; reconstructive surgery is not required but because of the malignancy risk gonadectomy is needed and although the timing is debatable it is now usually performed early. The patient needs to be told of longer-term issues including hormone replacement and fertility.

Patients with PAIS need an early joint medical and surgical assessment of the external genitalia. There is currently a lack of a reliable indicator as to whether an infant reared as a male will virilize at puberty. A pragmatic approach is to assess growth of the phallus after a trial of 2 or 3 monthly injections of testosterone enanthate 25 mg before finally deciding whether a severely undervirilized infant can be reared as a male. Birth registration and naming the child is delayed until a decision has been made.

Those reared as females require appropriate genital surgery and gonadectomy performed early, and oestrogen replacement at the time of puberty. In the male a severe hypospadias and undescended testes need attention. Preoperative androgen therapy may produce phallic growth and facilitate surgical reconstruction.

Diagnosis

Conditions that lead to ambiguous genitalia associated with life-threatening metabolic disturbances (e.g. CAH) must be diagnosed early and dealt with efficiently

The next aim is to make a fast and accurate sex assignment that leaves no doubts in the minds of distressed and often guilt-ridden parents. Often, as in CAH, the diagnosis may be reached rapidly but sometimes delay is inevitable and it may take all the skills of a paediatric endocrinologist and urologist, together with a geneticist, to decide the most appropriate sex of rearing and to help the parents over this difficult period.

The sex of the child must not be guessed and both naming and registration should await a correct diagnosis. If the situation is fully and kindly explained to the parents most will accept a period of uncertainty.

The following groups must be considered for investigation for intersex anomalies:

- Any child with ambiguous genitalia.
- Apparent females with clitoral enlargement.
- Neonates with inguinal masses or herniae.
- Apparent males with micropenis.
- Apparent males with severe hypospadias, particularly if associated with undescended testes.

- Apparent males with bilateral impalpable undescended testes.

Table 20.2 lists the main features of the history, physical examination, blood and urine analysis and other frequently useful investigations. It should be noted that ovaries are only very rarely palpable so that a gonad in the groin or scrotum is nearly always a testis. Although the presence of a uterus can sometimes be confirmed by rectal examination, an expert ultrasound examination is more accurate and gives the opportunity for more effective assessment of the internal organs.

A genitogram, performed by injecting contrast medium into the common opening of the urogenital sinus, is particularly informative

Table 20.2 Main features of history and investigations

History
Family
    Parental consanguinity
    Neonatal deaths
    Intersex
    Genital anomalies
    Primary amenorrhoea
    Infertility
Maternal
    Exposure to drugs or androgens
    Tumours
Neonatal
    Vomiting and/or diarrhoea

Physical examination
Dysmorphic features
Blood pressure
Pigmentation of genital and areolar areas
Size of phallus
Site of urethral/sinus opening
Palpability and symmetry of gonads

Blood analysis
Urgent chromosomal analysis
17-Hydroxprogesterone*
LH, FSH, testosterone
Urea and electrolytes
Cortisol and ACTH

Urine analysis
Adrenal steroids in CAH
Pre- and post-HCG stimulation, androgen precursors may
    be helpful in testosterone biosynthetic defects

Other investigations
Ultrasound of groins and abdomen
Genitogram
Laparotomy/laparoscopy and gonadal biopsy
Androgen binding studies ± androgen receptor analysis

*Serum must be saved so that other adrenal steroids can be measured if necessary.

for planning reconstructive surgery, as can be endoscopy of the sinus with a cystoscope. Laparotomy/laparoscopy is now usually reserved for suspected true hermaphroditism where a gonadal biopsy is essential for the correct diagnosis. However, it may be needed later in several other conditions for removal of inappropriate internal organs.

Karyotype

Chromosomal analysis is an initial investigation and the result should be available within 48 hours. Three distinct karyotype groups emerge – abnormal, 46XX and 46XY (Figures 20.4–20.6). Table 20.1 shows the clinical features of patients in each group.

Karyotype abnormal

Figure 20.4 shows the three main groups of karyotype anomalies in this gonadal dysgenetic group. Knowledge of the abnormal karyotype and the appearances of the external genitalia lead to a firm diagnosis of Turner's and Klinefelter's syndromes and mixed gonadal dysgenesis. The latter is the only one likely to present in the neonatal period. Laparotomy/

laparoscopy is needed to diagnose true hermaphroditism with a mosaic pattern.

Karyotype 46XX

Figure 20.5 shows the diagnostic possibilities when the chromosomal pattern is 46XX. Biochemical abnormalities identify CAH from other forms of female virilization. The rare 46XX male may have undescended testes or hypospadias but usually normal male external genitalia. Transplacental androgenic activity is now rare. Laparotomy/laparoscopy is necessary in the suspected true hermaphrodite with a 46XX pattern.

Normal females and some patients with pure gonadal dysgenesis have a 46XX pattern. This latter condition is not a neonatal problem.

Karyotype 46XY

Here there is undervirilization in all but the normal male child and those with hernia uteri inguinale (persistent mullerian duct syndrome [8,11] (Figure 20.6). 46XY associated with normal female external genitalia and palpable inguinal testes is typical of the complete androgen insensitivity syndrome. Patients with 46XY pure gonadal dysgenesis do not have palpable gonads and present later.

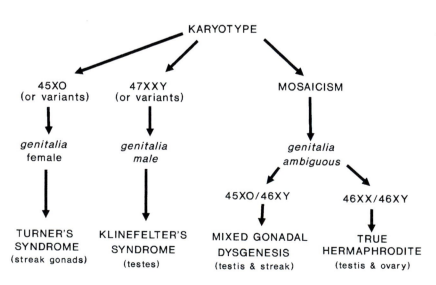

Figure 20.4 Diagnostic pathway for gonadal dysgenesis based on karyotype and genital appearances.

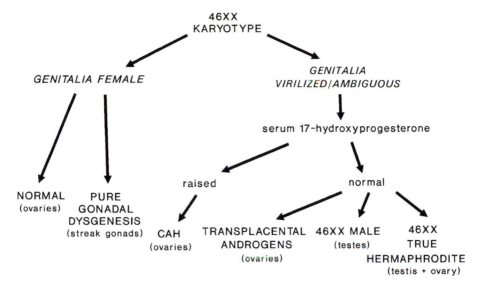

Figure 20.5 Diagnostic map for patients with 46XX karyotype based on genital appearances and biochemistry.

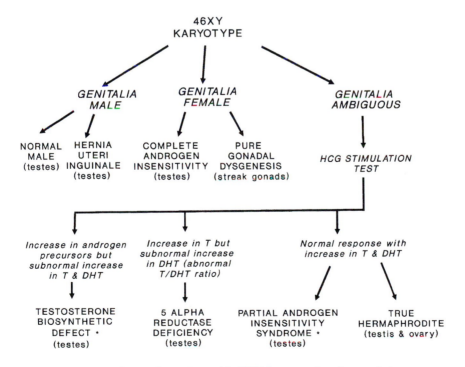

Figure 20.6 Diagnostic map for patients with 46XY karyotype based on genital appearances and HCG stimulation test.
*It may be necessary to access response of penis to 3 months of intramuscular testosterone before deciding sex of rearing.

Neonates with a 46XY karyotype and ambiguous genitalia who have either a testosterone biosynthetic defect, an inability to convert testosterone to DHT or resistance in the androgen-sensitive cells to the action of androgens can usually be distinguished by an HCG stimulation test [12] (Figure 20.6).

Less than 15% of true hermaphrodites have a 46XY pattern [5] and, as with all true hermaphroditism, laparotomy/laparoscopy is needed to make the diagnosis.

The three pathways shown in Figures 20.4–20.6 cover the diagnosis of all the conditions briefly described in Table 20.1. The broad approach described here is somewhat simplistic and does not cover a few rarer and more complicated defects.

Difficulties arise in the undervirilized male whose phallus is initially too small to be acceptable as a penis but the response to a trial of testosterone is as yet uncertain. Thus, in patients with partial androgen resistance or testosterone biosynthetic block, there may be an inevitable delay in diagnosis and choice of sex of rearing.

Sex of rearing

All 46XX patients with CAH, complete androgen insensitivity, Turner's syndrome and pure gonadal dysgenesis should be reared as female.

46XX males and patients with Klinefelter's syndrome should remain male, as they both have male external genitalia.

All the other conditions – mixed gonadal dysgenesis, true hermaphroditism, testosterone biosynthetic defects and partial androgen insensitivity – are associated with varying degrees of under- or overvirilization and the decision for sex of rearing is based on:

1. The size of the phallus and its potential for enlargement under androgen stimulation.
2. The presence and accessibility of a structure to provide a vagina.

Other factors that should be taken into consideration are the prospects for fertility and the potential for malignant change in the gonads. The only group with real potential for fertility is those with CAH and here the decision to raise as female is already made. There has been the occasional report of fertility in true hermaphroditism [8], but in other conditions unassisted fertility is unlikely.

The risk of malignancy in dysgenetic gonads associated with a Y chromosome is discussed below. It may occasionally influence the decision on sex of rearing, as in mixed gonadal dysgenesis.

Surgery in patients with intersex disorders

The following range of operations is needed according to the sex of rearing:

Genitoplasty

Genitoplasty, which involves clitoral reduction and vaginoplasty, reconstructs the genitalia to as near female appearances and function as possible [18–20]. The clitoris needs to be approximately normal size with preservation of its blood supply and sensation. The vagina must be functional and open onto the perineum in the correct position. Excess phallic skin is used to reconstruct the labia.

For social and psychological reasons the operation for low confluence of vagina and urethra (Figure 20.7(a)) should be performed as soon as possible after the child's general medical and metabolic state has been stabilized, perhaps between 3 and 6 months of age. However, when the confluence is high (Figure 20.7(b)) the procedure is more complicated and can be postponed until the age of 2–3 years.

Early in the history of genitoplasty, the clitoris was removed completely [21]. Alternatively, attempts were made to recess it under the pubic arch but this led to discomfort during sexual stimulation [22]. Now the best results are achieved by resecting the corporal bodies with preservation of the glans with its blood and nerve supply. The dorsal nerve of the phallus, a branch of the pudendal, is preserved together, ventrally, with the vascular mucosal strip which is the opened urogenital sinus.

A preliminary endoscopy of the sinus shows the level of the confluence of the urethra and vagina. A wide V-shaped incision is made with its base in the posterior perineum (Figure 20.8(a)). The flap of skin with its underlying fatty tissue is lifted until the thin sinus and its

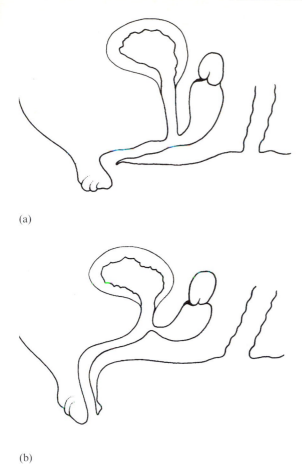

(a)

(b)

Figure 20.7 Low (a) and high (b) confluence of the vagina and urethra into the urogenital sinus.

overlying bulbospongiosus muscle are exposed. The sinus is then incised posteriorly until the urethra is identified (Figure 20.8(b), (c)). The incision is extended posteriorly up into the posterior wall of the vagina until its widest point is reached (Figure 20.8(c)). The flap is sutured to the apex and along the edges of the incision (Figure 20.8(d)).

The phallic skin is freed with a subcoronal incision and subsequently used to provide the labia minora and a hood over the newly sited clitoris. The glans is then isolated on the principle described above (Figure 20.8(d)). Dissection of the dorsal neurovascular bundle is difficult as it is firmly attached to the surface of the corpora. If in doubt, some tunica of the corpora can be left attached to it. Distally the nerves splay out and the dissection should stop 1 cm from the corona. Excessive bleeding from

the cut edge of the opened sinus can be prevented by a running catgut suture. After excision of the corporal bodies (Figure 20.8(d)), the glans is recessed under the pubic arch and fixed there with non-absorbable sutures between the periosteum and the remaining 1-cm stump of the corpora (Figure 20.8(e)).

Unless the glans is particularly large it is best not to trim it at this stage as some spontaneous diminution in size is inevitable. The vagina is packed with ribbon gauze coated in Vaseline or Proflavine and the bladder is drained with an indwelling catheter. Small drains are left in the labia minora for 24 hours. The catheter and the pack are removed after 48 hours and gentle dilatation of the vagina begun with a small plastic dilator. The dilatation technique is shown to the parents, who must continue with it until the vagina is completely healed, often 4–6 weeks.

There are three alternative techniques for the difficult vaginal reconstruction when the confluence of the urethra and vagina is high. A method was described by Hendren and Crawford [23] in which the small upper third segment of the vagina is located by a suprapubic approach and brought down to meet the exposed perineal dissection. Recently, Passerini has described a method of tubularizing the phallic skin and introducing it as a tube to provide a vagina [24]. The approach used by one of us (R.H.W.) has been to isolate the vaginal segment via a dissection behind the urogenital sinus with the aid of a Fogarty balloon placed in it endoscopically, and then to incise the vaginal segment at its anterior margin so that a flap of vagina can reach the posteriorly based flap of perineal skin. The bare anterior vaginal wall is covered with a sheet of phallic skin that extends beyond the urethral meatus and into the vagina [20].

Follow-up is essential and all these girls should have an examination under anaesthetic around puberty to make sure that the vagina is adequate. A revision operation may be necessary at that time. In the unlikely event of the glans being too large the lateral edges can be excised at any stage after the original operation.

Hypospadias repair

Extensive hypospadias repair is needed in many children reared as male using the usual

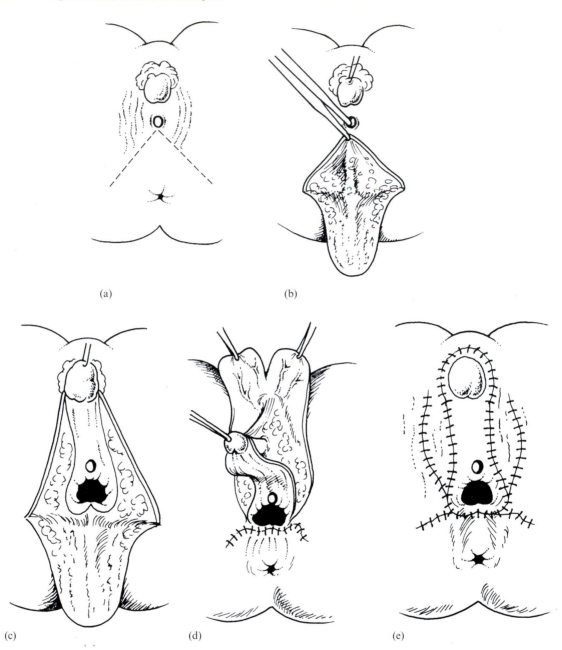

(a)   (b)

(c)   (d)   (e)

Figure 20.8 (a)–(e) Stages of genitoplasty (clitoral reduction and vaginoplasty).

techniques. Fistula or stenosis may occur in 5–25% of patients and will need further surgical attention. There is probably no need to perform a primary excision of a utricle if present, but there is a small but significant risk of infection and stone formation that may require action later if it is not removed.

Orchidopexy

Undescended testes in children reared as male need to be brought down into the scrotum unless the gonad is severely hypoplastic or a streak. If extensive dissection is needed it can be undertaken at the time of a laparotomy for excision of inappropriate internal genitalia.

Laparotomy/laparoscopy

In some patients, such as true hermaphrodites, it is essential to have knowledge of the internal genitalia for diagnostic purposes. In others such as mixed gonadal dysgenesis, there is no urgent need to know the nature of the internal genitalia, but it will be necessary to remove the inappropriate organs after the sex of rearing has been decided upon.

Mastectomy

Inappropriate breast development at puberty may call for a mastectomy in patients reared as male.

Gonadectomy

Gonads inappropriate to the sex of rearing should be removed because of inappropriate hormone secretion and because of the gonadal tumour risk that is discussed below.

Gonadal tumour risk

The association between gonadal neoplasia and disorders of sexual differentiation is well established [7,25]. Most tumours are of germ cell origin and range from the more common benign gonadoblastomas to malignant dysgerminomas/seminomas. The important predisposing factors are the presence, particularly in combination, of a Y chromosome and gonadal dysgenesis, but the latter is not essential as risk groups include true hermaphroditism and androgen insensitivity.

Thus, between a quarter and a third of patients with 46XY pure gonadal dysgenesis or mixed gonadal dysgenesis (45XO/46XY) will develop a gonadoblastoma in streak gonads and a proportion of these will progress to malignant dysgerminoma/seminoma [7]. However, in dysgenetic conditions where there is no Y chromosome, for instance Turner's syndrome (45XO) or pure gonadal dysgenesis (46XX), the gonads are not at an increased risk of tumour formation.

Patients with true hermaphroditism and a Y chromosome (46XY and 46XY/46XX) are also at risk, as are patients with androgen insensitivity, particularly the complete variety.

Although testicular undescent may play a role in the aetiology of the malignancy in the latter condition, it is more likely that there is an intrinsic gonadal abnormality and carcinoma-in-situ has been demonstrated in a number of patients with both CAIS and PAIS.

The exact increased risk of malignancy in patients with androgen insensitivity is unknown but the prevalence estimation of 2–5% [26] is many times higher that the overall risk for the adult male population.

Micropenis

A micropenis can be defined as having a stretched length that is smaller than more than 2.5 standard deviations below the mean for age [27]. Clinically the penis lacks the bulk of normal corpora cavernosa and is not merely short in length. There may be an adequate foreskin that gives the impression of a larger organ than really exists. The condition should not be confused with buried or hidden penis where there is normal length and bulk of the corpora, often concealed in pubic fat, but abnormal attachments of phallic skin so that the penis does not protrude to the normal extent.

As a micropenis is simply small but normally formed, the early stages of penile development must be normal (Figure 20.1). Hormone influence is lacking in later pregnancy.

Thus, the aetiology of micropenis [27,28] can be hypogonadotropic hypogonadism (defects at hypothalamic or pituitary level), hypogonadism alone (at gonad level) or a failure of the phallus to respond to available hormones (androgen insensitivity). In addition, in some cases, no aetiology can be identified and this idiopathic group is often the commonest group in *isolated* micropenis.

Hence micropenis is seen in hypogonadotropic hypogonadal syndromes such as Kallmann, Prader–Willi and septo-optic dysplasia, where there is a defect in fetal pituitary LH production. Examples of primary hypogonadism are Robinow's syndrome, Klinefelter's syndrome and X polysomatics (XXXY, XXXXY, XXYY). Although the cause is unknown, micropenis is also sometimes seen in other recognized syndromes such as Noonan, Down and Cornelia de Lange.

Investigation

General examination may reveal dysmorphic features suggestive of the conditions mentioned above. A karyotype is important to exclude Klinefelter's syndrome or other X polysomies which are associated with primary hypogonadism. During early infancy and at puberty it may be possible to differentiate hypogonadotropic hypogonadism from primary hypogonadism by measurement of LH, FSH and testosterone. In the first condition gonadotrophins and testosterone are both low, but in the latter condition low testosterone is associated with high gonadotrophins. High testosterone and high gonadotrophins indicate androgen insensitivity and further assessment by androgen-binding studies and molecular analyses is indicated. After infancy and before puberty (i.e. during childhood) gonadotrophin deficiency may be difficult to diagnose, but testicular function can be assessed using an HCG stimulation test.

Management

Sexual assignment depends on the degree of micropenis, the aetiology of the condition and the response to testosterone given as long-acting intramuscular testosterone enanthate. This is usually given as three injections at monthly intervals and the response noted. The response, however, does not allow prediction of the adult penile size. Growth is seen best in hypogonadotropic hypogonadism and in the idiopathic group [29].

In children with a minute penis a female sex of rearing may be more appropriate. Reconstructive surgery and oestrogen replacement at puberty will then be required.

Some of the least well sexually adjusted children are amongst this group with micropenis; if reared as male the penis may remain inadequate.

Hypospadias

It is clear from what has gone before in this chapter that any child with hypospadias and impalpability of one or both testes should be considered for investigation for intersex and a karyotype should be performed.

The routine management of idiopathic hypospadias is outside the scope of this chapter but the condition should be assessed carefully in the neonatal period so that the implications can be explained to the parents and surgery, if needed, planned well ahead. It must be emphasized to the parents that circumcision must not be performed at this early stage as all excess skin may be needed for a definitive repair. Very occasionally indeed, the meatus is too small for an adequate stream of urine and may need adjustment in the form of a meatotomy. This should be performed by the surgeon who will undertake the complete repair.

Circumcision

For centuries, throughout the world, the principle indications for circumcision in infants have been cultural and religious. The medical indications seen in older children, such as repeated balanitis or a tight fibrous foreskin, are almost never seen in the newborn period. However, when the time-honoured cultural habit of routine circumcision in the newborn in North America was questioned and partially abandoned [30], it was noted that urinary tract infections (UTI) were more common in uncircumcised boys [31] and such boys were 10 times more likely to require hospital admission for UTI.

The disadvantages of early circumcision are pain, bleeding, inflammation, psychological trauma and the very rare occurrence of death or severe mutilation of the penis. The advantages have been listed as a lower incidence of balanitis, carcinoma of the penis and carcinoma of the cervix in partners. In addition, it may promote better hygiene and give some protection from sexually transmitted diseases [32]. Despite critical appraisal of the dilemma both for [32] and against [33] circumcision, the issue remains somewhat unclear. A recent analysis of the question of greater prevalence of UTI in uncircumcised boys [34] suggested that the preferred choice is no circumcision unless there are other reasons to suggest that there is a considerable risk of UTI in the first year of life.

The benefits of early circumcision in the prevention of UTI in boys who are found on prenatal or postnatal ultrasound scanning to have congenital urological abnormalities, such as reflux or obstruction, would appear clear enough and such active intervention seems reasonable to the present authors.

Neonatal circumcision remains a parental choice after the advantages and disadvantages have been explained. Alternative methods for the prevention of balanitis and colonization of the preputial sac with pathogens have been judicious retraction [35] or active colonization with maternal bacteria [36].

References

1. Hughes IA, Pinsky L. Sexual differentiation. In: Collu R, Ducharme JR, Guyda HJ (eds) *Pediatric Endocrinology*, 2nd edn. New York: Raven, 1989; pp 251–293.
2. Sinclair AH, Berta P, Palmer MS et al. A gene from the human sex-determining region encodes a protein with homology to a conserved DNA-binding motif. *Nature* 1990; **346**: 240–244.
3. Miller WL. Immunoassays for human mullerian inhibiting factor (MIF): new insights into the physiology of MIF. *J Clin Endocrinol Metab* 1990; **70**: 8–10.
4. Donahoe PK, Budzik GP, Trelstad R et al. Mullerian-inhibiting substance: an update. In: Greep RO (ed) *Recent Progress in Hormone Research*, vol 38. New York: Academic, 1982; pp 279–330.
5. Lalau-Keraly J, Amice V, Chaussain JL et al. L'hermaphrodisme vrai. *Ann Pediatr Paris* 1986; **33**: 87–91.
6. Luks FI, Hansbrough F, Klotz DH Jr et al. Early gender assignment in true hermaphroditism. *J Pediatr Surg* 1988; **23**: 1122–1126.
7. Savage MO, Lowe DG. Gonadal neoplasia and abnormal sexual differentiation. *Clin Endocrinol* 1990; **32**: 519–533.
8. Blyth B, Churchill BM, Houle A-M, McLorie GA. Intersex. In: Gillenwater JY, Grayhack JT, Howards SS et al. (eds) *Adult and Pediatric Urology*, 2nd edn. St Louis: Mosby Year Book, 1991; chap 58, pp 2141–2171.
9. Walker J, Hughes IA. Adrenal disorders. *Curr Paediatr* 1992; **2**: 140–144.
10. White PC, New MI. Genetic basis of endocrine disease 2: congenital adrenal hyperplasia due to 21-hydroxylase deficiency. *J Clin Endocrinol Metab* 1992; **74**: 6–11.
11. Guerrier D, Tran D, Vanderwinden JM et al. The persistent mullerian duct syndrome: a molecular approach. *J Clin Endocrinol Metab* 1989; **68**: 46–52.
12. Hughes IA. The gonads. In: Hughes IA (ed) *Handbook of Endocrine Tests in Children*. Bristol: Wright, 1986; chap 6, pp 112–131.
13. Peterson RE, Imperato-McGinley H, Gautier J et al. Male pseudohermaphroditism due to steroid 5-alpha-reductase deficiency. *Am J Med* 1977; **62**: 170–191.
14. Peterson RE, Imperato-McGinley J, Gautier T et al. Urinary steroid metabolites in subjects with male pseudohermaphroditism due to 5-alpha-reductase deficiency. *Clin Endocrinol* 1985; **23**: 43–53.
15. Brown CJ, Goss SJ, Lubahn DB et al. Androgen receptor locus on human X chromosome: regional localisation to Xq 11–12 and description of a DNA polymorphism. *Am J Hum Genet* 1989; **44**: 264–269.
16. Batch J, Williams D, Davies H et al. Androgen receptor gene mutations identified by SSCP in 14 subjects with androgen insensitivity syndrome. *Hum Mol Gen* 1992; **1**: 497–503.
17. Batch J, Evans B, Hughes IA et al. Mutations of the androgen receptor gene identified in perineal hypospadias. *J Med Gen* 1993; **30**: 198–201.
18. Snyder HMcC, Retik AB, Bauer SB et al. Feminizing genitoplasty: a synthesis. *J Urol* 1983; **129**: 1024–1026.
19. Whitaker RH. Genitoplasty for congenital adrenal hyperplasia: anatomy and technical review. In: Spitz L et al (ed) *Progress in Pediatric Surgery*, vol 23, Berlin: Springer-Verlag, 1989; pp 144–150.
20. Whitaker RH. Genitoplasty for virilizing congenital adrenal hyperplasia. In: Frank JD, Johnston JH (eds) *Operative Paediatric Urology*. Edinburgh: Churchill Livingstone, 1990; chap 13, pp 123–132.
21. Gross RE, Randolph J, Crigler Jr JF. Clitorectomy for sexual abnormalities: indications and technique. *Surgery* 1966; **59**: 300–308.
22. Lattimer JK. Relocation and recession of the enlarged clitoris with preservation of the glans: an alternative to amputation. *J Urol* 1961; **86**: 113–116.
23. Hendren WH, Crawford JD. Adrenogenital syndrome: the anatomy of the anomaly and its repair. Some new concepts. *J Pediatr Surg* 1969; **4**: 49–58.
24. Passerini-Glazel G. A new 1-stage procedure for clitorovaginoplasty in severely masculinized female pseudohermaphrodites. *J Urol* 1989; **142**: 565–568.
25. Woodhouse CRJ. Late malignancy risk in urology. *Br J Urol* 1992; **70**: 345–351.
26. Verp MS, Simpson JL. Abnormal sexual differentiation and neoplasia. *Cancer Genet Cytogenet* 1987; **25**: 191–218.
27. Lee PA, Mazur T, Danish R et al. Micropenis. 1. Criteria, etiologies and classification. *Johns Hopkins Med J* 1980; **146**: 156–163.
28. Lee PA. Micropenis. Androgens in childhood. In: Forest MG (ed) *Pediatric Adolescent Endocrinology*, vol 19. Basel: Karger, 1989; pp 149–154.
29. Lee PA, Danish RK, Mazur T et al. Micropenis. III. Primary hypogonadism, partial androgen insensitivity syndrome, and idiopathic disorders. *Johns Hopkins Med J* 1980; **147**: 175–181.
30. Thompson HC, King LR, Knox E et al. Report of the ad hoc task force on circumcision. *Pediatrics* 1975; **56**: 610–611.

31. Herzog LW. Urinary tract infections and circumcision. A case-control study. *Am J Dis Child* 1989; **143**: 348–350.

32. Schoen EJ. Sounding Board: the status of circumcision of newborns. *New Engl J Med* 1990; **322**: 1308–1312.

33. Poland RL. The question of routine neonatal circumcision. *New Engl J Med* 1990; **322**: 1312–1315.

34. Chessare JB. Circumcision: is the risk of urinary tract infection really the pivotal issue? *Clin Pediatr Phil* 1992; **31**: 100–104.

35. MacKinlay GA. Save the prepuce. Painless separation of preputial adhesions in the outpatient clinic. *Br Med J* 1988; **297**: 590–591.

36. Winberg J, Bollgren I, Gothefors L et al. The prepuce: a mistake of nature? *Lancet* 1989; **i**: 598–599.

21

The prenatal and neonatal testis

P.A. Borzi

Embryology of the testis

An overview of the embryological development of the indifferent gonad into a mature testis is necessary to understand the abnormalities associated with the fetal and infant testis. Sexual differentiation is determined at conception with the inheritance of the 46XY genotype. Under the influence of Y chromosomal information, and in particular the SRY gene (testis-determining gene factor), the indifferent gonad develops into the fetal testis [1,2].

The primitive germ cells migrate from around the caudal yolk sac dorsally during the fifth week reaching the region of the mesentery and the mesonephros. Mesenchyme arising from the nearby mesonephros and the overlying columnar epithelium combine to constitute a genital ridge medial to the primitive mesonephros. With the arrival of the primordial germ cells the epithelial cells overlying the gonad form sex cords into the underlying mesenchyme. By the beginning of the eighth week visible male sex differentiation is occurring [3].

The sex cords continue to develop into seminiferous tubules and ultimately the testis. Leydig cells (probably derived from mesenchymal fibroblasts) appear around the eighth week and are known to increase in size and activity, secreting androgens by weeks 9–10. The functional fetal testis secretes testosterone and mullerian inhibitory substance (MIS). Involution of mullerian duct structures coincide with stimulation of wolffian deriva-

tives (vas deferens, epididymus and seminal vesicles).

The seminiferous tubules elongate and coil. They remain solid until at least the fifth to sixth month of gestation. The rete testis joins the ductules of the mesonephric duct, establishing continuity with the wolffian system. Between 12 and 15 weeks the testis has migrated from the genital region to the proximity of the deep inguinal ring under the influence of 5-hydrotestosterone. Penile differentiation and urethral tubularization is completed around week 14–15. The testis remains stationary until 26–28 weeks when the final inguino-scrotal descent takes place.

The cellular components of the testis mature at well-documented postnatal stages. Leydig, Sertoli and germ cells are essentially present and functioning by weeks 7–9. Fetal Leydig cells disappear by the fourth month and are gradually replaced by juvenile variants up to the end of the second year of life. With puberty further maturation occurs to adult Leydig cells and increased androgenosis. Primordial germ cells invade the mesenchyme between the sex chords and differentiate into gonocytes. Further maturation to fetal gonocytes occurs before birth. Subsequent transformation to type A spermatogonia (4 months postnatally) and B spermatocytes and primary spermatocytes (around 4 years) then allows the testis to remain dormant until puberty when spermatogenesis is stimulated. Testicular hormonal maturation is evident from early intrauterine life [5]. At term, cord blood testosterone levels have fallen and may be related to reduction in HCG levels in late pregnancy or increasing oestrogen concentration [5]. Following delivery there is a precipitous rise in plasma testosterone peaking at 2 months and gradually falling to levels consistent with later childhood by 6–7 months [6,7]. Coincident with this rise is an elevation of plasma LH which returns to the prepubertal range by 4 months of age [7,8]. This early increased testosterone activity and possibly male cerebral androgenic imprinting has implications for male children considered for sexual reassignment. It would appear that the pituitary testicular axis is activated early in the neonatal period. Abnormalities of this axis have been documented in cryptorchidism by some investigators [8,9], suggesting an important role in testicular descent.

Testicular undescent

Since Hunter's original descriptions on testicular descent no exact and complete mechanism has been established [10]. Few would argue that mechanical factors contribute to ensure the scrotal position of the developing testis (Table 21.1). This is confirmed by the higher incidence of cryptorchidism in children with abdominal wall defects, e.g., gastroschisis and prune belly syndrome [11]. Hormonal influence must play a major role in descent [12,13]. Children with GNRH deficiency (Kallman's syndrome), pituitary hypoplasia aplasia, anencephaly, and 5α-reductase deficiency (pseudovaginal perineoscrotal hypospadias) are commonly cryptorchid. Finally, no one has yet isolated androgen receptors within the guvernaculum. Recent findings in the animal model suggest that hormonal influences may act at a spinal level with a messenger neurotransmitter

Table 21.1 Influences on testicular descent

Mechanical
  Traction gubernaculum, cremaster
  Relative somatic growth
  Intra-abdominal pressure
  Epididymal enlargement[70]
  Genitofemoral nerve[71]

Hormonal
  Testosterone
  5-Hydrotestosterone
  Mullerian inhibitory substance[72]

---

released with a direct action on gubernacular contractility [13,14].

The gubernaculum testis by way of its anatomical placement must be involved, in some way, in the mediation of testicular descent extending from the developing testis to the internal inguinal ring. It changes morphologically during this stage. In the early phases of descent up to 15 weeks it becomes swollen distally especially within the inguinal canal and externally. From 26–28 weeks the gubernaculum shortens and is hollowed out by the advancing processus vaginalis while the inguinoscrotal descent occurs. It becomes a thin insignificant structure at the completion of testicular migration [4,10].

The incidence of testicular maldescent in newborn males is found to vary with birth weight and gestational age [15,16]. Scorer found that of 3612 newborns examined within 4 days of life, 2.7% of full-term (greater than 2500 g) and 21% preterm (less than 2500 g) boys had undescended testes. By 12 months the incidence had fallen to 0.8%, the majority descending by 3 months of age. This finding may be explained by the testosterone 'surge' seen in the first 3 months of life [6,7]. It would appear that no further descent occurs and agrees with the incidence found in US Army recruits [17]. An undescended testis in a baby less than 37 weeks' gestation or less than 2500 g is more likely to descend by 3 months [15].

Recent reviews [18] found an increased incidence of cryptorchidism. This may be affected by the definition of undescended testis (anatomical description versus clinical measurement and interobserver variants). Although testicular ascent in a previous descended testis has been documented [19], the finding is rare.

It is unresolved whether the morphological changes seen in the cryptorchid testis are secondary to increased body temperature or in fact a primary event. Scorer [16] noted that a testes that had not descended by 3 months of observation were always smaller than its normal partner. In recent years lightmicroscopic changes of reduced numbers of Leydig cells, decreased sizes of seminiferous tubules and growth of spermatogonia have been seen in testes of boys of 2 and 3 years of age [20–22]. In their second year these changes are more dramatic in the 'higher' undescended testes.

Given that most cryptorchid testes at birth have descended by 9–12 months of age, the optimal time to initiate treatment to restrict the histological damage and its effect on spermatogenesis should be in the second year of life. Ludwig and Potempa [23] showed that fertility rate was directly related to age of orchidopexy (1–2 years – 87.5%; 3–4 years – 57%; 5–8 years – 25%; greater than 13 years – 14%). Martin [24] found that malignancies were more likely to develop in children undergoing orchidopexies after 10 years of age. By implication the malignancy risk may reduce if orchidopexy was performed earlier. What is known is that orchidopexy done in late childhood and early adolescence results in low fertility rates [25]. As the trend to earlier infant surgery is recent, substantial benefit cannot be gauged for 15–20 years.

Clinical examination of a child with cryptorchidism aims to detect the presence or absence of the testis in question as well as the well-being of the contralateral testis. Anatomical absence, i.e., monorchia and anorchia, is rare [26]. Testicular tissue should be found in 95% of surgical explorations for maldescended testes. Over 20% of clinically impalpable testes are absent at operation.

Although surgical correction of undescended testis is the mainstay of treatment, hormonal treatment has been tried with variable success. Intramuscular human chorionic gonadotrophin (HCG) therapy over 3–4 weeks [21,27,28] has produced 20–50% success in achieving intrascrotal testes (bilateral and unilateral).

Interest has shifted to gonadotrophin releasing hormone (GnRH), as it can be administered intranasally as well as intramuscularly. Once again the results have been variable [29]. It would seem that combining HCG therapy to non-responders with GnRH improves the descent [30]. Response to hormone administration is dependent on the position of the undescended testis. Most agree that only retractile and high scrotal testes will attain an intrascrotal position. Hormonal therapy improves the surgical conditions for higher situated testes and cannot be expected to contend with the anatomical obstacles found by Hazebroek et al. [31] in these patients who failed two courses of LHRH nasal spray. Despite evidence of dysfunction in the pituitary testicular axis to support the theoretical benefit of hormonal therapy [32], others have failed to confirm this finding [28].

Preoperative intranasal buserelin (GnRH analogue) has been shown to improve testicular histology on biopsy at the time of orchidopexy [33]. This enhancement of germ cells and Leydig cell number has the potential to improve fertility in the cryptorchid testis.

Testicular torsion

Neonatal testicular torsion represents approximately 10% of all torsions. Since its earliest description in the literature [34], there still persists a division of opinion about the correct management of not only the affected testis but also the contralateral non-involved side [35].

A clear division of neonatal torsion into *in utero*/perinatal torsion (evident at birth) and postnatal torsion (initially a normal testis) is needed. A postnatal event is potentially salvageable, whereas rarely does a prenatal torsion when explored yield a viable healthy outcome. A recent review found approximately 70% of torsions were present on delivery and 30% occurred in the first month of life.

In utero/perinatal testicular torsion occurs as a result of excessive mobility in the testis and spermatic cord from its covering. This extravaginal torsion (outside the tunica vaginalis) differs from the more common intravaginal variant or 'bell clapper' type encountered in adolescents and adults as well as in a proportion of postnatal testicular torsion [36]. Contraction of the spiralling cremester muscle *in utero* or during delivery is thought to be the precipitating event to produce rotation of the hemiscrotal contents. Primary testicular infarction with secondary torsion has been proposed after finding contralateral ischaemia during scrotal exploration [37]. No experimental studies have surfaced to confirm this interesting postulate.

The usual clinical presentation of a perinatal torsion is as an asymptomatic firm testicular mass at the initial paediatric examination. Often this is indurated with loss of normal anatomical profile. A scrotal 'herald patch' or ecchymosis within the skin frequently overlies the testis [38]. The testicular mass may remain in the scrotum or ride high into the inguinal area. Translumination is unsuccessful unless an early associated hydrocele has developed. The typical infant who presents with perinatal testicular torsion is a term baby, large for dates (birth weight 75th–90th percentile) [39] and possibly an infant of a diabetic mother. It does not seem to be related to mode of delivery, birth trauma or prematurity [38].

Confirmatory incidence of infarction or compromised vascularity can be obtained with colour Doppler ultrasound and radioisotopic scintography [40–42]. Unfortunately due to the smaller size of the patient and other technical aspects, it is recognized that each technique is not completely reliable. Antenatal torsion has been detected and followed conservatively postnatally [43].

The differential diagnosis of a neonatal scrotal swelling must include a reducible inguinal hernia, hydrocele, tumour, macro-orchidism (e.g., ectopic adrenal, cortex or spleno-gonadal fusion), torsion of testicular appendage and meconium peritonitis [44]. Rarely polyorchidism (separate testicular artery, shared epididymis and ductus deferens [45,46] and cross testicular ectopia (separate testicular artery, epididymis and ductus deferens [47]) may be seen in this age group.

Epidydimitis is a common cause of acute scrotal swelling in childhood, especially in boys less than 2 years of age [48]. Although differential enlargement of the epididymis may be detected, earlier scrotal exploration is often the final arbiter. Generally epididymitis results from retrograde infection spread along the ductus deferens following a urinary tract infection. Developmental anomalies involving the ureter and the seminal vesicle and vas deferens (Wolfian duct derivatives) may underlie the propensity for urethrovasal reflux and subsequent epididymitis. Urethral instrumentation or indwelling catheters may predispose to retrograde infection [49]. Rarely epididymitis reflects a systemic infectious disorder and haematogenous dissemination.

In view of the increased evidence of epididymitis in children under 2 years and the associated structural abnormalities, radiological investigations are warranted [50]. Ultrasonography of the renal tract and bladder as well as micturating cystourethrogram (MCU) are necessary initial investigations. Cystourethroscopy and functional renal imaging should be seen as follow-on steps to preliminary findings.

The child born with a normal testis who subsequently develops acute torsion (postnatal) justifies acute scrotal exploration to preserve testicular mass. The management of prenatal or advanced torsion as well as the contralateral testis in both prenatal and postnatal torsion remains clouded in controversy and disagreement [35]. The lack of a uniform nomenclature and unclear operative findings prevents accurate comparison of recommendations and testicular outcome.

Salvage of a viable testis following prenatal torsion is uncommon. Most series report findings of non-viability but retain the testis *in situ*. Subsequent findings confirm non-viability with testicular absence or atrophy [51]. Two surveys have found 80–100% of affected testes were non-viable [11,35]. One out of nine testis explored by Longino and Martin were found to be of normal volume at 2 years follow-up [52]. Urgent exploration of an established testicular torsion is unlikely to prevent anatomical disruption. It may preserve some endocrine but not necessarily exocrine function [53], although La Quaglia et al. [54] found no significant Leydig cell function.

The contralateral uninvolved testes represents the only hope for normal fertility and testosterone production in the presence of an absent or atrophied ipsilateral torsion. Krarup [55] clinically documented impaired spermatogenesis in the contralateral testis following testicular torsion. Others [56,57] had postulated experimentally that autosensitization from disruption of the blood–testis barrier and exposure of testicular antigens may be the mechanism of action. Further experimental [58,59] and clinical studies [60] failed to induce such cellular damage by prepubertal torsion. The retention of an ischaemic testis does not appear to significantly alter the spermatogenic function of the contralateral testis. The contralateral histological changes are confined to postpubertal torsion and to date no specific antibody has been identified.

Abnormal fixation and investment of the testis and tunica vaginalis can be found in the majority of contralateral testes to ipsilateral intravaginal torsion [61]. Harris et al. [62] and Bellinger et al. [63] found contralateral 'bell clapper' deformities in over 80% of boys with unilateral anorhcia at surgical exploration. Similarly excessive mobility of the testis and its coverings within the hemiscrotum can persist beyond the first 7 days of life [51]. Therefore the potential exists for synchronous or asynchronous contralateral torsion of either anatomical variety in the adolescent [64], as well as the neonatal period [54,65,66].

In all cases of neonatal bilateral torsion, at least one testis was clinically involved at birth. La Quaglia et al. [54] found the asynchronous torsion occurred at 48 hours and 8 weeks of age. Given this finding, few would disagree that the contralateral testis must be protected at all costs. What is unclear is the timing of the orchidopexy. Relative risks of neonatal anaesthesia [67] argue in favour of delayed exploration at several months of age, relying on parental diligence to detect any abnormality in the interim. A short period of testicular torsion can produce ischaemic necrosis that would have potential detrimental effects on fertility and hormone production [68]. Although highly suggestive of advance non-viable torsion, the scrotal mass may resemble a testicular tumour and doubt may rest over its nature. In general these children are healthy term infants [39]. If anaesthesia is conducted in a suitable neonatal care facility the perioperative risks are minimized.

The 'early' ipsilateral detorsion and contralateral orchidopexy should be carried out through a scrotal incision unless an inguinal hernia is concurrently present. Bellinger et al. [63] showed experimentally dramatic testicular damage with suture fixation of the tunica albuginea to the scrotal septum. Dartos pouch fixation combined with eversion and fixation of the tunica vaginalis behind the cord is recommended. If suture fixation is deemed necessary, non-absorbable rather than absorbable sutures are suggested following documented cases of recurrent torsions after previous scrotal fixation [69].

References

1. Gubbay J, Collignon J, Koopman P et al. A gene mapping to the sex-determining region of the mouse Y chromosome is a member of a novel family of embryonically expressed genes. *Nature* 1990; **346**: 245–250.

2. Sinclair AH, Berta P, Palmer M et al. A gene from the human sex-determining region encodes a protein with homology to a conserved DNA-binding motif. *Nature* 1990; **346**: 240–244.

3. Gray SW, Skandalakis JE. The ovary and testis. In: *Embryology for Surgeons: the embryological basis for the treatment of congenital defects.* Philadelphia: WB Saunders, 1972; pp 563–582.

4. Backhouse KM. Embryology of testicular descent and maldescent. *Urol Clin North Am* 1982; **9**: 315–325.

5. Reyes FI, Winten JS, Faiman C. Studies on human sexual development: 1. Fetal gonadal and adrenal sex steroids. *J Clin Endocrinol Metab* 1973; **37**: 74–82.

6. Forest MG, Sizonenko PC, Cathiard AM, Bertrand J. Hypophysio-gonadal function in humans during the first year of life. *J Clin Invest* 1974; **53**: 819–828.

7. Winter JS, Hughes IA, Reyes FI, Faiman C. Pituitary–gonadal relations in infancy: 2. Patterns of serum gonadal steroid concentration in man from birth to two years of age. *J Clin Endocrinol Metab* 1976; **42**: 679–686.

8. Gendrel D, Chaussain JL, Roger M. Simultaneous postnatal rise of plasma LH and testosterone in male infants. *J Pediatr* 1980; **97**: 600.

9. Job JC, Gendrel D. Endocrine aspects of cryptorchidism. *Urol Clin North Am* 1982; **9**: 353–360.

10. Hunter W. *Observations on the State of the Testes in the Foetus and on the Hernia Congenita: medical commentaries*, Part 1, London: A. Hamilton.

11. Kaplan GW, Silber I. Neonatal torsion – to pex or not? In: King LR (ed) *Urological Surgery in Neonates and Young Infants.* Philadelphia: WB Saunders, pp 386–395.

12. Rajfer J, Walsh PC. Hormonal regulation of testicular descent: experimental and clinical observations. *J Urol* 1977; **118**: 985–990.

13. Hutson J, Beasley SW. Annotation: the mechanisms of testicular descent. *Aust Paed J* 1987; **23**: 215–216.

14. Larkins SL, Hutson SM, Williams MPL. Localisation of CGRP immunoreactivity within the spherical nucleus of the genitofemoral nerve. *Pediatr Surg Int* 1991; **6**: 176–179.

15. John Radcliffe Hospital Cryptorchidism Study Group. Clinical diagnosis of cryptorchidism. *Arch Dis Child* 1988; **63**: 587–591.

16. Scorer CG. The descent of the testis. *Arch Dis Child* 1964; **39**: 605–609.

17. Baumrucker GO. Incidence of testicular pathology. *Bull US Army Med Dept* 1946; **5**: 312–314.

18. John Radcliffe Hospital Cryptorchidism Study Group. Cryptorchidism: an apparent substantial increase since 1960. *Br Med J* 1986; **293**: 1404–1405.

19. Atwell J. Ascent of the testes: fact or fiction. *Br J Urol* 1985; **57**: 474–477.

20. Heckel WC, Heinz HA. Cryptorchidism and fertility. *J Pediatr Surg* 1967; **2**: 513–516.

21. Mengel W, Hienz HA, Sippe WG, Heckel WC. Studies on cryptorchidism: a comparison of histological findings in the germinative epithelium before and after the 2nd year of life. *J Pediatr Surg* 1974; **9**: 445–450.

22. Hadziselimovic F. Cryptorchidism: ultrastructure of normal and cryptorchid testes development. *Adv Anat Embryol Cell Biol* 1977; **53**: 3–10.

23. Ludwig G, Potempa H. Der Optimale Zeitpunkt der Behandlung des Kryptorchidismus. *Dtsch Med Wochenschr* 1975; **100**: 680.

24. Martin DC. Germinal cell tumours of the testes after orchidopexy. *J Urol* 1979; **121**: 422–425.

25. Chilvers C, Dudley NE, Gough MH, Jackson MB, Pike MC. Undescended testis: the effect of treatment on subsequent risk of subfertility and malignancy. *J Pediatr Surg* 1986; **21**: 691–696.

26. Levitt SB, Kogan SJ, Engel RM, Weiss RM, Martin DC, Ehklich RM. The impalpable testis: a rational approach to management. *J Urol* 1978; **120**: 515–520.

27. Garagorri JM, Job JC, Canlorbe MD. Results with early treatment of cryptorchidism with human chorionic gonadotrophin. *Pediatrics* 1982; **101**: 923.

28. Dickerman Z, Baumal B, Sandovsky V. HCG treatment in cryptorchidism. *Andrologia* 1983; **16**: 542–547.

29. De Huinck Keizer-Schrama S, Hazebroek F. Hormonal treatment of cryptorchidism: role of pituitary gonadal axis. *Semin Urol* 1988; **6**: 84–95.

30. Hadziselimovic F. In: Gillenwater (ed) *Cryptorchidism in Adult and Pediatric Urology* St Louis: Mosby, pp 2217–2243.

31. Hazebroek FWJ, De Muinck Keizer-Schrama SMPF, Van Maarschalker Weerd M, Visser HKA, Molenaar JC. Why lutenizing-hormone-releasing-hormone nasal spray will not replace orchidopexy in the treatment of boys with undescended testes. *J Pediatr Surg* 1987; **22**: 1177–1182.

32. Job JC, Gendrel D, Safan A, Roger M, Chaussain JL. Pituitary LH and FSH and testosterone secretion in infants with undescended testes. *ACTA Endocrinol (Copenh)* 1977; **85**: 644–649.

33. Hadziselimovic F. Hormonal treatment of the undescended testes. *J Pediatr Endocrinol* 1987; **2**: 1–5.

34. Taylor HR. A case of testicle strangulation at birth; castration recovery. *Br Med J* 1897; **2**: 88–89.

35. Das S, Singer A. Controversies of perinatal torsion of the spermatic cord: a review, survey, and recommendations. *J Urol* 1990; **143**: 231–233.

36. Muscat M. The pathological anatomy of testicular torsion. *Surg Gyn Obs* 1932; **54**: 758–762.

37. Burge DM. Neonatal testicular torsion and infarction: aetiology and management. *Br J Urol* 1987; **59**: 70–73.

38. Watson RA. Torsion of spermatic cord in neonates. *Urology* 1975; **5**: 439–443.

39. Reeves HH, Sigler RM, Hahn HB, Lynn HB. Torsion of the spermatic cord in the newborn. *Am J Dis Child* 1965; **110**: 676–692.

40. Lerner RM, Mevorach RA, Hulbert WC. Color Doppler use in the evaluation of acute scrotal disease. *Radiology* 1990; **176**: 355–358.

41. Mendel JB, Taylor GA, Treves S, Cheng TH, Retik A, Bauel S. Testicular torsion in children: scintigraphic assessment. *Pediatr Radiol* 1985; **15**: 110–115.

42. Haynes BE, Bessen HA, Haynes VE. The diagnosis of testicular torsion. *JAMA* 1983; **249**: 2522.

43. Hubbard AE, Ayers AB, MacDonald LM, James CE. *In utero* torsion of the testes: Antenatal and postnatal ultrasonic appearances. *Br J Radiol* 1984; **57**: 644–646.

44. Thompson RB, Rosen DI, Gross DM. Healed meconium peritonitis presenting as an inguinal mass. *J Urol* 1973; **110**: 634–635.

45. Wescott JW, Dykhuizen RF. Polyorchism. *J Urol* 1967; **98**: 497–500.

46. Mehan DJ, Chehval J, Ullah S. Polyorchidism. *J Urol* 1976; **116**: 530–532.

47. Beasley SW, Auldist AW. Crossed testicular ectopia in association with double incomplete testicular descent. *Aust NZ J Surg* 1985; **55**: 301–303.

48. Clift VL, Hutson JM. The acute scrotum in childhood. *Pediatr Surg Int* 1989; **4**: 185–188.

49. Kogan SJ. In: Gillenwater (ed) *Acute and Chronic Scrotal Swellings in Adult and Pediatric Urology* St Louis: Mosby. pp 2189–2215.

50. Williams CB, Litvak AS, McRoberts JW. Epididymitis in infancy. *J Urol* 1979; **121**: 125–127.

51. Guiney EJ, McGlinchey J. Torsion of the testes and spermatic cord in the newborn. *Surg Gyn Obs* 1981; **152**: 273–274.

52. Longino LA, Martin LW. Torsion of the spermatic cord in the newborn infant. *New Engl J Med* 1955; **253**: 695–697.

53. Bartsch G, Frank ST, Marbergen H, Mikuz G. Testicular torsion: late results with special regard to fertility and endocrine function. *J Urol* 1980; **124**: 375–378.

54. La Quaglia MP, Baven SB, Enaklis A, Feins N, Mandell J. Bilateral neonatal torsion. *J Urol* 1987; **138**: 1051–1056.

55. Krarup T. The testis after torsion. *Br J Urol* 1978; **50**: 43–46.

56. Nagler HM, White R. The effect of testicular torsion on the contralateral testis. *J Urol* 1982; **128**: 1343–1348.

57. Harrison RG, De Marval HJM, Lewis-Jones DI, Connolly RC. Mechanism of damage to the contralateral testis in rats with an ischaemic testis. *Lancet* 1981; **iii**: 723–725.

58. Henderson JA, Smey P, Cohen MS et al. The effect of unilateral testicular torsion on the contralateral testicle in prepubertal Chinese hamsters. *J Pediatr Surg* 1985; **20**: 592–597.

59. Nagler HM. Experimental aspect of testicular torsion. *Dialogues Pediatr Urol* 1985; **8**: 2–5.

60. Puri P, Barton D, O'Donnell B. Prepubertal testicular torsion: subsequent fertility. *J Pediatr Surg* 1985; **20**: 598–600.

61. Jones PC. Torsion of the testis and its appendages during childhood. *Arch Dis Child* 1962; **37**: 214–216.
62. Harris BH, Webb HW, Wilkinson AH, Stevens PS. Protection of the solitary testis. *J Pediatr Surg* 1982; **17**: 950–953.
63. Bellinger MF, Abromowitz H, Brantley S, Marshall G. Orchidopexy: an experimental study of the effect of surgical techniques on testicular histology. *J Urol* 1989; **142**: 553–555.
64. Benge BN, Eure GR, Winslow BH. Acute bilateral testicular torsion in the adolescent. *J Urol* 1992; **148**: 134–136.
65. Papadatos C, Moutsouris C. Bilateral testicular torsion in the newborn. *J Pediatr* 1967; **71**: 249–250.
66. Weingarten JL, Ganofalo FA, Cromie WJ. Bilateral synchronous neonatal torsion of spermatic cord. *Urology* 1990; **35**: 135–136.
67. Schreiner MS. Anaesthesia risk for neonates. *Dial Int Ped Urol* 1991; **14**: 2–3.
68. Smith GI. Cellular changes from graded testicular ischaemia. *J Urol* 1955; **73**: 355–358.
69. Vorstman B, Rothwell D. Spermatic cord torsion following previous surgical fixation. *J Urol* 1982; **128**: 823–824.
70. Hadziselimovic F, Kruslin E. The role of the epididymis in descensus testis and the topographical relationship between the testis and the epididymis from the sixth month of pregnancy until immediately after birth. *Anat Embryol* 1979; **155**: 191–196.
71. Beasley SW, Hutson JM. Effect of division of the genitofemoral nerve on testicular descent in the rat. *Aust NZ J Surg* 1987; **57**: 49–51.
72. Hutson JM, Donahoe PK. The hormonal control of testicular descent. *Endocr Rev* 1986; **7**: 270–283.

22

Genitourinary malignancies in the first year of life

R. Squire

Introduction

It is hard to describe the devastation experienced by parents on learning that their child has cancer. Of course, suspicion of malignancy strikes fear regardless of age, but extreme emotions often occur in response to cancer in infancy. Fortunately malignancy presenting in the infant under 1 year old is rare and so frequently these anxieties are misplaced. In the UK approximately 2% of all cancers occur in childhood, with an annual incidence of approximately 1.1 per 10 000 children [1]. Cancer diagnosed in the first year of life is slightly more frequent than in older paediatric age groups, and can be estimated at 1.5 per 10 000 live births.

Genitourinary malignancies account for nearly 10% of these tumours and 16% of paediatric genitourinary tumours occur before the first birthday. In summary, genitourinary malignancy under 1 year of age accounts for less than 2% of all childhood cancer, occurring in approximately 0.3 per 10 000 live births.

Overall survival for childhood cancer clearly varies depending on site and diagnosis, but infant genitourinary tumours fare relatively well, with a crude survival of 85%. This compares with approximately 80% long-term survival for all childhood genitourinary tumours, and approaching 70% for all childhood malignancy [2].

The first birthday does not represent a watershed in the presentation or management of genitourinary malignancy. However, there are aspects of genitourinary cancer peculiar to the infant, and these differences may influence the clinical approach. For example, there is an increased incidence of benign disease in the kidney (mesoblastic nephroma) and the ovary (benign follicular cysts). A testicular mass in the newborn may be due to testicular torsion, whereas a similar mass in an older child would almost certainly be due to a tumour.

As well as influencing management, some peculiarities may help shed light on the aetiology of cancer. As we develop increasing awareness of the genetic factors that predispose to malignancy, tumours occurring early in life take on a special interest. With a shorter latency period, there is less opportunity for environmental factors to come into play and it may be possible to document external influences more precisely as infants undergo regular screening examinations. The infant's prenatal environment must also be considered, and the relatively short interval between embryogenesis and tumour development may assist recollection of potential influencing factors.

Because of the rarity of genitourinary cancer in infancy, sound data on which to base management has been harvested from a variety of collaborations, carried out between major paediatric oncology centres around the world. It is increasingly likely that these conditions will become the preserve of the major specialist centre and this is likely to provide the best opportunity for future advances in management, as well as concentrating expertise and experience in the interests of optimum management of the individual.

Genetics

Processes that allow genes to influence the development of malignancy are slowly being unravelled and paediatric genitourinary tumours are at the forefront of this rapidly moving field. Logic would suggest that genetically determined tumours will present relatively early as the genetic influence is present from the beginning of embryonic development. This makes tumours of infancy and young childhood of particular interest. One of the most widely held theories endeavouring to explain the role of genes in cancer was developed using the epidemiology of Wilms' tumour as a mathematical model [3]. By comparing the incidence of unilateral and bilateral Wilms' tumour, Knudson and Strong proposed a 'double hit' theory, whereby cells become malignant as a consequence of two independent genetic mutations. They suggested that if a child is born with one mutation (or cancer gene) then only one further cellular mutation would be required, resulting in a higher risk of tumour development. This would also lead to a higher risk of bilateral disease, and earlier presentation in these children.

It is increasingly evident that at a molecular level, genetic mutations leading to aberrant cells play a crucial role in the final part of tumour development, but it is likely that only a few tumours develop in children with a germ line, or constitutional, cancer gene (i.e. present in every cell). A number of these cancer genes have now been identified.

Wilms' tumour

It has long been clear that at least some cases of Wilms' tumour are associated with cancer genes. One per cent of children with Wilms' tumour have a family history [4], and the risk increases to 10% for a twin. The mode of inheritance is uncertain, and is confused by a picture suggesting autosomal dominance, yet with siblings more commonly affected than parents.

Table 22.1 Congenital anomalies associated with Wilms' tumour

High risk	Low risk
Aniridia	Neurofibromatosis
Hemihypertrophy	Cryptorchidism
Beckwith–Weidemann syndrome	Hypospadias
Drash syndrome	Other genital anomalies
Pearlman nephroblastomatosis	

Wilms' tumour is associated with a number of congenital anomalies [5]. These are listed in Table 22.1. Chromosome 11 has become the genetic focus for attention in Wilms' tumour. The association with aniridia led to identification of a tumour suppressor gene at the 11p13 locus (WT1) [6]. More recent candidates for a second Wilms' tumour gene (WT2) have been identified, the 11p15 locus being the front runner. Wilms' tumour is thought to result from inactivation of the Wilms' tumour suppressor gene [7], resulting in failure to produce tumour suppressor proteins [8].

Rhabdomyosarcoma

The occasional association of rhabdomyosarcoma with congenital conditions such as fetal alcohol syndrome and neurofibromatosis clearly has genetic implications [9]. Furthermore, rhabdomyosarcoma in the urinary tract is associated with other urinary tract anomalies. Perhaps the most dramatic genetic association is with familial cancer, generally known as the Li–Fraumeni syndrome [10]. It is now clear that germ-line mutations in the p53 tumour suppressor gene on chromosome 17 are responsible for this hereditary predisposition to rhabdomyosarcoma, as well as breast, brain, lung and adrenocortical cancer [11]. A variety of chromosomal abnormalities have been demonstrated in rhabdomyosarcoma, but as of yet no specific genetic locus has been consistent [12]. Interestingly, it appears that adjacent to the 11p15 locus implicated in Wilms' tumour, is a tumour-suppressor gene relevant for rhabdomyosarcoma [13]. This association between Wilms' and rhabdomyosarcoma genes may explain the lower incidence of these two malignancies in the Asian population in the UK, as opposed to the higher or comparable incidence in most other paediatric tumours [14].

Germ cell tumours

There have been sporadic reports of familial germ cell tumours and it is possible that germ cell tumours are a rare component of the Li–Fraumeni familial cancer syndrome [15]. There is also an association with Klinefelter's syndrome. However, no germ-line mutations have been confirmed. Within the tumours a variety of chromosomal abnormalities have been reported, chromosomes 1 and 12 being implicated most frequently. It has been suggested that an abnormality on the short arm of chromosome 12 may be the primary event that leads to malignant transformation in a previously benign teratoma [16].

Environmental factors

There is no convincing evidence that environmental factors have a significant influence on the development of genitourinary tumours in infancy. It is of note that the Japanese experience with nuclear fallout in 1945 did not cause an increase in the incidence of paediatric solid tumours [17]. Regarding the pathogenesis of disease in infancy the dominant environment is that of the fetus or embryo rather than the neonate, and there is strong evidence that antenatal radiation increases the subsequent risk of leukaemia. However, even this malignancy presents in older childhood.

Case control studies in rhabdomyosarcoma have implicated paternal smoking (presumably causing sperm cell mutations) and possibly maternal toxaemia in pregnancy. Certain paternal occupations may also be of significance [18–20]. This is far less convincing than for adult sarcomas, where the exposure to many chemical carcinogens has been blamed.

In general, Wilms' tumour studies have not revealed an environmental aetiology, although again paternal occupation may be of minor significance [21,22]. Occupations implicated are machine workers, mechanics and jobs involving exposure to hydrocarbons or lead. A weak association has been demonstrated between Wilms' tumour and maternal anaesthesia using methoxyflurane during delivery [23]. This has not been verified.

It is interesting to note that geographical variations in the incidence of rhabdomyosarcoma and Wilms' tumour persist within indigenous racial groups even if they move to a different geographical location [14]. This may suggest that genetic factors outweigh those of the environment. However, studies for the effect of the environment on the incidence of rare conditions are inevitably weak. There are frequently a large number of variables with uncertain intensity of exposure. It is therefore inevitable that many potential environmental factors will be blamed for causing cancer in infancy on anecdotal evidence, and proof of innocence is difficult to find. In particular this applies to factors occurring during pregnancy, when the teratogenic risk is probably highest.

Prenatally detected urogenital masses

With increased use of third-trimester ultrasound scans comes an increase in prenatal diagnosis of abdominal masses. Cystic swellings tend to be picked up more often than solid masses, and the potential sensitivity of antenatal scans is high as amniotic fluid is a good medium for ultrasound.

Table 22.2 lists a differential diagnosis of prenatal cystic abdominal masses. Many of these conditions are extremely rare and in some it is impossible to make a precise diagnosis antenatally. There are seldom any indications for prenatal intervention. The main advantages of prenatal diagnosis are to warn the parents, so that they can be counselled, and to alert the clinician, so that correct postnatal management can be introduced. Nearly

Table 22.2 Cystic masses that may be identified prenatally

Renal area	Pelvis
Hydronephrosis	Obstructed bladder
Multicystic dysplasia	Ovarian follicular cyst
Polycystic disease	Sacrococcygeal teratoma*
Cystic nephroma	Hydrometrocolpos
Adrenal haemorrhage	Lymphangioma
Choledochal cyst	Anterior meningocele
Gastrointestinal duplication	Intestinal duplication
Intestinal atresia	Urachal cyst
Lymphangioma	Ovarian germ cell tumour*
Omental cyst	
Cystic neuroblastoma*	
Cystic teratoma*	

* Malignant lesions or lesions with malignant potential.

Table 22.3 Solid masses in the renal area that may be identified prenatally

Malignant	Benign
Neuroblastoma	Mesoblastic nephroma
Fibrosarcoma	Fibromatosis
Wilms' tumour	Nephroblastomatosis
	Nodular renal blastaema
	Horseshoe kidney

all of the lesions are benign and so a favourable outcome can usually be predicted.

Solid masses are liable to be of more concern, as the potential for malignancy is greater. Table 22.3 lists the differential diagnosis for prenatally diagnosed solid masses lying in the region of the kidney or in the pelvis. For a prenatal mass in the region of the kidney, by far the most likely diagnosis is neuroblastoma. It is worth noting that in this presentation neuroblastoma generally has a very good prognosis, and even some cases of fibrosarcoma respond remarkably well to chemotherapy.

Any lesion identified prenatally, whether cystic or solid, needs careful postnatal follow-up. This will generally involve repeating the ultrasound examination and possibly then proceeding to a CT or MRI scan.

Renal masses in infancy

Most renal masses in infancy are diagnosed incidentally, either during routine neonatal and developmental checks, or during medical examination for a concurrent illness. Renal tumours only account for about 5% of renal masses in infancy [24]. Table 22.4 lists the possible causes of a discrete mass in or around the kidney.

On occasions it can be surprisingly difficult to distinguish Wilms' tumour from neuroblastoma. Analysis of urine for catecholamine

Table 22.4 Renal masses in infancy

Wilms' tumour
Mesoblastic nephroma
Neuroblastoma
Nephroblastomatosis
Renal adenoma
Lymphoma
Horseshoe kidney

levels is mandatory in all these patients, but is not always elevated in neuroblastoma. CT or MRI imaging is generally fairly reliable but at the end of the day further investigation is directed by histological diagnosis. A tissue diagnosis is also necessary to discriminate Wilms' tumour from benign renal masses, such as mesoblastic nephroma.

Pelvic masses in infancy

The differential diagnosis of a pelvic tumour in this age group is considered in Table 22.5. Fortunately these lesions are all rare. Rectal examination should delineate the extent of the lesion in the pelvis, and initial investigations should include ultrasound, usually followed by MRI or CT scan. Cystovaginoscopy may be indicated in selected cases where there is clinical evidence of invasion of the bladder or vagina. Histology is usually required in order to make a diagnosis and in many incidences a limited biopsy (open or percutaneous) is the initial selection so that the role of preoperative chemotherapy can be considered. This improves the chance of preservation of bowel and bladder function. However immediate resection is usually indicated for neonatally presenting sacrococcygeal teratoma, and for ovarian masses.

Table 22.5 Pelvic masses in infancy

Rhabdomyosarcoma
Type IV sacrococcygeal teratoma
Germ cell tumour
Fibrosarcoma/undifferentiated sarcoma
Malignant ovarian tumour
Anterior meningo(myelo)cele
Chordoma
Lymphoma

Testicular masses in infancy

The management of a solid testicular mass in this age group is the most straightforward. Ultrasound examination is usually all that is required to confirm the clinical impression of a tumour, though it is not possible to distinguish whether the lesion is benign or malignant without histology. If a tumour is suspected then serum alpha fetoprotein (AFP) measurement should be carried out, more to aid follow-up than diagnosis. Reference to age-standardized charts from AFP levels is essential, as AFP is elevated in normal infants. The testicle should then be carefully delivered through an inguinal incision and a total orchidectomy carried out. If, on examination of the testicle, doubt about the diagnosis persists then the testicular vessels should be soft clamped, the testicle screened from the wound so that no spillage can occur and then a frozen-section biopsy can be carried out before proceeding.

However a different approach may be indicated for testicular swellings in the neonate, when testicular torsion can produce a hard swollen testicle, clinically indistinguishable from a testicular tumour. If neonatal torsion is suspected and the child is asymptomatic, then it is not unreasonable to observe the testicle for a few weeks. The torted testicle should progressively atrophy.

The commonest cause of a scrotal swelling in infancy is a hydrocele. It is important to remember that 25% of testicular yolk sac tumours present initially with a hydrocele [25]. Bearing this in mind, all infants with hydroceles should have a careful examination of the scrotum to make sure that the testicle within the hydrocele sac is fundamentally normal. If in doubt ultrasound examination of the testis should be carried out.

Wilms' tumour

Wilms' tumour, or nephroblastoma, is the dominant urogenital malignancy of childhood. As a result of large multicentre studies it has become one of the most well-understood paediatric malignancies. Therapy has consequently been refined to a high degree and outcome improved. The association between Wilms' tumour and various congenital anomalies (Table 22.1) is unique and has led to Wilms' tumour becoming an exciting model for the emergence of theories encompassing the aetiology of malignancy in general. Wilms' tumour is thought to be derived from the primitive metanephric blastaema. The tumours often contain tissues foreign to the normal metanephros, suggesting that the metanephric blastaema has potential not normally expressed in nephrogenesis.

Sarcomatous variants of Wilms' tumours occur rarely, and are distinctly unfavourable. Bone-metastasing renal tumours of childhood are not seen in infancy, but young boys, under 1 year of age, are peculiarly prone to develop rhabdoid tumours [26]. Renal cell carcinoma has not been reported in infancy.

Presentation

Prenatal presentation of Wilms' tumour is extremely rare, but it can present as a neonatal mass [27]. The peak incidence is in the third or fourth years of life, but over 15% occur before the first birthday [4]. Most commonly Wilms' tumour presents as an asymptomatic mass, and the pattern of presentation is largely the same regardless of age. Not uncommonly the mass is an incidental finding in a child attending for an unrelated medical examination, or is observed by a parent at bathtime. In 20–30% there are associated symptoms such as discomfort from the rapidly growing tumour, haematuria or poor feeding. At presentation 25% will have hypertension, usually due to renin secretion within the tumour [28]. Occasionally a child will be picked up through a screening programme based on identification of the risk groups identified in Table 22.1.

Management

Initial assessment should include ultrasound and CT or MRI scanning. The primary aim of the initial imaging is the identification of features which would suggest that surgery should be delayed until after adjuvant therapy. Indications for delayed surgery include the presence of metastases, intracaval tumour or bilateral disease. Doppler ultrasound may assist in identification of caval tumour, and rarely a cavogram may be helpful. CT scan of the chest is favoured for looking for pulmonary metastatic disease. The liver, regional lymph nodes and contralateral kidney should be included in the initial abdominal scan. Whilst the initial tumour work up is being carried out, blood pressure should be measured regularly. If the infant has hypertension, antihypertensive therapy should be introduced prior to any surgical procedure.

Therapy for Wilms' tumour combines surgery and adjuvant therapy in all cases, though the selection of adjuvant therapy is guided by the surgical and histological findings. The current staging system [29] should only strictly be applied following tumour resection and this is confusing in the light of the current debate on the role of primary chemotherapy in non-metastatic disease. While the results of current trials are awaited, some clinicians prefer to give primary chemotherapy in order to shrink the tumour and make the subsequent surgery less complicated. When primary chemotherapy is selected, a preliminary biopsy of the tumour is advised as misdiagnosis is not uncommon in the absence of histological confirmation. The rate of misdiagnosis in all age groups is approximately 5% [30], but is likely to be higher in children under 6 months where meso-blastic nephroma is more prevalent. Biopsy in theory ruptures the tumour and may therefore be an adverse factor, but this can be minimized by using a retroperitoneal (posterior) approach. Rupture may 'upstage' the tumour, resulting in an increase in adjuvant therapy, but this may be balanced by the potential for preresection chemotherapy to shrink the tumour so much that it is 'downstaged' by the time resection is carried out. This may result in a requirement for less adjuvant therapy over-all. Percutaneous needle biopsy is often ade-quate and if guided by ultrasound should safely identify solid areas of tumour for ade-quate histological definition.

Following resection of the tumour it is pos-sible to classify Wilms' tumour into favour-able and unfavourable histological types. Well-differentiated tumours, with a triphasic pattern consisting of blastaemal, epithelial and stromal cells, generally carry a much better prognosis, regardless of the stage of disease, than more anaplastic or undifferentiated tumours. How-ever on initial biopsy it is often not possible to comment on this aspect of the histology.

Chemotherapy regimens are fundamentally the same regardless of age, using vincristine, actinomycin-D and adriamycin, but early trials showed unacceptably high toxicity from chemotherapy in infants, so current protocols use reduced drug dosages under the age of 6 months [31].

Primary chemotherapy is preferred in meta-static disease or where there is caval or bi-lateral renal involvement. The timing of the surgery in these situations is not rigid. When there is metastatic disease the aim is to make sure that the metastases are controlled before attempting to resect the primary. If there is intracaval tumour the aim is to eliminate it so that there is no risk of tumour embolus. If the caval tumour persists despite chemotherapy, then cardiopulmonary bypass may need to be available to support the surgical resection.

The approach to bilateral disease differs, because nephron preservation is paramount. Bilateral minimal partial nephrectomy is the aim and preresection chemotherapy is manda-tory in order to reduce the tumour bulk, and allow preservation of as much of the normal renal parenchyma as possible. Bench surgery or renal transplantation may be required.

Prognosis

There has been a dramatic improvement in long-term survival in Wilms' tumour asso-ciated with refinement of chemotherapy regi-mens. However, more recent improvements may be falsely encouraging, as there has been a tendency to exclude the poor prognostic groups, such as the rhabdoid tumour. Local-ized tumours are associated with approxi-mately 90% 5-year survival, providing the histology is favourable. Lymphatic spread reduces this to 80%, and haematogenous metastases to 70%. Unfavourable histology tumours fare worse, with about 65% long-term survival. Only 20% of children with rhabdoid tumours will be cured. There is some data to suggest that younger patients do better, but this may well be because of inclusion of some benign tumours, such as mesoblastic nephro-mas, which are more prevalent in infancy.

Much attention is being paid to the long-term follow-up of patients with Wilms' tumour. The main issues are the long-term effects of nephrectomy, the side effects of adjuvant therapy and the risk of a second malignancy. The risk of hyperfiltration syn-drome resulting in long-term dysfunction of the remaining kidney remains uncertain, but current information would suggest that this problem is unlikely to have a major impact on the lives of children who have had a Wilms' nephrectomy [32]. Of more concern, perhaps, is the risk of a second malignancy following apparently successful treatment for Wilms' tumour. Extrapolation of early data suggests that approaching 10% of long-term survivors will develop a second cancer [33], though this figure may be lessened by the reduction of radiotherapy in current protocols. There is also a substantial population of children who develop symptomatic cardiomyopathy, particularly following treatment with adriamycin. This condition can have a major impact on the quality of life.

Nephroblastomatosis

Microscopic clusters of blastaemal cells have been recognized in the kidney for many years, and are undoubtedly potential precursors of malignancy. These clusters represent nephroblastomatosis. It is also clear that in many cases of nephroblastomatosis there is no progression, as these lesions can be found in approximately 1% of random perinatal autopsies, which is approximately 100 times the incidence of Wilms' tumour [34]. Nephroblastomatosis is usually perilobar but rarely intralobar, in the deep cortex or medulla. Examples of both of these two types are seen in the renal parenchyma of approximately 25% of Wilms' tumour cases. The precise clinical significance of nephroblastomatosis is uncertain but it is generally accepted that if multifocal lesions are seen in a resected Wilms' tumour kidney or are found on examination of a contralateral kidney, there is an increased risk of further tumour development. Management of nephroblastomatosis is debatable. Currently the most widely accepted approach is to avoid aggressive intervention, relying on close follow-up, possibly including regular ultrasound examination.

Cystic nephroma

This is a rare benign tumour that has been recognized as a discrete entity for over 100 years yet under 200 cases have been reported, described using a variety of names, including cystic adenoma and multilocular cyst. Cystic nephroma usually presents as an asymptomatic abdominal mass, but more recently it has been an incidental finding on ultrasound examination. Diagnostic criteria have been clearly defined as follows [35]. The lesion should be a solitary unilateral multilocular cystic abnormality, and the cysts should not communicate with each other or with the renal pelvis. On histological examination they should be lined with epithelium, with no renal parenchyma within the lesion itself. Most importantly the rest of the kidney must be normal. Recently bilateral cases have been described [36].

The aetiology of these lesions is uncertain. Similar abnormalities have been identified in association with both nephroblastomatosis and Wilms' tumour, and it remains possible that they are at the benign end of the Wilms' spectrum [37]. In the absence of a malignant component these lesions are almost certainly benign, but unfortunately imaging cannot reliably rule out a small adjacent focus of malignancy. Therefore excision is recommended. In view of the fact that they are usually benign, a nephron-sparing approach is appropriate and a partial nephrectomy is usually possible provided that careful attention is paid to the renal vascular anatomy [38].

Congenital mesoblastic nephroma

Congenital mesoblastic nephroma (CMN) is a rare, usually benign renal tumour occurring exclusively in infancy, first being recognized as a discrete entity in 1967 [39]. The tumour has distinctive morphology, characterized by bundles of spindle cells resembling fibroblasts or smooth muscle cells. However, congenital mesoblastic nephroma shares many histological features with Wilms' tumour and the distinction is confused by case reports of CMN which behave malignantly [40]. This may be influenced by the histological similarities some cases of CMN share with rhabdoid tumours of the kidney, which are aggressively malignant [41]. Like Wilms' tumour, CMN probably arises from the embryonal blastaema and some Wilms' tumour contain large regions which resemble CMN. Furthermore, cases of CMN with Wilms'-like cytogenetic abnormalities have been reported [42]. In all probability CMN is a 'cytodifferentiated' variant of Wilms' tumour, evolving at an earlier stage of renal development. This would account for the younger age group affected by CMN and possibly its different behaviour. CMN would therefore represent the benign end of a spectrum of disease.

Presentation

CMN is commonly diagnosed at birth, usually presenting prior to 3 months of age as an asymptomatic flank mass. Prenatal diagnosis is rare [43], possibly because cystic CMN is rare [44]. However, CMN has been reported in association with polyhydramnios leading to hydrops fetalis and intrauterine death [45,46]. It has been suggested that this is due to high urine output resulting from nephron trapping within the tumour. Haematuria and hypertension also occasionally occur at presentation, though less commonly than in Wilms' tumour. Other features at presentation include vomiting, jaundice and hypercalcaemia [47].

Management

Ultrasound and CT or MRI scanning should be considered as a preparation for surgery. Resection of the tumour is mandatory, despite the benign nature of the condition, as elements of nephroblastoma within the tumour cannot be excluded by biopsy alone. However, if an infant over 3 months of age has a large tumour with radiological features suggestive of Wilms', a preliminary biopsy may be considered as a prelude to adjuvant therapy (see management of 'Wilms' tumour', 'Management' above). If this biopsy suggests CMN then primary adjuvant therapy should not be given. Resection should be radical, as the tumour can project both into the otherwise healthy adjacent renal parenchyma and also into the perinephric tissues. Attempts have been made to define adverse prognostic features in the tumour, to identify patients who might benefit from adjuvant therapy following tumour resection. Cellular proliferation, high mitotic activity and, more recently, DNA aneuploidy are all associated with rare, aggressive CMN [48,49], and can be considered an indication for screening for metastases. The lung is the most common metastatic site. However, these adverse factors have not been reliable enough to provide a convincing argument for giving adjuvant therapy in the absence of metastases [50]. It remains debatable whether chemotherapy should be considered in children where there is evidence of residual disease following surgery. In these cases the age of the child and the presence or absence of adverse histological features may be factors to consider. Chemotherapy, if selected, is based on the Wilms' tumour protocols.

Prognosis

Radical surgery for CMN usually results in cure. However, local and metastatic recurrence can occur, usually but not exclusively in children presenting originally over 3 months of age [51]. Fortunately this is rare and in the literature more deaths have been reported as a complication of treatment (frequently overzealous) than as a result of disease progression.

Rhabdomyosarcoma

Rhabdomyosarcoma (RMS) is the predominant tumour of mesenchymal origin occurring in children. It is distinguished by the elements resembling striated muscle within the tumour. Overall paediatric RMS is a mixed bag of tumours, varying in behaviour with histological type, site of origin and age of patient. In the genitourinary tract of infants the tumour is usually of the botryoid type, a varient of embryonal RMS, arising in the bladder or vagina [52]. These tumours represent only a small percentage of all RMS and fortunately have a favourable outcome [53]. The less favourable alveolar and undifferentiated RMS are extremely rare in young children.

Presentation

Botryoid tumours usually present as a polypoid mass arising from the vagina or trigone of the bladder. The vaginal tumours may present as a prolapsing mass, while the bladder tumours will tend to cause haematuria. A mucosanguinous discharge may precede the appearance of a mass. On initial presentation ultrasound examination is of value to identify the gross features of a vaginal mass, or to investigate the renal tract if haematuria is the presenting feature. Biopsy generally precedes further investigation. The tumours are often very friable and if clean biopsies cannot be taken then haemorrhagic curettings will often yield enough tumour for diagnosis.

Management

Current management of RMS is initially biased towards organ preservation, with only unresponsive tumours needing a radical surgical approach [54,55]. Rarely, a small localized lesion may be excised completely but this is not usually the case, and radical excision at presentation is inappropriate. Once diagnosis is confirmed, a thoracic CT scan is required to look for pulmonary metastases and a CT or MRI scan of the abdomen and pelvis is used to define the extent of local disease, and to provide information on regional lymph nodes.

Treatment protocols depend upon organ of origin and histological subclassification. Chemotherapy is usually effective using a combination of agents such as vincristine, actinomycin D and ifosfamide (though ifosfamide is avoided in children under 3 months of age). Chemotherapy doses are calculated according to patient size, but are further reduced in infancy because of the greater risk of adverse effects. Residual disease can be often assessed endoscopically, and if it is deemed resectable without major functional damage to adjacent organs then surgery is the best option. If resection is likely to leave a permanent disability then radiotherapy should be employed first. Brachytherapy (using local radioactive implants) appears to be an exciting alternative to external beam therapy [56]. Brachytherapy can reduce the total dose employed and in particular reduces the toxicity in adjacent healthy tissues.

Eventually surgical excision of residual disease may be required, although in some cases chemotherapy and radiotherapy leave no evidence of tumour. Indication for radical surgery, such as cystectomy, is limited to circumstances where adjuvant therapy has failed to control the tumour or where there is evidence that more limited surgery has left inadequately treated disease. In this latter circumstance further adjuvent therapy may be considered first followed by a period of careful observation for signs of recurrence.

Prognosis

Treatment for urogenital rhabdomyosarcoma in infancy is usually effective, but problems with drug toxicity have resulted in poor survival figures [57]. With dose reduction 60–80%

event-free survival can be predicted, depending on the extent of disease at presentation [55].

Side effects are common, and are generally worse with more extensive resections and following radiotherapy. For instance, the combination of alkylating agents (ifosfamide) and radiotherapy can cause a severe haemorrhagic cystitis. Particular long-term problems are bladder dysfunction and vaginal stenosis, for which further intervention may be required, while gonadal dysfunction from both chemotherapy and radiotherapy may result in infertility in both sexes, and amenorrhoea in females. Perhaps most worrying is the risk of developing a second malignancy, associated with a higher than normal incidence of early malignancy in family members [58]. This raises ethical issues that have not yet been resolved. In some families there may be an indication to look for abnormalities in the p53 gene, in order to identify family members for whom measures to reduce risk of cancer should be considered [10,11].

Neuroblastoma

Neuroblastoma is the most common solid tumour in infants under 1 year of age, and accounts for 50% of cancers in the newborn. Although it is not a urogenital tumour, it is relevant in this context because of the confusion it can cause at diagnosis. Arising most commonly in the adrenal gland, it can also occur at other neuroectodermal sites. Peak incidence is in the third year of life, but there is a distinct population with tumours in infancy. Infant neuroblastoma is a unique entity and, in most cases, may be biologically different from the tumour seen in older children. Infant neuroblastoma is the most commonly spontaneously regressing tumour in man [59] and remarkably this spontaneous regression can even occur in the presence of massive and widespread metastases. Interestingly, random fetal autopsies reveal foci of adrenal neuroblastoma in otherwise healthy adrenal glands far more commonly than anticipated from the incidence of neuroblastoma in infancy [60]. This finding is called 'neuroblastoma *in situ*, and is presumably of little clinical significance, regressing spontaneously in nearly all cases.

Presentation

Neuroblastoma has been rarely diagnosed prenatally by ultrasound [61]. This presentation
differs from neuroblastoma *in situ* by the fact
that there is a lump within the adrenal gland.
Fetal neuroblastoma is sometimes associated
with maternal pre-eclampsia and hydrops
fetalis. The presence of these symptoms usually
indicates metastatic disease, similar to congenital 4S neuroblastoma presenting postnatally.
Presentation of abdominal neuroblastoma in
the infant may be due either to the abdominal
primary or due to metastatic spread. The
abdominal primary may be adrenal or para-
aortic and is often difficult to delineate from a
renal tumour on imaging. Raised urinary catecholamines suggest neuroblastoma, but normal
levels are unhelpful. Non-metastatic (localized)
neuroblastoma in infancy is increasingly likely
to be picked up incidentally on ultrasound
examination, neonatal screening examinations
or as part of a neuroblastoma screening programme.

Metastatic neuroblastoma in infancy typically presents as a small occult primary
tumour, with overt metastases in the liver,
bone marrow and/or skin. The liver involvement may result in massive hepatomegaly.
In extreme cases this can result in IVC compression, respiratory embarrassment or heart
failure. A bone scan must be performed, as the
presence of bone metastases is an important
adverse prognostic indicator.

Neuroblastoma screening

Recently considerable interest has been
expressed in the potential of screening for
infant neuroblastoma by testing for urinary
catecholamine excretion [62]. The intention of
screening is to detect cases of neuroblastoma
at an earlier age or stage, when prognosis is
better. Large studies, predominantly in Japan,
have demonstrated that it is possible to pick
up increased numbers of infant neuroblastoma
and these cases of screened neuroblastoma
have an excellent prognosis. Unfortunately
screening has not resulted in a reduction of
either the overall mortality or the incidence of
advanced disease [63]. We must therefore
assume that screening identifies asymptomatic

cases which are biologically benign, and which
previously remained undiagnosed.

Management

Localized neuroblastoma has traditionally
been treated with resection, followed by
chemotherapy if there is evidence of residual
disease. More recent studies suggest that in
infancy treatment of residual disease is often
unnecessary [64]. The data from screening
imply that many infant-localized tumours do
not even need excision, but unfortunately we
are currently unable to define the biology of
individual tumours reliably enough to decide
which ones are safe to leave. Excision of the
tumour still remains the standard therapy, and
also provides tumour for biological studies to
help address these issues. However resection
should be carried out without damage to adjacent organs. Large primary tumours which
extend across the midline are treated as for
older children, with initial intensive chemotherapy and surgery for residual disease.
Young age confers a better prognosis, and so
even in these infants surgery should not be
over-zealous.

A small primary associated with non-osseous
metastases in an infant has been classified
distinctly from the usual stage 4 (metastatic)
neuroblastoma and is called 4S [65]. The S
stands for special, indicating that these
tumours have a remarkably good prognosis,
and initial treatment is only required if the
bulk of the disease is compromising the child.
However the presence of bone metastases, or
very dense bone marrow involvement, unfortunately still indicates a very poor progress, even
in children under 1 year of age, and aggressive
therapy is then recommended. There are also
occasionally tumours which initially appear to
be 4S, but subsequently behave like stage 4
tumours, presumably due to poor biological
characteristics. An increasing number of characteristics can now be identified from tumour
specimens which will predict the behaviour of
the tumour. The most established of these are
N-myc oncogene amplification [66], and deletion of the short arm of chromosome 1 [67].
Even in 4S tumours it is advisable to excise the
primary tumour eventually, as otherwise there
is a risk of recurrence with a more aggressive
tumour.

Prognosis

Localized small tumours in infancy are associated with nearly 100% survival. Larger tumours (crossing the midline) fare worse, but the large majority still survive. Over 90% of infants with 4S disease will survive, but this falls to approximately 20% for stage 4 disease.

Germ cell tumours

Germ cell tumours are derived from primordial germ cells. They may be benign or malignant. Yolk sac tumour is the predominant malignant germ cell tumour of infancy, while differentiated teratoma is the benign presentation. However, teratomas may be of variable differentiation, and benign but poorly differentiated teratomas may undergo malignant transformation. Germ cell tumours are usually classified by their site of origin and nearly all genitourinary tumours are gonadal. In infancy testicular tumours predominate, ovarian teratomas being more common in the older age group. Approximately 1% of yolk sac tumours arise in the vagina. The most common non-gonadal site is sacrococcygeal. This is not strictly a urogenital tumour, although many of the longer-term implications of this tumour are urological [68,69].

Presentation

Testicular tumours present as a painless testicular mass, often associated with a hydrocele [25]. Vaginal tumours may present as a prolapsing vaginal mass, or a pelvic mass causing constipation or bladder dysfunction. They can be easily biopsied per vagina. Raised serum AFP levels indicate that a germ cell tumour is malignant. Once malignancy is confirmed the lungs and abdominal lymph nodes should be screened for metastases, usually with CT scanning.

Management

Benign, mature teratomas require excision only. Malignant germ cell tumours may require adjuvant chemotherapy, dependent upon the extent of spread and the presence of metastases. Chemotherapy combinations include bleomycin, etoposide and a platinum agent. Residual vaginal lesions require wide excision, but the chemotherapy is usually so effective that there is only minimal residual disease, such that the surgery does not need to be mutilating. Early follow-up with regular serum AFP measurement is recommended, as this can give warning of occult recurrence.

Prognosis

The published data for malignant germ cell tumours report long-term survival exceeding 75% [70], and current data suggest that this may be improving to over 90%. However the chemotherapy regimen has considerable toxicity, with particular adverse effects on kidney and lung function. Long-term follow-up, monitoring the function of these organs, is advised.

References

1. International Agency for Research on Cancer. In: Parkin DM, Muir CS, Whelan SL, Gao Y-T, Ferlay J, Powell J (eds) *Cancer Incidence in Five Continents*, vol VI. IARC Scientific Publication No 120. Lyon: IARC Scientific Publications, 1992.
2. Stiller CA, Bunch KJ. Trends in survival for childhood cancer in Britain diagnosed 1971–85. *Br J Cancer* 1990; **62**: 806–815.
3. Knudson AG, Strong LC. Mutation and cancer: A model for Wilms' tumor of the kidney. *J Natl Cancer Inst* 1972; **48**: 313–324.
4. Breslow NE, Beckwith JB. Epidemiological features of Wilms' tumor: results of the National Wilms' Tumor Study. *J Natl Cancer Inst* 1982; **68**: 429–436.
5. Miller RW, Fraumeni JFJ, Manning MD. Association of Wilms' tumor with aniridia, hemihypertrophy and other congenital malformations. *N Engl J Med* 1964; **270**: 922–927.
6. Francke U, Holmes LB, Atkins L, Riccardi VM. Aniridia–Wilms' tumor association: evidence for specific deletion of 11p13. *Cytogenet Cell Genet* 1979; **24**: 185–192.
7. Haber DA, Buckler AJ. WT1: a novel tumor suppressor gene inactivated in Wilms' tumor. *New Biol* 1992; **4**: 97–106.
8. Wheeler TT, Ziao JP, Dowdy SF, Stanbridge EJ, Young DA. Suppression of tumorogenicity of a Wilms' tumour cell line is associated with a decrease in synthesis of two proteins. *Oncogene* 1991; **6**: 1903–2007.

9. Warrier RP, Kini KR, Shumaker B, Schwartz G, Raju U, Raman BS. Neurofibromatosis, factor IX deficiency, and rhabdomyosarcoma. *Urology* 1986; **28**: 295–296.

10. Li FP, Fraumeni Jr JF. Rhabdomyosarcoma in children: epidemiologic study and identification of a familial cancer syndrome. *J Natl Cancer Inst* 1969; **43**: 1365–1373.

11. Malkin D, Li FP, Strong LC, Fraumeni Jr JF et al. Germline p53 mutation in a familial syndrome of breast cancer, sarcomas, and other neoplasms. *Science* 1990; **250**: 1233–1238.

12. Whang-Peng J, Knutsen T, Theil K, Horrowitz ME, Triche T. Cytogenetic studies in subgroups of rhabdomyosarcoma. *Genes Chrom Cancer* 1992; **5**: 299–310.

13. Loh Jr WE, Scrable HJ, Livanos E et al. Human chromosome 11 contains two different growth suppressor genes for renal rhabdomyosarcoma. *Proc Natl Acad Sci USA* 1992; **89**: 1755–1759.

14. Stiller CA, McKinney PA, Bunch KJ, Bailey CC, Lewis IJ. Childhood cancer and ethnic group in Britain: a UKCCSG study. *Br J Cancer* 1991; **64**: 543–548.

15. Hartley AL, Birch JM, Kelsey AM, Marsden HB, Harris M, Teare MD. Are germ cell tumors part of the Li-Fraumeni cancer family syndrome. *Cancer Genet Cytogenet* 1989; **42**: 221–226.

16. Murty VV, Dmitrovsky E, Bosl GJ, Chaganti RSK. Nonrandom chromosome abnormalities in testicular and ovarian cell tumor lines. *Cancer Genet Cytogenet* 1990; **50**: 67–73.

17. Miller RW, Boice Jr JD. Radiogenic cancer after prenatal or childhood exposure. In: Upton AC, Albert RE, Burns FJ, Shore RE (eds) *Radiation Carcinogenesis*. New York: Elsevier, 1986; pp 379–386.

18. Grufferman S, Wang HH, Delong ER, Kimm SYS, Delzell ES, Falletta JM. Environmental factors in the etiology of rhabdomyosarcoma in childhood. *J Natl Cancer Inst* 1982; **68**: 107–113.

19. Hartley AL, Birch JM, McKinney PA et al. The Inter-Regional Epidemiological Study of Childhood Cancer (IRESCC): case control study of children with bone and soft tissue sarcomas. *Br J Cancer* 1988; **58**: 838–842.

20. Magnani C, Pastore G, Luzzatto L, Carli M, Lubrano P, Terracini B. Risk factors for soft tissue sarcomas in childhood: a case control study. *Tumori* 1989; **75**: 396–400.

21. Olshan AF, Breslow NE, Daling JR et al. Wilms' tumor and paternal occupation. *Cancer Res* 1990; **50**: 3212–3217.

22. Bunin GR, Nass C, Kramer S, Meadows AT. Parental occupation and Wilms' tumor: result of a case-control study. *Cancer Res* 1989; **49**: 725–729.

23. Lindblad P, Zack M, Adami H-O, Ericson A. Maternal and perinatal risk factors for Wilms' tumor: a nationwide nested case control study in Sweden. *Int J Cancer* 1992; **51**: 38–41.

24. Medicow MM, Uson AC. Palpable abdominal masses in infants and children: a report based on a review of 653 cases. *J Urol* 1959; **81**: 705–712.

25. Exelby PR. Testicular cancer in children. *Cancer* 1980; **45**: 1803–1809.

26. Palmer NF, Sutow W. Clinical aspects of the rhabdoid tumor of the kidney: report of the National Wilms' Tumor Study Group. *Med Pediatr Oncol* 1983; **11**: 242–245.

27. Ritchey ML, Azizkhan RG, Beckwith JB, Hrabovsky EE, Haase GM. Neonatal Wilms' tumor. *J Pediatr Surg* 1995; **30**: 856–859.

28. Voute PA, Van der Meer J, Staugaard-Kloosterziel W. Plasma renin activity in Wilms' tumour. *Acta Endocrinol* 1971; **67**: 197–202.

29. Farewell VT, D'Angio GJ, Breslow N, Norkool P. Retrospective validation of a new staging system for Wilms' tumor. *Cancer Clin Trials* 1981; **4**: 167–171.

30. D'Angio GJ, Avans AE, Breslow N et al. The treatment of Wilms' tumor: results of the National Wilms' Tumor Study. *Cancer* 1976; **38**: 633–646.

31. Corn BW, Goldwein JW, Evans I, d'Angio GJ. Outcomes in low-risk babies treated with half-dose chemotherapy according to the third National Wilms' Tumor Study. *J Clin Oncol* 1992; **10**: 1305–1309.

32. Argueso LR, Ritchey ML, Boyle ET, Milliner DS, Bergstralh EJ, Kramer S. Prognosis of children with solitary kidney after unilateral nephrectomy. *J Urol* 1992; **148**: 747–751.

33. Breslow NE, Norkool PA, Olshan A, Evans A, D'Angio GJ. Second malignant neoplasms in survivors of Wilms' tumor: a report from the National Wilms' Tumor Study. *J Natl Cancer Inst* 1988; **80**: 592–595.

34. Bennington JL, Beckwith JB. Tumors of the kidney, renal pelvis, and ureter. In: *Atlas of Tumor Pathology*, 2nd series, Fascicle 12. Washington DC: Armed Forces Institute of Pathology, 1975.

35. Powell T, Shackman R, Johnson HD. Multilocular cysts of the kidney. *Br J Urol* 1951; **23**: 142–152.

36. Ferrer FA, McKenna PH. Partial nephrectomy in a metachronous multilocular cyst of the kidney (cystic nephroma). *J Urol* 1994; **151**: 1358–1360.

37. Beckwith JB. Precursor lesions of Wilms' tumor: clinical and biological implications. *Med Ped Oncol* 1993; **21**: 158–168.

38. Thomas DFM, Androulakakis PA, Ransley PG. Conservation of the kidney following an unusual presentation of multilocular cyst in a 7 year old child. *J Urol* 1982; **128**: 363–365.

39. Boland RP, Brough AJ, Izant RJ. Congenital mesoblastic nephroma of infancy. *Pediatrics* 1967; **40**: 272–278.

40. Beckwith JB. Mesenchymal renal neoplasms of infancy revisited. *J Pediatr Surg* 1974; **9**: 803–805.

41. Weeks DA, Beckwith JB, Mierau GW, Zuppan CW. Renal neoplasms mimicking rhabdoid tumor of kidney: a report from the National Wilms' Tumor

Study Pathology Center. *Am J Surg Pathol* 1991; **15**: 1042–1054.

42. Roberts P, Lockwood LR, Lewis IJ, Bailey CC, Batcup G, Williams J. Cytogenetic abnormalities in mesoblastic nephroma: a link to Wilms' tumor. *Med Pediatr Oncol* 1993; **21**: 416–420.

43. Appuzio JJ, Unwin W, Adhate A, Nichols R. Prenatal diagnosis of fetal renal mesoblastic nephroma. *Am J Obstet Gynecol* 1986; **154**: 636–637.

44. Vujanic GM. Congenital cystic mesoblastic nephroma: a rare cystic renal tumour of childhood. *Scand J Urol Nephrol* 1992; **26**: 315–317.

45. Angulo JC, Lopez JI, Ereno C, Unda M, Flores N. Hydrops fetalis and congenital mesoblastic nephroma. *Child Nephrol Urol* 1991; **11**: 115–116.

46. Blank E, Neerhout RC, Burry KA. Congenital mesoblastic nephroma and polyhydramnios. *JAMA* 1978; **240**: 1504–1505.

47. Shanbhogue LKR, Grey E, Miller SS. Congenital mesoblastic nephroma of infancy associated with hypercalcaemia. *J Urol* 1986; **135**: 771–772.

48. Barrantes JC, Toyn C, Muir KR et al. Congenital mesoblastic nephroma: possible prognostic and management value of assessing DNA content. *J Clin Pathol* 1991; **44**: 317–320.

49. Gailland D, Bouvier R, Sonsino E et al. Nucleolar organiser regions in congenital mesoblastic nephroma. *Pediatr Pathol* 1992; **12**: 811–821.

50. Howell CG, Othersen HB, Kiviat NE, Norkall P, Beckwith JB, D'Angio GJ. Therapy and outcome in 51 children with mesoblastic nephroma: a report of the National Wilms' Tumor Study. *J Pediatr Surg* 1982; **17**: 826–830.

51. Beckwith JB, Weeks DA. Congenital mesoblastic nephroma. When should we worry? *Arch Pathol Lab Med* 1986; **110**: 98–99.

52. Raney Jr RB, Tefft M, Hays DM, Triche TJ. Rhabdomyosarcoma and the undifferentiated sarcomas. In: Pizzo PA, Poplack DG (eds) *Principles and Practice of Pediatric Oncology*, 2nd edn. Philadelphia: Lippincott, 1993; pp 769–794.

53. La Quaglia MP, Heller G, Ghavimi F et al. The effect of age at diagnosis on outcome in rhabdomyosarcoma. *Cancer* 1994; **73**: 109–117.

54. Hays DM. Bladder/prostate rhabdomyosarcoma: results of the multi-institutional trials of the Intergroup Rhabdomyosarcoma Study. *Semin Surg Oncol* 1993; **9**: 520–523.

55. Stevens MCG, Oberlin O, Rey A, Praquin M-T. Non-metastatic rhabdomyosarcoma: experience from the SIOP MMT 89 study. *Med Pediatr Oncol* 1994; **23**: 171.

56. Flamant F, Gerbaulet A, Nihoul-Fekete C, Valteau-Douanet D, Chassagne D, Lemerle J. Long-term sequelae of conservative treatment by surgery, brachytherapy, and chemotherapy for vulval and vaginal rhabdomyosarcoma in children. *J Clin Oncol* 1990; **8**: 1847–1853.

57. Raney Jr RB, Gehan EA, Hays DM et al. Primary chemotherapy with or without radiation therapy and/or surgery for children with localized sarcomas of the bladder, prostate, vagina, uterus, and cervix: a comparison of results from the Intergroup Rhabdomyosarcoma Studies I and II. *Cancer* 1990; **66**: 2072–2081.

58. Heyn RM. Late effects of therapy in rhabdomyosarcoma. *Clin Oncol* 1985; **4**: 287–297.

59. Everson C, Cole WH. Spontaneous regression of neuroblastoma. In: Everson TC (ed) *Spontaneous Regression of Cancer*, Philadelphia: WB Saunders, 1966; pp 88–163.

60. Beckwith JB, Perrin EV. *In situ* neuroblastoma: a contribution to the natural history of neural crest tumours. *Am J Pathol* 1963; **43**: 1089–1104.

61. Jennings RW, LaQuaglia MP, Leong K, Hendren WH, Adzick NS. Fetal neuroblastoma: prenatal diagnosis and natural history. *J Pediatr Surg* 1993; **28**: 1168–1174.

62. Sawada T, Todo S, Fujita K, Iino S, Imashuku S, Kusunoki T. Mass screening of neuroblastoma in infancy. *Am J Dis Child* 1982; **136**: 710–712.

63. Bessho F, Hashizume K, Nakajo T, Kamoshita S. Mass screening in Japan has increased the detection of infants with neuroblastoma without a decrease in cases in older children. *J Pediatr* 1991; **119**: 237–241.

64. Matthay KK, Sather HN, Seeger RC, Haase GM, Hammond GD. Excellent outcome of stage II neuroblastoma is independent of residual disease and radiation therapy. *J Clin Oncol* 1989; **7**: 236–244.

65. Brodeur GM, Seeger RC, Barrett A et al. International criteria for diagnosis, staging, and response to treatment in patients with neuroblastoma. *J Clin Oncol* 1988; **6**: 1874–1881.

66. Brodeur GM, Seeger RC, Sather H et al. Clinical implications of oncogene activation in human neuroblastoma. *Cancer* 1986; **58**: 541–545.

67. Fong CT, Dracopoli NC, White PS, Merrill PT, Griffith RC, Housman D. Loss of heterozygosity for the short arm of chromosome 1 in human neuroblastoma: correlation with N-myc amplification. *Proc Natl Acad Sci USA* 1989; **86**: 3753–3757.

68. Malone PS, Spitz L, Kiely EM, Brereton RJ, Duffy PG, Ransley PG. The functional sequelae of sacrococcygeal teratoma. *J Pediatr Surg* 1990; **25**: 679–680.

69. Boemen TML, Van Gool KD, De Jong TPVM, Bax KMA. Lower urinary tract dysfunction in children with benign sacrococcygeal teratoma. *J Urol* 1994; **151**: 174–176.

70. Heidermann P, Jurgens H, Neithammer D. Improved survival of malignant germ cell tumors in children with BEP/VIP chemotherapy. *Proc Am Soc Clin Oncol* 1991; **10**: 316.

23

Ethical aspects of prenatal diagnosis

J.G. Thornton

Introduction

Prenatal diagnosis causes moral dilemmas because it often leads to a conflict of interest between mother and baby. There is no difficulty over fetal treatment with maternal consent, but problems arise when a mother requests abortion, or refuses an intervention which is thought to be in the fetal interest. Since abortion is so central to the ethical dilemma, its consideration forms the earlier part of this chapter. Less commonly, a conflict arises between mother and baby because a fetal intervention is refused and this is covered in the latter part. Readers whose clinical contact with renal disease patients begins only after birth should find the discussion relevant, since some of the arguments about fetuses *in utero* also apply to newborn infants, and any clinician might have to advise the parents of an abnormal baby about abortion and so should be aware of the philosophical issues.

It is illuminating to discover that many senior medical students and junior doctors condone or even perform abortion, but simultaneously believe that it is morally equivalent to murdering a young child. Often, such doctors justify their position with arguments such as 'the abortion would be done by someone else anyway', or 'a liberal policy will prevent maternal deaths from illegal abortion'. Such reasons would hardly justify child killing. Clinicians, who can perform an act morally equivalent to killing young children on these grounds, are at risk of either becoming brutal-ized by what they are doing, or of losing their self-respect. They may arbitrarily limit their service in an attempt to salve their consciences, and are poorly equipped to resist any future eugenic pressure that there should be certain 'indications' for abortion for the sake of some greater good. Nevertheless, this state of affairs is perhaps hardly surprising when neither undergraduate textbooks of gynaecology [1,2], or postgraduate texts [3,4], or books on clinical genetics and fetal medicine [5,6], or even books devoted to the clinical aspects of abortion [7], give any account of the philosophy behind the pro-abortion position.

Abortion

Most people learn at their mother's knee that killing humans is wrong, and if they consider the matter at all, feel that killing an unborn fetus is particularly wrong, because the child is both innocent and defenceless. Nevertheless, most societies tolerate abortion, and England and Wales are no exception with 186 912 abortions in 1990 [8,9]. Since only a minority of women undergo more than one abortion, it has been estimated that at least 1 in 3 of the cohort of women entering puberty today will have an abortion during their lifetime [10,11]. Are we, as some anti-abortionists claim, living in the midst of a holocaust comparable to the Nazi slaughter of the Jews, or can this killing be justified?

I propose to begin by stating the case against abortion as precisely as possible, and then to examine two pro-abortion arguments which I will call the 'personhood' and 'women's rights' positions. Although these encompass the views of many pro-abortionists, they are unlikely to convince those whose opposition to abortion is based on religious revelation, and many non-religious people find them counterintuitive. Nor are they the arguments used by parents to justify the abortion of their own loved and wanted but abnormal child. I will therefore also describe a third method for deciding about the morality of abortion, by appeal to a principle that can be accepted by believer and non-believer alike, the Judeo-Christian Golden Rule – act towards others as you wish them to act towards you.

The case against abortion

This is commonly stated thus:

Proposition 1. Killing innocent people is wrong.
Proposition 2. The fetus is a person.
Therefore – the fetus should not be killed/aborted.
BUT
Proposition 3. People should be allowed to do as they like with their own bodies.
Proposition 4. The mother is a person.
Therefore – the mother should be allowed to empty her uterus and have the abortion.
Proposition 5. Where one person's right not to be unjustly killed conflicts with another person's right to do as they wish with their own bodies, the right not to be unjustly killed takes precedence.
Therefore – Abortion is wrong.

Personhood arguments

Most criticism of the argument above is directed at proposition 2. Although the fetus is undoubtedly a member of the species *Homo sapiens*, it is claimed that it is not a person in the sense of an individual who may not be unjustly killed. The reason (it is argued) that it is wrong to kill people is because they value their lives, they are conscious beings aware of themselves having a continuous existence over time, and because they would be deprived of something which they are able to value (their

future life) by being killed [12]. Assuming we do not wish to be arbitrarily killed, we cannot be consistent and also kill other people similar to ourselves. However, the fetus is different from us in morally important ways. It is not conscious, or self-aware, and is deprived of nothing which it values by being killed. It therefore fails this test of personhood and can be killed. To permit the killing of animals, but to save fetuses, would therefore be speciesism [13] (discrimination according to an arbitrary irrelevant criterion, membership of a species). A consequence of using this definition of a person is that killing higher animals such as gorillas and dolphins would also be wrong, if we believed that they were self-aware and valued their lives.

Many people have difficulties with this kind of argument since, in the actual world as we know it, only one species, *Homo sapiens*, is a serious contender for personhood. The arbitrariness of defining personhood as membership of the species *Homo sapiens*, is not immediately obvious. However philosophers have offered a number of thought experiments to draw attention to the problem. Imagine that one day we meet creatures from outer space. How should we decide whether to have them for dinner in one sense or the other? Most of us would use behaviour, rather than membership of our species, or appeal to divine revelation, to decide, especially if we remember that the alien may also be deciding whether it is morally permissible to eat us! Similar decisions may one day have to be made about computers that behave intelligently, and apparently value their existence.

This line of reasoning appears to lead to the counterintuitive conclusion that not only may fetuses be killed, but so also may newborn babies and the mentally handicapped, who also fail this test of personhood. Some philosophers have gone so far as to argue that infanticide is indeed sometimes permissible [14], although its side effects, such as the offence caused to other persons, mean that it would rarely be permitted in practice. On this view the personhood of a newborn infant is a social construct which society does not choose to bestow on unborn fetuses. We can imagine societies, such as the Spartans, whose members withhold personhood from newborns, or yet others who bestow it on unborn fetuses (these are the societies which do not permit abortion).

The arbitrary nature of such a social construct is disquieting to many, but it is surely no more arbitrary than membership of a species, or the possession of a soul indicated by religious revelation.

Such discussions of the personhood of newborns are not entirely academic. It is easy to imagine that with advances in neonatology there may one day be so many tiny babies needing support, that people able and willing to care for them will be scarce. We would not force nurses to work in neonatal units against their will, and if no one else could be found to staff such units, society might well decide that some killing of newborns was acceptable. If our definition of personhood is correct, the only people wronged by such killing would be the other adults involved.

Women's rights arguments

The other point at which pro-abortionists engage the prolifer is at premise 5. They argue that even if the fetus is to be regarded as a person who may not normally be unjustly killed, the mother should not be forced to carry it for 9 months against her will. It may be kind of her to do so, but she should be allowed to escape the burden. We do not expect people to give even a pint of blood against their will to save other people's lives.

This line of argument has been put most forcefully by the American philosopher Judith Jarvis Thompson in a famous paper [15]. She drew an analogy with forcing someone to give aid to a paradigm person, in her example a famous violinist. The analogy was with pregnancy resulting from rape, but it can easily be modified to include other cases of unwanted pregnancy.

Imagine that a world-famous violinist at the height of his powers develops a fatal kidney disease. His doctors state that unless he is connected to the circulation of another person he will die, but that the disease is self-limiting, and that after 9 months of circulatory connection he will recover to full health. Unfortunately, he has a rare blood group and no one can be found of that group who is also willing to be connected to him. A society of music lovers resolve to search the world for a suitable person, and find you. Of course you may not agree to their proposal, so they simply kidnap you one day as you are walking home, anaes-thetize you, transport you to the clinic in the Swiss alps, connect you to the violinist's circulation and wake you up. When the clinic director explains what has happened you are outraged and demand to be disconnected. The director reminds you that you only need to stay connected for 9 months and that if you disconnect the violinist, he will die. Must you remain connected? Thompson's intuition and my own are that while it would be kind of you to stay connected, strong personal reasons, such as career and family needs, would justify disconnection. Moreover, disconnection would still be justified if your behaviour had to some extent led to your kidnap. For example, you might have been well aware that the music lovers were searching for a person to kidnap, but nevertheless persisted in going home by a secluded route because you wanted the pleasure of viewing the sunset. By analogy, taking sexual pleasure does not commit you to bearing the unwanted pregnancies which occasionally result. Anyone who wishes to understand the strength of feeling of a woman bearing an unwanted pregnancy should read Thompson's forceful paper.

These women's rights arguments are not unanswerable. Many individuals maintain that their intuitions are different from Thompson's; you should remain connected, and the rape victim should bear the child [16]. Moreover, neither 'women's rights' nor 'personhood' arguments carry much force with the parents of an abnormal child who want a baby. They don't see the fetus as a non person who can be killed like an animal, and they want to bear a baby. Why do they want the abortion and how can they justify it?

Abortion and the Golden Rule

The following is condensed from Hare [17], another classic contribution to the abortion debate, which, like Thompson's, is widely anthologized and worth reading in the original. Hare claimed that the most fundamental moral principle was that of consistency, that we should treat like cases alike. He is in good company. Philosophers have formulated this principle in many ways, most notably Immanuel Kant's categorical imperative, 'act only according to that maxim which you can will should be a universal moral law', or the

Golden Rule, formulated many times in history, but which is most familiar to us from Christ's Sermon on the Mount – 'do unto others as you would they do unto you'. Hare claimed that abortion is a problem, not because of anything intrinsic to the fetus at the time the abortion is done (for reasons given above), but because of the potential of the fetus to become a human person. This potentiality argument is usually dismissed by philosophers on two grounds. First, we do not normally treat things according to their potential state, but rather according to their actual state. I cannot treat you as if you were dead, although you are inevitably going to be in that state one day. More seriously, philosophers imagine that acceptance of the potentiality argument would commit them to also treating sperms and eggs as potential people, and maximizing fertility at all costs. We will see shortly that this need not be the case.

Hare's first move was this. We should do as we were glad was done to us. If we are glad that we were not aborted, we should not abort the fetus. If there was only one fetus/potential person to consider, that would be the end of the matter and abortion would be wrong. However, if we take potentiality seriously, there is not just the fetus of this present pregnancy to consider, but also all the other potential babies which this mother may have if her present pregnancy is ended. These other fetuses may later be glad that the abortion took place. For simplicity, consider a woman carrying an abnormal fetus who plans a particular family size. There are two potential people to consider, the abnormal fetus and the, probably normal, replacement fetus which will only come into existence if the abortion is done. The abnormal fetus would wish that the abortion does not happen. However the replacement fetus will only come into existence at all if the abortion is done, and therefore would presumably will the abortion. We resolve the conflict by a thought experiment, by asking what we would choose if we were forced to live through both potential people's lives. If we chose no abortion, we would have one handicapped life and one non-life (the replacement fetus will not be conceived because its mother will be busy caring for her handicapped child). If we chose the abortion, we would have one non-life (the abortion) and one healthy life (that of the replacement fetus). Surely, even

from this potential person perspective, we would choose that the abortion takes place. Consistency, and the Golden Rule, indicate that we should act as we would wish done to ourselves, and do the abortion.

This argument has good philosophical reasons to support it. It appeals to a principle, the Golden Rule, with which anyone can agree, rather than to intuitions which often conflict, and those of us who wonder if our intuitions are indeed correct can use this principle against which to test them. At a practical level it captures the feelings of parents of a handicapped fetus much better than the personhood and women's rights arguments. They love and want to bear their baby, and if they kill it will grieve severely. They will frequently say that they are acting in the child's interest to avoid a life of suffering. If the abnormality is relatively mild, outside observers who consider only the present abnormal child, may find the parents' attitude hard to accept, since the child is still likely to have a life of more value than no life at all. Only a few abnormalities are so severe that it can be confidently said that no life would be better than an, albeit imperfect, affected life. However, parents usually see clearly the choice between the perfect child of their dreams, which they will still probably bear if they undergo the abortion, and the handicapped child they are carrying. If both these potential people are considered it is not difficult to support the abortion even from the fetus's perspective.

There are thus at least three separate lines of argument that individually justify abortion. Taken together there would seem to be overwhelming justification for abortion at the mother's request for severe fetal abnormality. To claim otherwise we must not only provide a reason for treating human fetuses in a special way by virtue of their humanness, but also impose this belief on a mother who believes otherwise. This will be difficult in a religiously tolerant society if the specialness of the fetus rests on religious belief. We must also believe that it is justifiable to force women to give aid to fetuses, even if the pregnancy arose through no fault of their own, and explain why we do not expect men to give even a pint of blood if they do not wish to. Finally, we must be prepared to argue that the woman with an abnormal fetus, who says that she can only look after one child, should bear and look after this one, rather than bearing and looking after another healthy child.

There is one other bad anti-abortion argument that is still sometimes heard in the context of abortion for abnormality; the claim that handicapped children should not be aborted because of the joy they bring to others. Although this view is often heard from the handicapped themselves, and no one would dispute that they do indeed usually lead worthwhile lives, and often enhance the lives of those with whom they come in contact, it is still fallacious. We can test its force by considering a case in which the handicap and abortion issues are separated [18].

Imagine that a woman carries a child with spina bifida, and that a simple medicine has been discovered that will heal the defect. She only has to take a tablet. However the mother declines the tablet, saying that the last handicapped child she bore made her, and all who came in contact with the child, so happy that she intends to have another. The outrage we would feel towards that mother indicates that the happiness from other people's misery argument has no independent force apart from its anti-abortion element.

Prenatal diagnosis

This lengthy digression about the morality of abortion is a necessary prelude to the ethics of prenatal diagnosis. If prenatal diagnosis was limited to improving treatment of abnormal fetuses, there would be little dispute about its morality. However, in practice the most frequent therapeutic option to follow a prenatal diagnosis is pregnancy termination. It is therefore legitimate to ask what are the real aims of prenatal diagnosis and how are they justified?

Prenatal diagnosis could be justified in two ways, either by the claim that it had the effect of reducing the amount of suffering in the world, or because it increased individual parents' freedom of choice. I shall call the former the utilitarian reason. It does not stand up to close scrutiny and would be a dangerous path for society to follow. The freedom of choice reason is justified, if abortion is justified, and has its own inbuilt safeguards against abuse.

The utilitarian argument for prenatal diagnosis

It might be claimed that if abnormal fetuses were terminated, the total amount of suffering in the world would be reduced. With respect to some programmes, such as serum screening for neural tube defects [19], this may well be correct. However, there is no generally agreed method for making such a calculation in practice. How can the loss of a normal child by accidental abortion be weighed against the suffering of a child with spina bifida? It is difficult enough for individuals to make these calculations, for society as a whole it would be impossible. If it were attempted, a list of conditions severe enough to justify abortion could perhaps be drawn up, and abortion permitted only for these conditions.

However, the implications of taking such a list seriously are unpleasant. Living people with handicap whose disabilities were on the list would justifiably feel that society did not value them. The parents of babies with conditions on the list could hardly fail to feel some social pressure to have an abortion. What would be allowed for parents of a child affected with a mild handicap not on the list, who had other reasons, perhaps handicap themselves, that made them unable to bring up the child? Respect for parental autonomy would soon take second place to utilitarian calculations in such a programme, and power would be put in the hands of the doctors. Since it is so difficult to decide how much handicap justifies abortion, there would be a risk that one day doctors would decide on eugenic grounds. The history of eugenic movements does not inspire confidence that someone would not one day argue that certain racial groups, the socially disadvantaged, or those with mild handicap should be added to the abortion justified list [20].

Freedom of choice

A better way to justify prenatal diagnosis is by appealing to its ability to increase parental choice and the exercise of autonomy. If we believe that there are good arguments for permitting abortion, then prenatal diagnosis needs no more justification than that it provides information for parents on which to exercise choice. Parents, not doctors, should decide what abnormality is severe enough to justify abortion, since they will usually bring up the child, and it is the mother who undergoes the abortion. Parents can usually be relied on to decide in the best interests of their children. Even if we occasionally disagree with individual decisions, it is very unlikely that parents will ever make systematically unjust decisions on, for example, racial grounds or for trivial handicap, because they come from all social backgrounds, and belong to all racial groups. In prenatal diagnosis, the overall result of many different people making their own personal decisions, and living with the consequences, will always be preferable to one expert group deciding. In a similar way many individuals making their own decisions in a free market invariably outperform any planned economy [21]. There is no slippery slope towards eugenic abortion for racial subgroups or the socially disadvantaged unless the groups involved actually choose it.

Mild abnormalities or low risk of severe abnormality

If prenatal diagnosis is provided in this way with the aim of increasing parental choice, it is inevitable that parents will occasionally request abortion for reasons that seem to their doctors to be trivial. It is tempting to draw a line and perform abortion for, say, Down syndrome, or neural tube defect, but refuse it for, say, Turner's syndrome, or low risks of severe abnormalities. Imagine the following urological case. A woman is carrying a fetus with bladder outflow obstruction secondary to urethral valves. At 22 weeks the liquor volume and urinary sodium are normal. Good prospective data are limited, but let us assume that after neonatal resection of the valves, 95% of such babies will have full health, but that 5% will ultimately develop renal failure necessitating dialysis or transplantation in childhood. Does this justify termination if informed parents request it? The answer must be yes, if we agree that abortion is a permissible choice for parents, and we wish to maximize choice. To argue otherwise means going down the utilitarian route with all its discriminatory effects and eugenic risks.

The above appears straightforward but if freedom of parental choice is taken to its logical conclusion, it also may have some unattractive consequences. For example, is abortion justified for parental preference for fetal sex? The feeble response of the liberal who does not wish to go that far is usually to claim that it is either an offence to the doctor's own autonomy, or society's disapproval that justifies refusal. Neither position is satisfactory. The offence to the doctor's autonomy should not prevent others from offering sex selection if they wish. The idea that it is social disapproval that prevents us offering abortion for sex selection leads us back to the utilitarian list of conditions justifying abortion, with sex selection just not making it. Is there any defensible point at which the liberal can draw the line?

One approach is to remind ourselves that reasons for abortions for 'abnormality' fall along a continuum from 'strong' (Tay Sach's disease), through 'weak' (Turner's syndrome), 'very weak' (sex preference) to 'extremely weak' such as preference for a handicapped child. We would have no difficulty refusing a request to terminate a normal fetus because the mother wanted an abnormal child, perhaps because it would always be dependent on her. Our reason would be that we also had a duty to the future child. If parents requested prenatal diagnosis to select a chess prodigy, or football player, we again could legitimately refuse in the future child's interest. The future child's interest in abortion for sex selection is unclear. It is difficult to argue convincingly that in an individual case the resulting child would be harmed, although it is generally presumed that there would be a preference for male children, and various adverse effects are possible if it became a widespread practice. These include a lowering of the status of females and an increase in homosexuality, war and violent crime. However, there may also be good demographic effects, and the status of women might rise as a result of their relative shortage. Since there are no empirical data, and given the general presumption that we need a strong reason to prohibit an action, I believe that sex selection should be permitted*. From this perspective, abortion for minor handicap or low risk of handicap is clearly in the future child's interest, and should be performed at the parent's request.

The ethical position sketched out here is strongly pro-choice. The acceptance of it has the practical consequence that the counselling given to parents of an abnormal fetus must be non-directive. The parents should be helped to decide in accord with their own values without the doctor's/counsellor's values intruding. This is not easy. Even risks can be presented in a value-laden way. Fortunately, the effects of presentation on understanding are fairly well understood and with care biases can be minimized [22]. It is even more difficult for parents to incorporate the values they place on different outcomes in decision making, and here again they are vulnerable to outside influence. Techniques such as lotteries to measure utilities, and decision analysis to incorporate them systematically into the overall decision, may be helpful [23].

A more serious criticism has recently been levelled against liberal non-directive counselling [24]. Clarke argues that the fact we usually refuse termination for sex selection, but permit it for minor abnormalities, indicates that society has already decided that minor abnormalities do justify abortion, and that offering prenatal diagnosis inevitably involves imposing these utilitarian conclusions on parents. If Clarke is correct, we have already fallen into the utilitarian trap, are discriminating against the handicapped and are in danger of sliding towards eugenics. Clarke's preferred solution would seem to be to accept this, and stop pretending that we are giving parents a completely free choice. He wants clinical geneticists to protect themselves from the charge that they are thus discriminating against the living handicapped, by returning to a greater involvement in the clinical care of the handicapped. This option is hardly practicable for obstetricians involved in prenatal diagnosis, and since I would not like to administer even a socially derived utilitarian list of justified reasons for abortion, I would prefer to find an adequate reason for refusing sex selection or, in the absence of such a reason, to accept the

consequences of permitting sex selection.

Parental refusal of fetal therapy or abortion

Finally, I turn briefly to the other type of feto-maternal conflict; the situation where a fetus would benefit from treatment *in utero* but its mother refuses such treatment, and the very rare situation where the fetal disease is so awful that continuation of the pregnancy would cause the fetus more suffering than abortion, but where the mother still insists on carrying it. Although it is tempting to follow the pro-choice line here, and allow parents complete freedom to refuse fetal therapy or to continue an abnormal pregnancy, there is an important difference between this and a parental request for abortion against a doctor's better judgement. After abortion there is no baby, but after maternal refusal of therapy or continuation of an abnormal pregnancy, there will be a handicapped child and later a handicapped adult. That future person has an interest in a treatment decision in a way that a fetus does not have an interest in an abortion decision. If the future child will be harmed, that harm should be weighed against the mother's right to refuse therapy. Such considerations have led some philosophers [25] and judges [26] to support interventions for fetal benefit against the mother's wishes. The most common intervention forced on mothers has been caesarean section with 21 cases in the USA up to 1987 [26] and there has been a recent case in the UK [27]. At the present state of knowledge similar arguments could be used to justify compulsory fetal blood transfusion for rhesus disease and in future might justify many other types of *in utero* surgery.

If we could be satisfied that fetal benefit from the intervention was clear, that maternal risk was small, and that the mother was acting either against or with disregard for the fetal interest, I believe such compulsory interventions would be justifiable. Even the most ardent libertarians accept that the state may act to restrain its citizens from harming other citizens [28]. However, in practice these conditions are rarely if ever fulfilled. Doctors are often wrong, there are significant maternal risks from most interventions, and mothers simply do not refuse treatment because they wish to harm their baby, or do not care what

*Since I am a clinician who performs abortion, I should record that I also understand that abortion for sex selection is illegal in the UK and therefore I do not offer it. However, if the law was one day changed to permit abortion on demand at an early stage of pregnancy, I would find it difficult to restrict it to women who did not know the sex of their baby.

happens to it. There are also important side effects of compulsory treatment; other women would be made fearful, and might harm their babies by avoiding medical care altogether. Compulsory surgery might discriminate against certain racial groups and the socially deprived; most reported patients in the USA have been either single or members of minority groups, and some have not spoken English [26]. It is likely that communication difficulties and cultural factors led to the disagreement between patient and doctor.

I conclude that compulsory intervention for fetal benefit is not wrong in principle if the alternative is an avoidably damaged person, but in practice the benefits rarely if ever justify the side effects. Similar arguments apply to compulsory abortion, and since it is both very unusual for it to be better for a person to be aborted than to have lived at all, and the adverse side effects of compulsory abortion would be even greater than those of compulsory fetal treatment, I believe it would never in practice be the correct course of action. It is of interest that similar arguments have recently led some American appeal court judges to move away from supporting compulsory intervention [29].

Summary

Prenatal diagnosis raises two kinds of feto-maternal conflict. In general, abortion for handicap is morally justifiable on maternal request, and a liberal policy should be followed even for mild abnormalities. Doctors offering prenatal diagnosis should concentrate on being non-directive. Their activities are justified because they increase parental choice, not because they reduce suffering. Abortion for sex preference is at the borderline of permissibility but unless we believe that the children resulting from such action have been harmed by it or that there is some overriding adverse social consequence, it should be allowed. Abortion with the express aim of causing a handicapped child to be born, or refusal of treatment with the avoidable consequence of causing a child to be handicapped, are both morally wrong, because of the consequences for the resulting person. The former should not be permitted, but because of the uncertainty of medical knowledge, the side effects of compulsory treatment and the knowledge that they have been applied unjustly in the past, compulsory interventions would very rarely if ever be justified in practice.

References

1. Lewis TLT, Chamberlain GVP. *Gynaecology by Ten Teachers*, 15th edn. London: Edward Arnold, 1990.
2. Symonds EM (ed) *Essential Obstetrics and Gynaecology*, 2nd edn. London: Churchill Livingstone, 1992.
3. Whitfield CR (ed) Dewhurst's textbook of obstetrics and gynaecology for postgraduates. 4th edn. Oxford: Blackwell, 1986.
4. Tindall VR. *Jeffcoate's Principles of Gynaecology*, 5th edn. London: Butterworths, 1987.
5. Harper PS. *Practical Genetic Counselling*, 3rd edn. London: Wright, 1988.
6. Harrison MR, Golbus MS, Filly RA. *The Unborn Patient. Prenatal Diagnosis and Treatment*, 2nd edn. Philadelphia: WB Saunders, 1990.
7. Potts M, Diggory P, Peel J. *Abortion*. Cambridge: Cambridge University Press, 1977.
8. OPCS. *Abortion Statistics 1990*, Series AB No 17. London: HMSO, 1991.
9. Botting B. Trends in abortion. *Popul Trends* 1991; **64**: 19–29.
10. Clarke M. Unsafe sex: the case for a primary health care initiative. *Contemp Rev Obstet Gynaecol* 1989; **1**: 261–265.
11. Drife J. One in three. *Br Med J* 1991; **33**: 653.
12. Glover J. *Causing Death and Saving Lives*. Harmondsworth: Penguin, 1977.
13. Singer P. *Animal Liberation*. New York: Avon Books, 1975.
14. Tooley M. Abortion and infanticide. In: Cohen M, Nagel T, Scanlon T (eds) *The Rights and Wrongs of Abortion*. Princeton: Princeton University Press, 1974.
15. Thompson JJ. A defense of abortion. *Philos Public Affairs* 1971; **1**: 47–66. (Reprinted in: Rachels J (ed) *Moral Problems*. New York: Harper, 1979.)
16. Finnis J. The rights and wrongs of abortion: a reply to Judith Thompson. *Philos Public Affairs* 1973; **2**. (Reprinted in: Cohen M, Nagel T, Scanlon T (eds) *the Rights and Wrongs of Abortion*. Princeton: Princeton University Press, 1974.)
17. Hare RM, Abortion and the Golden Rule. *Philos Public Affairs* 1975; **4**. (Reprinted in: Rachels J (ed) *Moral Problems*. New York: Harper, 1979.)
18. Harris J. *The Value of Life*. London: Routledge.
19. Cuckle HS, Wald NJ. The impact of screening for open neural tube defects in England and Wales. *Prenat Diagn* 1987; **7**: 91–99.
20. Gould SJ. *The Mismeasure of Man*. London: Pelican.
21. Hayek FA. *The Constitution of Liberty*. Chicago: University of Chicago Press, chap 2.

22. Tversky A, Kahnemann D. Judgement under uncertainty: heuristics and biases. *Science* 1974; **185**: 1124–1131.

23. Thornton JG, Lilford RJ, Johnson N. Decision analysis in medicine. *Br Med J* 1992; **304**: 1099–1103.

24. Clarke A. Is non directive genetic counselling possible? *Lancet* 1991; **338**: 998–1001.

25. Kluge E-HW. When Caesarian section operations imposed by a court are justified. *J Med Ethics* 1988; **14**: 206–211.

26. Kolder VEB, Gallagher J, Parsons MT. Court ordered obstetrical interventions. *New Engl J Med* 1987; **316**: 1192.

27. Dyer C. British court orders caesarean section. *Br Med J* 1992; **305**: 978.

28. Nozick R. *Anarchy, State and Utopia.* Oxford: Blackwell, 1974.

29. Curran WJ. Court-ordered Cesarean sections receive judicial defeat. *New Engl J Med* 1990; **323**: 489–492.

Index